Encounters between Patients and Doctors

MIT Press Series on the Humanistic and Social Dimensions of Medicine

Stanley Joel Reiser, general editor

Encounters between Patients and Doctors

An Anthology

edited by John D. Stoeckle, M.D.

The MIT Press
Cambridge, Massachusetts
London, England

This book was set in Baskerville by Asco Trade Typesetting Ltd., Hong Kong, and printed and bound by Halliday Lithograph Company in the United States of America.

Library of Congress Cataloging-in-Publication Data

Encounters between patients and doctors.

(MIT Press series on the humanistic and social dimensions of medicine; 5)
Includes bibliographies and index.
1. Physician and patient.   2. Interpersonal relations.   I. Stoeckle, John D.
II. Series. [DNLM: 1. Communication.   2. Physician-Patient Relations.
W1 MI938M v.5/W 62 E558]
R727.3.E52   1987   610.69′52   86-10387
ISBN 0-262-19235-7
ISBN 0-262-69097-7 (pbk.)

This book is for Olivia Finlay; also J.B.E. and A.Y.S.

Contents

4

Client Control and Medical Practice   *179*
Eliot Freidson

5

Negotiating Reality: Notes on Power in the Assessment of Responsibility   *193*
Thomas J. Scheff

6

Behavior in Private Places: Sustaining Definitions of Reality in Gynecological Examinations   *215*
Joan P. Emerson

7

The Captive Professional: Bureaucratic Limitations in the Practice of Military Psychiatry   *235*
Arlene K. Daniels

III

THE NATURE OF THE COMMUNICATION

Introductory Comments   *255*

8

Gaps in Doctor-Patient Communication: Patients' Response to Medical Advice   *259*
Vida Francis, Barbara M. Korsch, and Marie J. Morris

9

Explanatory Models in Health-Care Relationships: A Conceptual Frame for Research on Family-Based Health-Care Activities in Relation to Folk and Professional Forms of Clinical Care   *273*
Arthur Kleinman

IV
BARRIERS TO COMMUNICATION: WHY CARE DIFFERS

10
Who Is Really Ignorant—Physician or Patient?
John B. McKinlay

11
Variations in Patients' Compliance with Doctors' Advice: An Empirical Analysis of Patterns of Communication
Milton S. Davis

12
Problems of Communication, Diagnosis, and Patient Care: The Interplay of Patient, Physician, and Clinic Organization
Irving Kenneth Zola

V
STUDYING THE RELATION: CAN IT BE RESEARCHED?

13
Information Control and the Micropolitics of Health Care
Howard Waitzkin in association with John D. Stoeckle

14
Chinese-Style and Western-Style Doctors in Northern Taiwan
Emily M. Ahern

VI
THE GOOD RELATION

Foreword

This collection of readings on relations between patients and doctors addresses issues that have always been central to the practice of medicine. The growing power of medical science and technology during recent decades has tended to turn the attention of physicians and medical educators away from these meetings of persons through which needs of the patient are recognized and met. Some critics have suggested that medical scientists are, at best, uninterested and, at worst, neglectful of this reality.

This volume contains compelling evidence against that view. One of the first readings is L. J. Henderson's important essay on "Physician and Patient as a Social System," published in 1935. Henderson's interests were by no means confined to the social and personal dimensions of medicine. He was one of the pioneers in the application of the concepts and techniques of physics and chemistry to biology and medicine. His monograph on the "Fitness of the Environment" is as thoughtful an exposition of the importance of the physiochemical circumstances of the earth for living as his essay on physician-patient relations is on the significance of social and personal circumstances in health care. Henderson and many other contributors to this volume recognized that the science and art of medicine are, or should be, complementary and cooperative rather than antagonistic and competitive.

John Stoeckle has rendered a service not only to the medical students who will learn from these readings but to all persons who want to become more familiar with the structure, dynamics, nature, modes of communications, investigation, and goals of the relations between doctors and patients. Throughout his professional career, Dr. Stoeckle has lived his commitment to improving the quality of medical care. Like Francis Peabody, his predecessor at the Harvard Medical School, he has long recognized that "the secret of caring for the patient is to care for him." By offering original papers in the field rather than didactic summaries, Stoeckle allows each student the opportunity to learn in his or her own way about discoveries in this important part of health care. In this sense the book makes a statement about teacher-student relations that bears an interesting analogy to the commentaries on doctor-patient relations. In both cases the emphasis is on a binary relationship between learners, not on a unilateral exposition by an expert. This book reaches toward both good medicine and good education.

Daniel C. Tosteson, M.D.
Dean
Harvard Medical School

Preface

This small book of readings is on the relationships of people seeking medical aid to those who try to help. It is dedicated to all bed, home-bound, and walking patients and to all practitioners in their everyday medical work with patients.

Counted among the practitioners (either in yesterday's egalitarian idiom, the health workers, or in today's professionalization of everyone, the health professionals) are generalist MDs as family doctors, GPs, internists, pediatricians, and gynecologists-obstetricians, along with the specialty consultants in medicine and surgery; then, alongside these MDs, RNs, pharmacists, social workers, nurse practitioners, physician assistants, aides, LPNs, office assistants, and those reflective administrators who have become part of our medical institutions but not yet wholly committed to "bottom-line" corporate thinking; finally, but not least, all of the students training for all those future jobs in practice and for the leadership they must bring to the relationship if patients are to continue to have personal care.

Of all bed, home-bound, and walking patients, those going to the doctor in the office deserve special mention. In this recent era of hospital expansion (now coming to a close), ambulatory patients have received little attention in the literature on patients, even though their visits to doctors' offices mark the beginning of their career in seeking help. In these readings and commentary such out-of-hospital encounters take their proper place.

Presenting these readings also acknowledges those new goals and old values that may renew practice, education, and the everyday contracts of doctors and patients: (1) patient-centered practice that uses appropriate technologies, that attends to the tasks of care, and that provides comprehensive services with both prevention and rehabilitation; (2) education that joins the technical and humane for learning the medical tasks, organized in practices outside as well as in the hospital; (3) interprofessional work that is more collaborative than hierarchical.

Unlike books on disease topics in medicine, this volume is not a current annual review of the research literature on the doctor-patient relation. The appearance of literature on this subject is erratic, certainly not like those annual reports and publications from medical research laboratories with their newness and promise of constant progress, promoted by science reporters as "medical advances." These selections come out of publications far older than the professional journals issued today. Despite their past, the readings do address contemporary issues in this age of technological medicine. I hope they will stimulate and sustain interest in the plain, difficult, and satisfying tasks of care while reviving memories of those unique encounters that begin at the very first visit with a patient—or a doctor.

For assistance in organizing the collection and text, I thank Sarah Bollinger, Florence Zamcheck, Meryl Sommer, Kelly Gritz, and Philip Stoeckle. For advice, both old and new, I am grateful to several colleagues, now at other institutions, with whom I have been privileged to work: George Abbott White, Eliot House, Harvard College; John McKinlay, Boston University; Stanley Reiser, University of Texas Medical Center; Howard Waitzkin, Medical School, University of California at Irvine; Andrew Twaddle, University of Missouri; and Irving Zola, Brandeis University. Moreover, I want to acknowledge my many colleagues on the medical, psychiatric, and surgical services of the Massachusetts General Hospital who, even if not interested in these doctor-patient themes, have supported, if not stimulated, my interest in this topic through consultations, gossip, instruction, supervision, listening, and their own personal accounts of relationships. Among those lending that essential support are the several chiefs of the medical service. As the hospital expanded and medical subspecialization grew, they kept alive what many institutions did not, the idea and tradition of a general medical clinic: Drs. Walter Bauer (deceased), Robert Ebert, in particular Alexander Leaf, and John Potts; from outside of medicine, the chiefs of the psychiatric service, Drs. Eric Lindemann (deceased), Leon Eisenberg, and Thomas Hackett.

Practitioner colleagues who should be mentioned include Aaron Lazare in particular, along with Benjamin Gill, Jerome Weinberger, Gerald Davidson, Arthur Barsky, Arthur Kleinman, Sherman Eisenthal, Harold Bursztajn, Bernard Levy, Robert Coles, and Michael

McGuire, all of whom came from the psychiatric service to consult on, treat, and study medical outpatients while teaching medical students; then, as medical colleagues, Roger Sweet, Walter St. Goar, John Irwin, Jerome Grossman, Gerald Foster, Steven Levisohn, Lawrence Wood, Richard Pingree, James Dineen, Joseph Gardella, J. Andrew Billings, Charles Weiss, John Goodson, Terrence O'Malley, Allan Goroll, Albert Mulley, James Richter (and all the members of the Internal Medicine Associates and the General Medicine Unit); then further away Lawrence May (now at U.C.L.A.) and Robert Lawrence at the Cambridge Hospital. To this list I must add over a decade of Harvard Medical School students and MGH medical residents including their patients whose encounters I have been privileged to review by video-tape; and, finally, colleagues in the social service department and nursing service, with whom I have shared the care and discussion of patients in and out of the clinic, hospital, and MGH health centers—in this instance Ruth Sittler, Alice Rogers, Barbara Noonan, Sharon Follayttar, and Mary Ryan.

John D. Stoeckle, M.D.
Primary Care Program (General Medicine Unit),
Massachusetts General Hospital
Division of Primary Care, Harvard Medical School

Encounters between Patients and Doctors

Introduction

Medicine's task is patient care. In that work, nothing is more important than the doctor-patient relation. Some would say that in these assertions alone there is sufficient reason to present a collection of readings on encounters between patients and doctors, though many would disagree. Critics outside the medical profession, such as Ivan Illich (1976) in *Medical Nemesis*, view the relation as an obstacle to more appropriate self-treatment or as altogether unnecessary because much medical care is unneeded, ineffectual, actually harmful, or threatening to the autonomy of the individual. Documenting the medicalization of everyday life, sociologists of the profession decry the social control of the doctor (Zola 1972). Inside the profession, which is seldom of one mind on this or other subjects, views understandably differ.

Despite the traditional professional homage that is always paid to the relation, many do not consider it central to care.

Physicians often grant technology that central position because they define medicine more by the science it uses than by its actual task of care. When professional ideology defines medicine as scientific, professionals may assert that medicine *is* science, forgetting that science provides only a *method* for the study of illness. Or they may mistake medicine's technologies of diagnosis and treatment for science, forgetting they are only the products of scientific knowledge and that they are often applied irrationally in practice. With these common misperceptions, only technology, not the doctor-patient relation, is held important—a view frequently repeated in older commentaries.

As if diagnosis without specific treatment was not useful at all, L. J. Henderson, a physician and the Abbott and James Lawrence Professor of Chemistry at Harvard University, was quoted in the 1920s as saying (presumably in reference to Erlich's treatment of syphilis with arsphenamine) that "somewhere between 1910 and 1912 . . . a random patient with a random disease, consulting a doctor chosen at random, had, for the first time in the history of mankind, a 50–50 chance of profiting from the encounter." A decade later, before the era of antibiotics, William R. Houston (1936), a medical practitioner, in *The Art of Treatment* proudly wrote: "The practicing physician ... is the retail distributor of the achievement of scientific discovery." In the same period, the distinguished Committee on the Costs of Medical Care (1932), using a less commercial metaphor, espoused a similar idea about doctoring: "The physician is the first 'contact man' between medical science and the people. He occupies the front line trenches in man's warfare with disease." While the doctoring relation might be seen as only instrumental for the use of technology, more cynical observers would have us believe it is even less, merely a bedside manner added on to medication. The old-fashioned professional mixture of doting paternalism, cheery optimism, and quick sympathizing, however, no longer appears comforting and soothing; indeed, to many today it appears authoritarian, false, and sexist.

As these older comments suggest, any assertion that the relation is central will be challenged. Perhaps the relation will always appear to follow and complement medicine's scientific-technical development simply because the profession and the public only view the improvement of care as a technical change, since medical technologies are so easily visible and tangible to everyone, for example, in the direct physical experience of modern medical tests and subsequent treatments of the body. In contrast, that new modes of relationships through personal communication, new attachments, or changes in doctors' behaviors and explanations of illness might also improve treatment is an entirely uncommon thought.

From still another professional perspective the relation may seem peripheral. Medicine is often viewed as a system of cures that reduces disease morbidity and mortality, promising longer lives and freedom from illness. If medicine has these powerful consequences, then the doctor-patient relation itself can hardly be important. At best, it may be instrumental for those medical cures, ensuring that patients "take their pills" and "have their operations," at worst, it may seem to be an archaic piece of "magic" or inconsequential trifle healing touch, a mere "holding hands of lonely old ladies at the office." However, if the powerful claims made on medicine's behalf are ill-founded, then the relation may have significance of its own.

Such is the actual but quite unacknowledged case; morbidity and mortality have been reduced by economic development and public health, certainly not by medical treatment alone, as so many modern critics have convincingly argued (McKeown 1971; Cochrane 1972; Fuchs 1974; Powles 1973; McKinlay and McKinlay 1977). And yet the commonplace thinking persists that all of medicine's therapies must have these aggregate outcomes rather than the relief of the illness of a patient. Moreover, making the larger claim remains useful in garnering public support for medicine, especially today, when the sophisticated technologies for individual treatment have become so expensive that the patient cannot directly pay for them and even the state and industry (which do pay) have begun to question their cost if not their efficacy. Perhaps modern therapies cannot be financed unless these larger public-health outcomes are attributed to them—a false rationale that may be used to justify further the expansion of technologies regardless of their effectiveness.

As a consequence of such exaggerated claims for medical treatment, the recognition of medicine as a system of patient *care* whose functions are the relief and control of illness is obscured, and the importance of the doctor-patient relation ignored. But when medicine is understood and valued as patient care, these functions of relief and control become apparent and the relation may again seem central. In this latter view, medicine is defined not only as the cure of a disease but also as the all-encompassing care of the patient's discomfort, distress, disability, and dying; functions in which the doctor has several tasks: the diagnosis and treatment of medical and psychological illness; the communication of information about the illness, its diagnosis, its treatment, its prevention, and the prognosis; the personal support of patients of all backgrounds in all stages of illness; the optimal maintenance of the chronically ill; and the prevention, where possible, of the patient's disease and disability through education, persuasion, and preventive treatment (Stoeckle 1979). For these very *caring* tasks, medicine's claims are more modest, though no less essential. The medical-social help provided is rarely curative, but it may be preventive, rehabilitative, or useful for relief and maintenance of the patient. The communicative, educational, persuasive, supportive, and caring behaviors of the doctor with the patient are central to the provision of such help. The relation is the care of the patient; it is care that technology cannot by its nature provide.

Despite its crucial position in care, attention to the relation may still be diverted by popular interest in the expansion and cost of the "health-care system." However, all consideration of the relation is not lost amid these policy concerns about size and costs. Since the expanded system presses against the humanistic values of the relation, attention to the encounter between doctor and patient is being regained as well as refocused. Actually, the growth of the "system's" technology, specialization, treatment organizations, and practitioners has created the ground for modern issues about the relation: its substitution by technology, its subdivision with specialization, its attenuation within large practice organizations, and its expansion through multiple health practitioners. These issues and events deeply concern the public, which views them less as large issues of distant public policy and more as immediate everyday hassles in the seeking and experiencing of medical help.

This book of readings on medical encounters does not address these large issues directly as matters of policy; rather, it addresses them at the common level, where they touch on the lives of patients and doctors. It also examines six general features of the doctor-patient relation:

• the structure (what are the ground rules for interaction?)
• the dynamics (how does the interchange take place?)
• the nature of communication (what goes on?)
• the barriers to communication (why care differs?)
• the study of the relation (can it be researched?)
• the good relation.

To provide perspective on these readings and topics, a profile of the doctor-patient relation in modern medical practice is first sketched, and the sources of the literature on this subject briefly reviewed.

A Profile of Doctor-Patient Encounters

Quantity

Nowadays nearly everyone goes to see the doctor at some time and, what with the chronic nature of disease, the modern search for the healthy body, and the easy availability of medical services, some people go all the time. In *The Uses of Literacy*, Richard Hoggart (1961) notes that in Great Britain the doctor is the educated person with whom the working class has the most personal contact, even when the number of educated persons and the other experts in the "service professions" have so greatly increased.[1] Lawyers, engineers, schoolteachers, and college professors each outnumber the practicing doctors, but unlike the doctor, they are not consulted by so many people throughout their lifetime. Since only a stubborn 3 percent of adults resists going to the doctor, encounters are bound to be numerous (Kessel and Sheppard 1969).

Statistics on office visits show the working-class and poor have 4–5 physician consultations per year, as many as those in the middle and at the top; additionally, more than 80 percent of the population consults the doctor each year, a distinctly modern situation, since medical visiting was not always so popular and prevalent. In 1930 only 50 percent of the population saw the doctor, and there were only 2.6 visits per person per year (Peterson 1972). Today the rate of visits per person per year is 4–5, quite similar in all developed countries (Bice and White 1965; Kohn and White 1976) except the USSR and Israel which have much higher visiting rates (Knaus 1972; Antonovsky 1972). In the USSR the figure is some 10 visits per year and in Israel it is 12 visits per year, presumably because many more doctors are available and because, as Judith Shuval and her colleagues (1970) note from their case study of Israeli medical practice, the doctor is more directly involved in the culture and is used for many "latent" as well as strictly medical functions.

In Israel, as everywhere, doctors sanction failure to cope, enhance status, supply "scientific" explanations of illness, promote catharsis, and give out, as in every welfare state, certification of sicknesses and handicaps that may bring patients a variety of benefits, such as time-off slips, examination and jury-duty excuses (Singleton 1982), special housing, taxi and ambulance transportation, home health aides, compensation, welfare assistance, retirement, and disability income. In the case of disability, Deborah Stone (1979) has, like the sociologist Talcott Parsons, characterized doctors as "gate keepers" to such awards. Access to disability benefits as one form of "transfer payments" of the welfare stare (Stone 1979; Stone 1983) requires a medical visit and the doctor's OK or, some would argue, the doctor's moral judgment on the patient's worthiness for disability benefits. In this connection, note the following examples from the files of medical practice:

Dear Doctor:
Your patient has applied for Title II and/or Title XVI disability benefits and has listed you as a treating source.
    Your report must contain....
Sincerely,
Disability Determination Service

Dear Sir or Madam:
This is to certify that Mrs. A. Jones is under care and treatment for degenerative arthritis, arteriosclerotic heart disease, and diabetes mellitus.
    Her examination and medical studies reveal....

Because of her multiple medical handicaps she is totally and permanently disabled for work. Any assistance you can provide her will benefit her overall health.

Sincerely,

Dr. X

Yet doctors may also close gates. Tough-minded medical examiners, out to eliminate those they perceive to be undeserving compensation seekers or to cut their program costs, may restrict access to such transfer payments by using overly technical, so-called objective criteria in disability decisions, as those turned down well know.

Now, if the USSR and Israel are at the upper extreme of physician use, developing countries are often at the very opposite, because, among other things, they do not have many doctors. In large areas of such Third World countries, visits to a doctor are seldom a practical possibility or a perceived necessity. The ratio of medical doctors to population is too small to make many office visits possible. Only a tiny minority can consult when, for example, Kenya has but one MD per 10,000 population, and Nigeria one per 30,000 (Janzen and Ackinstall 1978)—ratios considerably smaller than Israel's one per 412 and the USSR's one per 220 persons, a situation where the doctor may actually be waiting for patients to attend.

Statistics on national and regional variations in doctors per population and in office visit rates are abundant, but these statistics alone provide an incomplete account of all doctor-patient contacts. Few studies include the doctors' visits to hospital patients although these are sizeable since, in 1980, one out of seven persons was admitted to the hospital as an inpatient and then was visited daily an average of eight times, eight days being the average length of stay (American Hospital Association 1985).[2] Calculating all the medical encounters in the United States in 1980, patients made no less than a billion visits to physicians' offices, and doctors made still another 400 million visits to patients in acute and chronic hospitals. And this estimate is conservative. Looking at physicians' reports of visits in 1977 rather than at when and where patients reported they went and how long they were attended, Robert C. Mendenhall (1981) obtained similar figures: 1.14 billion face-to-face patient encounters by 225,091 physicians, in and out of the hospital. In contrast, I have taken the number of days of patient care in short-stay hospitals (272.6 million) and assumed that each patient was visited by the doctor at least once a day (Haupt 1983). Similar assumptions were made about the 150 million patient-days stayed by chronic patients in hospitals and the visits they required.

Generally, these daily visits were necessary in order to collect a fee. (A qualification should be added about doctor visit fees. In contrast to the daily fees of medical specialists, surgeons only collect a fee for the operation, but that surgical fee, nonetheless, is usually large enough incentive for the surgeon to make those daily visits, even without itemized tabulation of or payment for them.) These hospital figures are also conservative, because many patients are visited by more than one doctor—particularly those in teaching hospitals, where patients are visited by consultant specialists besides the personal doctor, also by resident physicians (65,000) and by clinical fellows (5,846) in training (Butler 1980).

One datum on the magnitude of these hidden visits from consultants comes from insurance payments to doctors. Of patients hospitalized in Massachusetts under Blue Shield insurance in 1974, 16 percent had other consultants in addition to their own doctor; in 1985 the percentage was 35. The actual visits by other hospital consultants are probably even greater than the percentages would suggest. Since insurance does not pay for all consultants, or, if it does, pays for but a fraction of their visits, many consultant encounters simply do not appear in these actuarial accounts (personal communication, Blue Cross–Blue Shield of Massachusetts 1980) and yet even with these consultant additions still other visits by resident physicians and clinical fellows are not included. Among the nation's acute care hospitals residency training is attached to 15 percent, which contain 40 percent of the beds (446,302); thus, given 374,969,431 inpatient days, residents may visit patients 149,987,772 times, often in groups rather than singly [*Hospital Statistics, 1984* (Chicago: AHA, 1984)]. These visits by physicians in training are hidden by the usual surveys. Moreover, visit surveys (National Center for Health Statistics 1984) do not include those encounters with anesthesiologists, radiologists, clinical teachers, and researchers, all of whom may attend hospitalized patients though they are not the "personal" doctor.

Physicians also visit patients in nursing homes and chronic-care facilities, but when they do, they visit them less often than in acute-care hospitals (Solon and Greenwalt 1974). According to a 1975 survey by the Massachusetts Department of Public Health approximately 60 percent of nursing-home patients were visited at least once within an 8-week period, the remainder less often (Commonwealth of Massachusetts 1975). Patients in chronic-care hospitals may have fared better than those in nursing homes since they were visited more often, nearly 50 percent once within a week, the remainder at least once within 4 weeks. Such minimal visiting rates were initially required by public law and regulations, but since 1977 those same regulations have required daily visits in chronic-care hospitals and monthly visits in nursing homes (Commonwealth of Massachusetts 1983), essentially administrative demands for still more visits. Without periodic doctor visits these medical facilities cannot obtain approval for their charges to patients, so that doctor-patient encounters are ensured, though we know nothing of the discourse or what such mandatory consultations do or mean for long-term institutional patients.

Until recently this enormous quantity of encounters between medical practitioners and patients has been growing, as have the numbers of encounters with dentists, nurses, social workers, nonphysician health workers, and "nonprofessional" and professional counselors of all kinds. Yet a word of caution, since some medical encounters decreased in number in 1983 and 1984, and, for certain doctors, even before. Careful studies by Haggerty et al. (1975) in Rochester, New York, for example, indicated that visits per child to pediatricians were declining. Similar trends have been reported for general practice in Great Britain (March 1968; Fry and Roy 1972; Fry 1980). Moreover, with new regulations for payment by diagnosis (DRGs), overall visits to hospitalized patients have now begun to drop, this in the wake of declining hospital admissions and shorter stays, from 7.0 days in 1983 to 6.6 days in 1984 (American Hospital Association 1985). An American Medical Association survey shows that total visits to MDs declined from 1.553 billion in 1982 to 1.524 billion in 1983 (AMA Center for Health Policy 1984). These trends suggest, significantly, that visit growth has stopped, if not declined. Even so, going to the doctor remains popular though some of the public may have the means to go, and some others have stopped going so often for reasons well worth the profession's attention.

Patients' contacts with other health-care professionals in the "greater health profession" are notably less numerous than their encounters with MDs. Visits to dentists number 1.2 per person per year, and the combined rate of contact with other practitioners outside the hospital (nurses, pharmacists, optometrists, midwives, podiatrists, medical social workers) is reported to be 2.6 (Kohn and White 1976).[3] Outside the "greater health profession" (but pressing to be inside) are still other practitioners providing medical help. The 18,000 chiropractors in the United States are visited by no less than 3.6 percent of the population each year (Silver 1980; Wardwell 1976). From an even larger perspective, a 1928–1931 survey (Falk et al. 1933) found that 21.3 percent of the population saw some "nonphysician practitioner" in a 12-month period; by 1980 that percentage had grown to 35.1 (U.S. Department of Health and Human Services 1985). These figures should give comfort to those who live in fear of a "physician monopoly."

Now, there are those who would still contend that the medical connections of the doctor to the public are so numerous only because licensure and health insurance give the professional a state- and industry-subsidized monopoly on medical care (Baron 1982). But this is only a partial truth. People everywhere seek medical help from multiple sources, and certainly from "healers" other than MDs. Those other practitioner-healers work in what Kleinman (1973), Loudell (1974), and other medical anthropologists have referred to as the "three systems of care": the popular, the folk, and the professional systems. Even in modern societies, it must be acknowledged, people go to various doctors (generalists and specialists) and *also* to relatives, friends, medical advice books (Stoeckle 1984), "hot lines," self-help and support groups (Gartner and Riessman 1984), and to many other so-called "marginal practitioners" and "alternative healers" as well as to those very new professionals that now include holistic practitioners and behavioral therapists, none of whom are included in the more conventional surveys.[4]

Much as counseling and psychotherapy have proliferated outside the profession of psychiatry, medical help has also gone "popular" and commercial (that is, has gone outside the dominance and control of the formal medical profession), as a quick glance through the personal ads of local newspapers and counterculture magazines will demonstrate. Especially explicit ads, such as those found in Boston's *Phoenix* or the *Whole Earth Times*, offer medical advice and cures for anyone in search of that illusive state, bodily health. Moreover, social scientists and epidemiologists are quick to remind us that self-help and contacts for medical aid in the popular, folk, and alternative systems clearly outnumber doctor visits in the professional system, judging from the number of illnesses that are not brought to medical attention. In community and household surveys, something of an iceberg of distress that goes without professional medical aid is repeatedly revealed. White et al. (1961) and Hannay (1979) have reported that, out of 1,000 reported illnesses, only 250 were brought to a doctor; even this doctor attendance figure some advocates, like People's Medical Society (1985), would want to reduce further through the abolition of licensure and the promotion of self-care and popular health education. Such educational efforts, however, may well be frustrated, even among the "educated." Since health education may increase perceptions of bodily distress, and since not all physical complaints will be contained by self-treatment, those repressed intentions to see a doctor may well be overcome. Despite the rational reassurance of health education and the relief that may be obtained through self-treatment with over-the-counter remedies, the patient's attribution that "gas" might, after all, be the cancer mother had may trigger a decision to visit the doctor after all!

Acknowledging all the helping encounters that can be found in the lay and folk systems and that may never have been counted with accuracy, this book nevertheless focuses on medical aid in the professional system and on the doctor-patient encounters. In the United States, these encounters take place with 527,900 medical practitioners, including osteopaths (U.S. Department of Health, Education and Welfare 1978; Wilson and Newhauser 1974; Health Policy Institute 1982; U.S. Department of Health and Human Services 1981, 1985). Left out of this account of the professional system are all the other practitioner-patient encounters in and outside the hospital with the nation's 1,152,000 nurses, 144,000 pharmacists, 126,000 dentists, 47,300 social workers, 22,000 optometrists, 15,000 physical therapists, 12,000 dieticians, 8,700 podiatrists, 4,200 lay midwives, 5,000 physicians' assistants, 10,000 nurse-practitioners, and 18,000 chiropractors (U.S. Department of Health and Human Services 1985; Stambler 1979), and with medical technicians of all kinds. Setting these vast numbers aside, the rationale for restricting attention to the encounters between doctors and patients is not that MDs are necessarily more important to patients in this age of collaborative care[5] but, more, that such encounters have had the most intensive and formal analysis and, happily, have many features in common with all the others (Zola 1972).

Places To Meet: The Office and the Bedside

Contrary to the media's overly dramatized image, most encounters begin outside the hospital and take place privately (that is, in offices with the doors closed); however, even in this period of seeming medical affluence, many still do not. Encounters still occur in spaces behind thinly curtained examining tables or in stark hallways and bare waiting rooms. Curtained cubicles are found in some of the former free clinics of the 1970s converted to health centers and in old outpatient departments and emergency rooms that were built with the idea that the space of a "clinic" had similar uses as a hospital "ward" (Thompson and Golden 1975). The ward was meant to be an economical open area where 15–20 of the "sick poor" could be easily observed and treated by nurses. Then only bodily care and easy visibility for the nurse was deemed important; personal communication and privacy were not. With the same assumptions that medical treatment was largely silent and did not (for the "sick poor," anyway) require personal communication, the dispensary and the clinic were made open too. At best they were divided by curtained-off examination tables, quite in contrast with the firmly separated examination and consultation rooms in a private doctor's home office. But nowadays, when personal communication and the status that comes with privacy and space are deemed important by everyone, these older group-treatment facilities are gradually being modernized, "privatized" into single-room offices that can be used not just by doctors but also by nurse-practitioners, social workers, and physicians' assistants for "their" patients. This provision of individual offices for the encounters of all members of the hospital staff and all their patients is part of a general social (and political)[6] trend of expanded amenities and privacy, except where patients are deliberately seen in groups because of newer group-treatment or health-education strategies.

The view from inside the practitioner's office today will show, in addition to the old examining table, a desk and two chairs of varying degree of "quality"; for the room is a place to sit and to exchange and record looks, information, and feelings (though the latter may not be the expected agenda of a patient or doctor) as well as to have a physical examination (Gammock 1982; Schwartz 1981; Cox and Groves 1981; Malkin 1982). These simple props for the stage of the medical office are similar for practitioners of many other healing arts and cults—acupuncturists in China, cuvanderos in the Azores (Robert Like, Department of Family Medicine, Rutgers Medical School, personal communication, 1983), pulse doctors in Taiwan (Kleinman 1980), and homeopaths, chiropractors, and holistic MDs in the United States—all of whom engage in some form of interrogation (and listening) followed by some examination of the body (if only looking or pulse taking) before applying their own special treatment techniques. All offices of healers have the same basic plan and fixtures. In the offices of some medical doctors, the consultation and examination areas are separate. Whether to increase their efficiency (or status) by examining one patient while another undresses or gets a "shot" or simply to separate their detached tasks of questioning and listening from the physically close bodily examination (and the undressing for it), some doctors continue to maintain an "office" for interviews and an "exam room" for doing those "complete physicals" and tests on patients.

Separate rooms for these separate functions of discourse and examination were the tradition in private offices located in homes or office buildings until a combined consultation-examination office (14 feet, 9 inches by 9 feet, 9 inches) was developed for Minnesota's Mayo Clinic in 1914 by the architect Eberle (Kirk and Sternberg 1955). The concern then was efficiency but of another kind. Every doctor in that group practice could not have two rooms, one unoccupied some percentage of the time. For modesty, the privacy of disrobing with the doctor present and the shielding of the physical exam from the intrusion of others, a sliding curtain surrounded the exam table or the undressing space, separating the room as in older hospital wards and clinics.

Today, neither the consultation area nor the examination area is large, nor is either expanding; indeed, they are getting smaller. When architects recommend the size of a doctor's work space in an old office building that is being renovated or converted, it is usually 10 by 12 feet—smaller than the older home-based offices. Those dimensions have remained standard for all rooms in old buildings, since that is the way they have always been built and divided up (Cowan 1964). In comparison with the office of the doctor who practiced out of the first floor of his home or of a converted town house (from the 1850s to the 1930s), the arena for the visit has continued to diminish over the years, from a spacious 16 by 20 or 18 by 18 feet (George Anteblian, 209 Beacon Street, Boston, MA, floor plans, 1980), to the 8 by 10 or 9 by 10 feet consultation-exam room in the modern professional office building [*Planning Guide for Physicians' Medical Facilities* (Chicago: AMA, 1979)]. Moreover, since Eberle's innovation, new offices more often than not also contain the examining table. The case for these new combined consultation-examination offices at 8 feet by 10 feet is that they cost less to build when construction is expensive and they are cheaper and easier to rent.[7]

In the past, it could be argued that, when rooms even smaller than 8 by 10 feet were constructed, little attention was being given to the interaction itself; cost containment was the main consideration, and users were accorded low status. Such spaces can still be seen in the clinics of some university and municipal hospitals. They were designed for, and are tolerated by, the disadvantaged poor and their salaried resident doctors (who work but one 3-hour session per week in the clinic). Such differentials in office space, and the presence of benches rather than chairs in the waiting room, distinguished then and may still today the full-time "private" doctor from the part-time "clinic" doctor, the solo practitioner from the institutional group, the private patient from the charity or welfare case. Hidden architectural

1932 SOLO PRACTICE

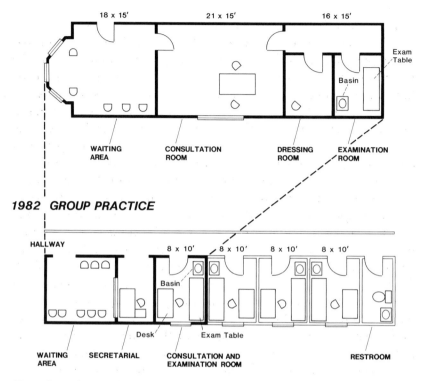

1982 GROUP PRACTICE

Floor plans of 1932 solo practice and 1982 group practice. Courtesy of Medical Art Department, Massachusetts General Hospital.

messages about class and care were and are not lost on either patients or the staff. That is, the private supervisors of such clinics have remarked for years that they would never work in such accommodations to treat their "own patients" (not to mention themselves), and patients in clinics have often asked the doctor "Could I see you in your private office?" Such is the importance of the accommodations to the status of both doctor and patient; spatial differentials for different patients and staff members also served the institution when separate private offices were provided, but away from the teaching clinic. Private staff in their "faculty practice" offices were thereby excluded from possible control of the educational practices and training environment, commonly termed "the teaching service beds" and "the clinic offices." Additionally, in today's consumer-oriented private settings carpeting and fashionable furnishings have become essential. The elegant physical ambiance now substitutes in part for the doctor's declining authority, at the same time signaling the patient that the practice must also be as technically up-to-date as the modern office decor.

The small office is not only low in status; it is also impersonal when used by ten doctors per week rather than one and necessarily devoid of any personal mementos that might suggest the individuality of the practitioner: Dr. X with her diplomas, her family pictures, her special books, her hobbies, trophies, and knickknacks—relics of a personal past and present that make the office, as doctors are prone to remark, "my den," with a distinctive order or clutter that bespeaks the practitioner's personality. Even in today's private group practices and clinics, professional self-disclosure in an office is rare and difficult to maintain. Like the operating room (OR) scheduled for operations by all types of surgeons, institutional office space is often standardized, aseptic in appearance, and devoid of anything that might reveal the doctor's human qualities to the patient; the proper distance that medical authority seems to require is maintained while clues that might bring the doctor closer to less desirable patients are banished. Indeed, the layout of many medical clinics and group practices is often just like that of the surgical operating room. That waiting room out front is separated by a reception counter from the doctor's office-exam rooms out back, an arrangement that effectively screens the doctor, nurse, and patient from mutual glimpses and glances before they meet. After the wait, the patient is greeted and escorted back to the office by a secretary or nurse (seldom by the doctor) for an interview and physical, which are verbal and manual "operations" of the medical practitioner. Like a surgeon, the doctor often has a personal office, that den somewhere else, at home or in the hospital and, therefore, much as a surgeon "goes to the OR," the doctor will "go to the clinic." The office waiting rooms and lobbies of medical office buildings are less and less distinguishable from those of airports, corporate offices, bus stations, and hotels, as Norman Mailer tartly observed in *Armies of the Night* and as the French director Jacques Tati spoofed in the movie *Playtime*; moreover, the waiting rooms of treatment institutions may be similarly used as places to meet, gossip, sleep, or "kill time," like hotel lobbies, but by far more down-and-out people (Stoeckle and Zola 1964). In addition, the first floors of many hospitals and clinics, with their automated banking services, flower shops, stores, and cafeterias, now resemble suburban shopping centers, a transformation of a once religious institution into a modern commercial building for "secular" consumers as well as patients.

After viewing the offices in the new mental health clinics of the 1960s and 1970s, Fred Bloom argued in "Psychotherapy and Moral

Culture: A Psychiatrist's Field Report" (1977) that the office standardization he saw was not merely bureaucratic public economy but was cultural, at least in its implication for the psychotherapeutic relations between doctor and patient. In a culture noted to be increasingly narcissistic and impatient with suffering of any kind, long-term relations and therapies are not expected; instead, brief relationships and quick cures, such as operations, are the desired norm. For short-term treatment, the office now need not reveal something of the doctor's background as it did in the past, when both the doctor and the patient were engaged in long-term efforts at change and when the topic of self-disclosure was explicitly addressed.[8]

A century ago, D. W. Cathell (1882) addressed the topic of self-disclosure, though with a quite different intent, in a charming essay entitled "The Physician Himself and What He Should Add to His Scientific Acquirements." During that century, doctors' own sense of professionalism and technical competence was shaky, and the public knew it. Cathell pointedly advised them to enhance their professional status and ideal through appropriate office decor:

If possible have an office that is not used for a family parlor or any other purpose. Show aesthetic cultivation in its arrangement, and make it look fresh, clean, and scientific. Flowers, either in bouquets or growing, are pleasing to every eye, and denote culture and refined taste on the part of the physician and those about him.

It is not unprofessional to keep at hand your library, miscroscope, and other aids to precision; also your diplomas, certificates of society membership, pictures of eminent professional friends and teachers, anatomical plates or anything else that has associations in your mind; but it is better to have such only as have relation to you as a student or as a physician. Professional relics and keepsakes whose history is connected with your medical studies, such as the human skeleton, either entire or in parts, pathological or anatomical specimens, and mementos of your dissections, are both appropriate and useful. A cabinet of minerals is also in good taste. Let no sharks' heads, impaled butterflies, miniature ships, stuffed birds, or anything else be seen that will place you in any other light before patients than that of a physician. Endeavor to lead every observer to think of you as a physician only.

Display neither political nor religious emblems, portraits, etc., about your office; these relate to your personal statements, while your office is a public place of every class of people, and no matter what kind of partisan or sectional pictures you might display, they would surely be repugnant to some.

Between Bloom's critique of today's democratized but depersonalized offices (which ignores the gain in privacy and patient status that individual treatment rooms for everyone provide) and Cathell's 19th-

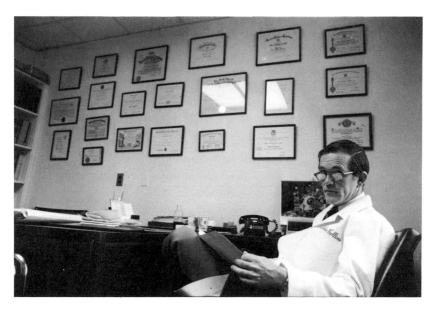

The office of a surgeon. Reprinted from Mark L. Rosenberg, *Patients: The Experience of Illness* (Philadelphia: Saunders, 1980), with author's permission.

century advice (which promoted pseudo-secientific professionalism over personal and political disclosure) lies the newer, modernistic waiting room along with each doctor's carpeted office, his or her den. Erving Goffman (1959) might argue that these seemingly more elegant amenities are but shallow "impression management," designed to lure the customer, disclosing only modern affluence to conceal the diminished status of the profession. Yet no matter how "low" or "high" the taste, the decor and personal effects at least give the patient important clues for knowing the doctor that standardized rooms do not (Coble et al. 1982). For example, the contents of the waiting room may reveal something of the political position of the doctor; perhaps there are pamphlets on free enterprise, on dealing with Medicare, or even on the hazards of nuclear war along with the popular magazines and the latest health-education literature on diet, exercise, smoking, heart disease, and cancer. Oppressive standardization has come about not only for reasons of economy in the public sector that financed mental health centers, it should be noted, but in the private medical sector too. Medical suites *need* joint occupancy (when Dr. A is in the hospital, Dr. B can use the office), and there is more shift work (Dr. C works 1 or 2 days in one office followed by 3 or 4 days in another, or stays at home for child care on some days).

Despite Bloom's perceptive travel account of clinic offices, a few qualifications should be made. It is hard to find offices entirely unadorned even if they are not personally owned or no rent is paid. Besides bureaucratic memoranda on walls, such other office emblems as calendars, posters, and prints (tacky as they might be) are often pasted up—admittedly not quite as rich a display as in personal offices, where family photographs on desks or walls disclose a bit of the doctor. These and other uses of photographs have depicted the different sides and changing character of the encounter.

If photographs of the doctor's family adorn the office, photographs of patients are quite a rare find in many wanderings through medical suites. As office adornments or views of the relationship, I know of only one office wall containing pictures of the doctor's adult patients—in this instance of celebrity professional athletes who had undergone successful surgery of injured joints. Such an exhibit is, in effect, a visual endorsement of the doctor, like the signed photographs of celebrity patrons restaurants display. Other photo displays of patients are those snapshots of babies delivered or infants treated (Candib 1982; Selwyn 1984), mementos of the earliest professional attachment, put in an office album or on the bulletin board for review on visits with the child and parents. The intent of these displays is unlike another custom of "before and after treatment" photographs that used to dot old medical records, meant to show the benefits of plastic and orthopedic surgery to other doctors, those "body shots" of skin rashes, of deformities from endocrine disorders, and the congenital "freaks" that made a permanent photographic physical exam for hospital records (Apple 1984). Photoillustrations from those earlier relationships disappeared in the 1960s because they came to be considered potentially discriminatory.[9] Yet in some areas of medicine the use of pictures of patients has returned, though now for other purposes. Sometimes patients are photographed so they can be quickly recognized in the waiting room (C. C. Wang, Radiation Clinic, Massachusetts General Hospital, personal communication, 1982), and newly pregnant women can now get ultrasound pictures of their babies *in utero* for family albums. While Mayo Clinic internist John Berkman once showed anorexia nervosa patients photos of their emaciated bodies as part of his anaclitic therapy (Giffin et al. 1957), today, psychotherapists and clinical instructors show the videotaped encounter to the patient for treatment and to the student for learning the interview. On the doctor's side of the relation, photo identification of another kind is now often demanded of the hospital staff. In large treatment institutions, just as in banks, factories, and universities, the

staff—including the doctors (who now are so often employees)—
must carry photoidentification cards simply to assure the plant security they are not trespassers.

If patient photographs are out of fashion in the medical record, so
too is the old tradition (mentioned by Cathell) of posting pictures of
one's mentors on the office wall. Pictures of professors, teachers, or
colleagues are now uncommon even in the offices of academic doctors. Mentors of a professional career are now so numerous and
pedagogical relationships so diluted that a single picture would probably not suffice, nor is it the present custom to acknowledge these
former subordinate relationships.

At another extreme is the displaying of photos of the medical staff
in the waiting room of a group practice ("Photo gallery introduces
staff," *Patient Care*, March 30, 1979). From this photo gallery patients
can then recognize doctors other then their own, perhaps expanding
their attachments to the group. This photographic presence of the
modern doctor at the office encounter is quite unlike the "live presence" of the general practitioners that D. W. Winnicott, the British
pediatrician and child psychoanalyst, considered so important in the
relationship between patient and doctor, as when he wrote:

The value of a general practitioner in a village is largely that he is alive, that
he is there and available. People know the number of his car, and the back
view of his hat. It takes years to learn to be a doctor, the training may absorb
all of a father's capital; but in the end the really important thing is not the
doctor's learning and skill, but the fact that the village knows and feels he is
alive and available. The doctor's physical presence meets an emotional
need.   (Winnicott 1978)

For the doctor's real presence (as in this nostalgic account), and for
that emotional need, photographs will never substitute. However,
more of them are likely to appear as advertising becomes a norm in
the business of medical practice, as medical service becomes a commodity, and as the doctor and the patient are relabeled as *the health
care provider* and *the consumer*.

The beginnings of such advertising are already here. Television
advertising by "health professionals" for medical and dental services
accounted for expenditures of $62 million in 1984 (*American Medical
News*, 1985). Dentists appear in pictures in ads on New York subways
and local Boston suburban newspapers, and medical doctors appear
in radio and TV spots and in those mailed flyers seeking patients for
HMOs and walk-in clinics with "We Care" slogans. This pro-
motional trend (now legal) was anticipated by two earlier develop-

ments. The first were photographs of doctor-authors that accompanied clinical articles written for colleagues in "throwaway" medical journals or catalogs of drug advertisements, and second were the airline posters and magazine ads in which a celebrity heart surgeon (like a celebrity ball player) promoted flying, and, in front of "his hospital," promoted himself with his own bronze bust.

Pictures of doctors and patients together are rare, and when they do occur, they are not displayed in offices. The earliest photos of a doctor operating on an anestheized patient were publicly displayed to celebrate the hospital and its surgical practice; those that followed were for medical texts, showing the doctor demonstrating the technique of physical examination (Burns 1980; Cabot 1927). Ordinary photographs of both doctor and patient in the office, similar to those in the FSA collection of the 1930s (Stoeckle and White 1985), have become a very common scene in drug advertisements, though the home visiting scenes in the FSA photos or those of W. Eugene Smith (1986) have not yet been imitated. With glossy color photos, the encounter is now a backdrop for the writing of a prescription—antidepressants for the attractive but sad aging housewife; birth control pills for the erotic young woman; and anti-inflammatory drugs for the muscular male athlete.[10]

Quite aside from decor and photographs, the office has functions and uses. It comfortably contains the traditional dyadic exchange between one patient and one doctor, though hardly big enough to accommodate the whole family or even a patient and escorts—unless, of course, they all crowd up on the examination table. Yet students of proxemics, such as Edward Hall (1968) and Robert Sommer (1969), would be pleased to note that the usual up-to-date 10 by 8 foot furnished office does have its benefits. By necessity, the dimensions make for the intimate communication these writers delineate; the doctor and patient are now put close together. With the furnishings in place, the doctor and the patient can hardly be more than 5 or 6 feet apart, and when seated, are closer to the 3 feet that is considered the optimal distance for intimate exchange, whether they are facing each other across the desk or across one of its corners. (The latter is said to be the very best position and propinquity for personal exchange.) As one looks at these smaller offices, it is obvious that the desk can no longer be comfortably placed between the doctor and the patient but must be in a corner or against a wall to assure more open space. Those desk placements that now put the patient and doctor across the corner of the desk are a cost-dictated architectural squeeze that robs the modern doctor of the previous authoritarian position and interpersonal distance. Furthermore, maintaining the benefits of close dyadic exchange when an interpreter (or an escort) is also in the office requires that the interpreter be seated beside or behind the doctor, thus eliminating triangular exchanges in which looks, questions, and responses are passed between the patient and the interpreter before actually reaching the doctor.

Architects, such as Kirk and Steinberg in the classic *Doctors' Offices and Clinics*, also write about the office space (Kirk 1955), as does the ophthalmologist B.J. Sachs when he closely examines the dynamics of an ophthalmologist's work (Sachs 1975), including his waits on slow-moving old people before and after ocular exams, fees for service, space for equipment, and the scheduling of visits. Sachs notes the extra space needed for the patient's escort,[11] the position of the secretary needed to maintain visual control of the patients in the waiting room, and the 12–15 square feet per patient needed for "comfortable" waiting (16–19 feet is even more "comfortable"). In spite of its obvious importance, few write about the effects that the physical layout of the office may have on communication between doctor and patient.

One who does is Paul Goodman (1959) in his essay "The Meaning of Functionalism." With clarity and vividness, Goodman observes that seating varies with the type of public or private function, from the Greek theater to the psychoanalytic couch. The patient on the couch and the therapist seated out of sight is the psychoanalytic setting meant to promote the patient's free association; the Sullivanian school for treating psychotic patients calls for the doctor and the patient seated in chairs face to face across a desk, an arrangement meant to facilitate discussion of current reality problems; the characteranalysis school of Wilhelm Reich had the patient on a couch, nearly naked, with the actively poking therapist sitting alongside attempting to break down the defenses of the patient and focus on his resistance to therapy; the Gestalt school paid no attention to fixed seating arrangements, for "their aim is to heighten awareness ... and to find new possibilities of 'creative adjustment' to it, rather than to repeat the archaic habits that the patient has fallen into to avoid excitement." Psychotherapist Leston Havens (1976) has observed that sitting side by side, both doctor and patient looking ahead, is the true Sullivanian position, acknowledging that the patient's problems are produced "out there by others" (not inside the patient) and that by sitting beside the patient, also looking out, the doctor acknowledges the patient's interpersonal perception of victimization. In medical practice, the seating is like Goodman's description of the Sullivan school, but with variations in the position of the desk which, in turn, reflect differences in closeness between the doctor and the patient. No matter about closeness, for the doctor is looking, if not staring, at the patient in joint acknowledgment that what is wrong is *inside* the patient. The disease producing the distress is in the body or the mind. The patient is the object of clinical observation, as Stanley Reiser (1977) has written, and the earliest mode of this observation is visual: the doctor looks only at the countenance and habitus of the dressed patient for clues to the diagnosis of disease.

Considering the room again, the Gestalt tactic of moving the desk, the chairs,[12] and the table around seems to have no measurable influence on communication, but it has rarely been tried or studied (Rosenbaum 1975). In a note, "Why Not Discard the Desk?," P. W. Short (1980), a British general practitioner, reports that 41 percent of his patients did not care when he discarded the desk, 46 percent liked the arrangement without the desk, and 13 percent wanted the desk back. Of office furnishings, we should note that the doctor's chair is invariably different from the patient's, the former an executive swivel armchair that is movable and larger than the straight back that fixes the patient in one place, thus signaling the dyadic differences in authority, control, and movement in the office encounter.

In Japan, medical office furniture is still different, for there the patient and the doctor commonly sit directly oppoiste each other without an intervening desk, and often closer than 3 feet[13]; the patient is on a fixed but rotating stool that is used for a sitting up physical examination as well as for the interview; the doctor again has an executive-style swivel (Yonezo Nakagawa, Medical School, Osaka University, personal communication; and author's personal observation, 1982). This rotary staging of the patient certainly makes the medical acts of interview and examination move faster, as it was once done in the United States by chest and ear-nose-throat specialists. Then and now, queries could be brief and quick "physicals" limited to the head, neck, or chest could be performed with the patient on the stool, the otolaryngologist standing, the ptysiologist sitting, neither changing positions by going to an exam table after the interview.

In the functions of the office, closing the office door remains decidedly important. It is a visible guarantee of privacy that facilitates communication by supporting the confidential aspects of the doctor-patient relation. And yet, as Kenneth Clute's (1963) survey of Canadian general practice showed, guaranteed privacy was then less than

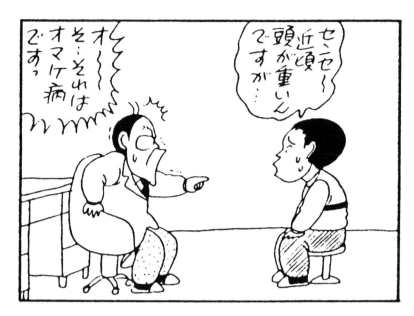

Cartoon illustrating positions of doctor and patient in Japanese office encounter.

certain, even with the door closed. In his travels through Canadian provinces, Clute found some doctors' offices with such poor acoustics that patients in the waiting room could easily hear all the complaints and medical advice going on inside the office. Even later, in the 1980s, such acoustical leakage can still be found in urban and suburban American professional office suites, where it may be muted only by the background noise of air conditioning, the traffic of the office staff, and in some instances by music.

While the office remains a private space for communication, the accommodations in hospitals, despite the greater number of private rooms, are becoming more public as more and more staff attend the patient. Most encounters take place at the bedside. Now the doctor is often standing up, the patient lying down. Rarely does the doctor sit except to take the initial history, and that narrative frequently has been taken by the doctor standing up at the bedside or stretcher in emergency rooms prior to admission. The patient's bed is usually in a one-, two-, or four-bed room, rarely in the old-fashioned ward with its 15–20 beds for the "sick poor." Big wards are out of fashion; hospital accommodations have become private in response to the wishes of the hospital managers and the public, and because of federal regulations. (Private rooms may also be more profitable than lower-cost ward accommodations, especially if they are supported by the reimbursement rates of federal and private insurance.) A decade after the enactment of Medicare and Medicaid, the American Hospital Association (1975) reported that 22.6 percent of hospital beds were in one-bed rooms, 60.9 percent in two-bed rooms, and only 16.5 percent in rooms with three or more beds (usually four).[14] Even with more privacy of space, the actual bedside encounter in today's more spacious one-, two-, three-, or four-bed room is really more public, since so many more staff now attend the patient than the patient's personal doctor alone and the patient's record is read everywhere in many separate departments and laboratories, if not by transport staff as well.[15]

Lying comfortably bedded in their private rooms, however, patients are quite uneasy about being alone. A walk down hospital corridors will quickly show a row of open doors to all those private rooms. Patients keep their doors open so as not to be neglected by the staff, whose attention and visible relationship they do not want to miss. "This room is dangerously unguarded," wrote the poet L. E. Sissman (1978) during his hospital stay with Hodgkin's disease. Here Sissman poignantly expressed for the patient what Florence Nightingale advocated for nurses (and patients) in 1861: mutual visibility. The Nightingale ward, with its central nursing station looking out over an open ward of 50 beds, promoted mutual supervision and observability of the patients and the nurses (Thompson and Golden 1975). Moreover, for nurses, the large ward was efficient. In their single rooms today, few patients can obtain that same degree of supervision and observability, unless they can afford a private-duty nurse or be observed by a television monitor (which then of course robs them of the visual exchange with the nurses).

Despite these trends toward single, "closed" hospital rooms, some open space for encounters is likely to persist because the long-sought conversion of the hospital into a private world of single rooms meant to imitate the personal bedroom at home (as in the Phillips House of Massachusetts General Hospital, built in 1922) will be difficult to complete, less for socio-economic than for technical reasons (Thompson and Golden 1975). If large wards are "out" for the poor, and semi-private or private rooms are "in" for everyone, the social and economic reasons are apparent: Hospital insurance began to cover single rooms in the 1950s, and in the 1960s the general social-political press for more equal care in society led to Medicare's specification of semi-private accommodations. Nonetheless, common wards (though smaller ones) continue to be reinvented for everyone, but now for technical reasons rather than for reasons of social class or payment differences. Occasionally, treatment strategies, implicit or explicit, may also influence design, as rehabilitation wards are common grounds for sharing pain and reinforcing self-sufficiency among patients. But the main reason for the resurgence of common wards is the economic need to share the high-tech equipment and labor-intensive personnel for acute care and to facilitate easy observation of and access to patients. Thus, two modern "wards" for patients with respiratory failure and heart attacks each have their own shared equipment and staff, although nowadays these and other "wards" like them are called by a host of invented names: respiratory, coronary, neurological, critical, or intensive-care "units." Considered to offer the very best care, they at least offer the most expensive; at the Massachusetts General Hospital, such critical-care units account for only 94 beds (8.6 percent) of the total 1,094, while using 30 percent of the nursing staff. Patients, on the average, spend 3.4 days in such open "public" units before being transferred to private or semi-private rooms, if they recover (Thibault et al. 1980). These modern labor-intensive wards with machines, doctors, and nurses constantly at the bedside are in stark contrast to their historical predecessor, the 50-bed ward staffed by two nurses.

The bedside is not the only place where a hospital patient may meet a doctor; it is, however, the most celebrated location. Healing is traditionally equated with bed rest, and professionals have their strongest attachment to the patient in bed. Compared to other encounters, the patient in bed is the "sickest" and most dependent (Van der Berg 1967), and the doctor is most in control (or at least the patient's supine position reinforces that illusion) when she or he stands. Additionally, it could be argued today that the percentage of doctor-patient encounters in which the patient is in bed has increased because of technological interventions of treatment that require the patient to be there and because of hospital insurance that pays the physician more per hour in this setting than in the office (Blumberg 1979). As a result, the doctor's other encounters with "walking patients" and those wheeled away from the bedside are often viewed as less intense, less rewarding, and, hence, less important by doctors, patients, and public alike. Nonetheless, these other hospital encounters are worth attention, as they now take up a larger portion of the patient's brief 6.6 days of institutional life.

Looking at hospital contacts away from the bedside, the surgeon and anesthesiologist may meet the patient in the operating room, the radiologist in the imaging room or darkened fluoroscopy suite, and the physician in the laboratory that tests heart, lung, and circulatory functions when the testing techniques (or the professional control of them) require a doctor rather than a technician to "invade" the body with needles, potentially toxic drugs, and catheters. On meetings in these three settings away from the bedside there is little literature. Such encounters are often very technical, brief, and not repeated; the doctor-patient relation has been inflated to a procedure or test. Yet the distinctive relationship between the anesthesiologist and the patient has been reformed (Egbert et al. 1964). Because anaesthesiologists' contacts with patients in the operating room were so technical, and because they and their treatment were so unobservable to their patients, for some time they have reported on the advantage of talking to patients in advance of anesthesia, at the bedside the night or day before they are to be transported "to the OR to be put to sleep."[16] The reasons are not singularly to discuss the choice of anesthesia; more important, with psychological preparation for the procedure and postoperative pain, the patient's postoperative anxiety and pain can be somewhat reduced. Radiologists, too, sometimes visit patients at the bedside; some of their procedures (such as angiograms and radiation therapy) have become more complex, occasionally hazardous and liable to malpractice claims, so that direct prior contact with the patient and informed consent have become more important. Other health professionals also search for personal contact with patients; for example, operating-room nurses, now unmasked, promise to make visits to patients, now conscious, after their operation (Perioperative Nursing Committee, Department OR Nursing, Massachusetts General Hospital, Letter to Patients [Morris Waters], 1985).

While visits by anesthesiologists and radiologists are becoming more common, such professional contacts (at or away from the bedside) are never counted in official statistics on doctor visits in hospitals and they are not subject to much professional reflection or comment. The radiology literature contains only an occasional remark about the meeting of radiologist and patient. In one, "The Patient and His Problem," a paper on the radiographic examination of the gastrointestinal tract, Jack Dreyfuss (1971) noted there is "something about an X-ray examining room that stimulates most patients to be exceedingly brief and direct in stating their symptoms. It is in such a situation that a patient may occasionally offer a very helpful clue. The clue is particularly likely to be given to the radiologist in the down-to-business atmosphere of an X-ray room, immediately prior to starting an examination." In the kind of encounter described here, the radiologist and the patient are quickly talking about something that is personal: how the patient's body feels and works. The situation may be no different from many other fleeting relations and brief encounters with strangers, like Fred Davis's (1959) account of taxi drivers and their fares, in which the time pressure to communicate is great and the consequences of self-revelation not an interpersonal hazard because so limited. A strictly similar sort of urgent impersonal communication takes place in emergency wards, where the patients are often brand-new, strangers to the staff, and quick to disclose themselves.

In contrast, the commentary of surgeons differ as does their situation. Nowadays they write about operations and their complications. They rarely, however, write about the relationship except for the communication of information about cancer. Few surgeons even address the issues of taking care of the dying cancer patient. That was not always the case. Dying with cancer, a theme that surgeons once addressed extensively from personal experience, has become a specialized topic of oncologists and thanatologists, perhaps because the surgeon now attends fewer terminal patients. When surgery fails today, the radiotherapist and the oncologist with radiation and chemotherapy become the patient's doctors, providing these "curative," "palliative," and "adjunct" therapies, often until the very end. Despite these few examples of in-hospital contacts away from the bedside by anesthesiologists, radiologists, and surgeons, most of the anecdotes and literature are still derived from bedside and office encounters.

While the current perspective of life inside the hospital is one where doctor-patient interaction is conducted with more staff in attendance, that same situation is developing in office encounters. More staff attend the patient, as the health-care team of doctor, nurse, and social worker that began in the 1900s for the care of the "sick poor" (Cabot 1907) expands to include everyone. For example, in a hospital-based general medical practice, patients made 28,500 visits to doctors but also 4,992 visits to nurses, 2,247 to social workers, and 2,732 to dieticians (Stoeckle et al. 1981). The team of doctor, nurse, social worker,[17] and dietician is becoming a common treatment mode in both solo and group practices, but the old delegation of tasks it implies for working "under the doctor" is no longer acceptable as new professionals are seeking their own autonomy through collaborative rather than dependent relationships with the doctor, or by working on their own.

Putting these others on the team might seem like a loss in the therapeutic intensity of personal doctoring outside the hospital, a dilution of clinical attention that diminishes the doctor's importance and the attachment of the patient to the doctor or to any particular therapist. Perhaps. But there are gains in the multiple contacts of task delegation in practice, even though these gains are far too often unacknowledged, misstated, or only rationalized economically because they might be "cheaper" than the MD, not because they might enhance care. The literature on physicians' assistants (PAs) and nurse-practitioners (NPs) is peppered with studies and essays to prove how they are at least as good as or better than MDs (and cheaper), perhaps intended to persuade adminstrators, physicians, and the public (who cling to the old idea of isolated therapeutic responsibility) that non-physician health workers can be of real use in personal care, traditionally the doctors' domain, closed to intruders from other health professions (Ramsey et al. 1982; Yankauer and Sullivan 1982). Thus, it should not be surprising that PAs, NPs, and other health professionals, in turn, aspire to precisely the same claims about their special relationship with the patient and about their distinctive skills while also wanting to do more of care all alone and at lower cost. The gains realized through task delegation and team care are not technical and economic alone, however, they are also social. As a social task, care can be enriched when a variety of helpers bring additional support and stimulus to patients. This collaborative practice among doctors, nurses, PAs, and social workers is particularly beneficial to older persons who have been left with few and sometimes no social or family connections while having to cope with chronic diseases and handicaps. Care by a variety of persons of both genders and of different personalities and backgrounds diminishes dependency on only one helper and provides a richer complementarity in care that is not possible with a single practitioner.

Office, Home, and Telephone Encounters

Office Encounters
Encounters not only require a space, but space that is part of some larger "territory." Today the meeting of doctor and patient often takes place in a territory the doctor controls (the doctor's "own" office or hospital) rather than in the home, a territory the patient controls. This shift in the site of care from home to office, which began in the early 1900s, has made doctors more distant physically, if not psychologically, from the personal and social lives of their patients.

The location of the professional office is also less private in every instance, no longer exclusively located in the doctor's home or, as a private suite, in the professional "downtown" office or bank buildings with their mix of lawyers, real estate agents, dentists, and optometrists.

More and more often, patients are meeting doctors in larger treatment organizations, in medical group practices where their doctor works with other doctors: the hospital outpatient departments, private group practices, health-maintenance organizations, free clinics, surgi-centers, health centers, and industrial medical clinics (Stoeckle 1975). For example, in 1972 patients made some 520 million visits to doctors in solo practice, 180 million to doctors working in outpatient departments, 160 million to private and prepaid group practices (HMOs), 8 million to health centers, 7 million to doctors in factory clinics, and 1 million to free clinics. A decade later, Milton Roemer, in his survey *Ambulatory Health Services in America* (1981), reported similar figures but found that group practices, outpatient departments, and HMOs handled over 50 percent of all medical visits. Moreover, by that time the group-practice mode was sought by three of five younger doctors (H. J. Kaiser Foundation 1981).

At the same time that more doctor-patient encounters are taking place in larger practices, these, in turn, have become increasingly centralized in office buildings near or on hospital grounds. This centralizing trend is hidden by the fact that official statistics of ambulatory visits to hospitals count only those to outpatient departments, not those to private offices that are located in the hospital, on its grounds, or on a nearby campus. However, the centralization of practice can be perceived from studies of the location of doctors' offices, from the growth of academic medical centers, and from the expansion of hospital-based office buildings (Dorsey 1969; Kaplan and Leinhardt 1975; Beeson 1975). Nearly two-thirds of practitioners, including solo practitioners, are now located at or near hospitals (Stoeckle and Grossman 1977). Of organized group practices, only health centers, free clinics, some private group practices, and industrial clinics are purposefully located away from hospitals. This suggests the beginning of a marketing trend in which medical practices, like branch banks, will add similar units for suburban and neighborhood clienteles. Indeed, walk-in, fast-service, free-standing, doc-in-a-box, medical-surgical centers offering bits and pieces of the medical exam and discourse for immediate medical relief have begun to locate in the ubiquitous multipurpose suburban shopping centers (Tanner 1982).

While these several practice locations are the territorial sites for ambulatory visits, they do not include all the other sites where doctors may meet and examine patients, especially the 2.5 million persons who are institutionalized (U.S. Bureau of Census 1985). After those previously mentioned medical contacts at offices, acute- and chronic-care hospitals (7,678), and nursing homes (22,000) come several other institutional meeting places where doctors may work or be called to see patients: schools and homes for the deaf, the blind, the physically handicapped, the mentally retarded, and the emotionally disturbed (4,760); homes for the aged; prisons and jails (5,616 state and local, 68 federal); the dispensaries of public schools, colleges, summer camps, and cruise ships (Taylor 1981); and, finally, not to be forgotten, the numerous outpatient departments of the military hospitals. In hospitals and medical practices doctors have almost full control, but in educational or penal institutional settings the treatment and the relation will depart from the norm of practice in the community (Waitzkin and Waterman 1974; University of Pennsylvania Law School 1973; Selwyn 1980). For example, in prisons, visiting rates to the dispensary rise from the national average of 5.0, reaching 7–8 per prisoner per year (Twaddle 1976), while reports of the encounter describe a very altered relationship:

Inmates did use sick call to escape a boring job and see friends as well as to get treatment for illness.... At sick call the doctors asked the nature of the inmate's complaint and either sent him back to his assignment or to his cell after dispensing whatever medicine he thought was appropriate.... The time and effort necessary to explain, to help provide insight, to gain acceptance to achieve confidence was absent. (Becker and Della Penna 1975)

Collections of patients in special institutions and such divergent uses of medical aid aside, overall centralization of practice has resulted, in large part, from fast and easy transportation that has altered the distance and time to the encounter. Medical geographers (Weiss and Greenlick 1970; Eyles and Woods 1983), health planners, management consultants, patients, and doctors know that the distance, but not necessarily the time, to the encounter has increased as practices have centralized. However, so very few persons are carless (only 13 percent of the employed and 36 percent of the unemployed, the latter chiefly older women) and so few households (20 percent) are without cars that most persons can drive to the office or be taken there (Paaswell and Recker 1970). Regular patients in a practice may come from as far as 20 miles away from the office, while in rural areas they may come from 40 or 50 miles away and sometimes still farther. Yet, significantly, both rural and urban patients use the same amount of time, 30–60 minutes, in travel. Overall, 50 percent get to the office in 15 minutes, 80 percent in 30 minutes, and less than 5 percent in 45 minutes or more (Verbrugge 1979). Similarly, most doctors now drive to office encounters that are no longer held in their homes or near their patients, taking up to one hour (10 percent) of their working day (Shannon 1980; "Compare your work-load with 300 other physicians," *Physician Management*, January 1979, p. 53).

Besides the modern convenience of a car that can be readily driven to the doctor's office, even urban mass transportation, bad as it can seem, did something for the popularity of going for medical visits— particularly to the outpatient departments of hospitals, where modern, centralized, large-scale group practice first began. From the 1900s, the rising use of the outpatient department at Massachusetts General Hospital, among both old and new immigrants to Boston, was attributed as much to its close, one-block proximity to the Charles Street transit station as to the clinic's free or 25 cent admission fee, to the reputed distinction of its staff of medical and surgical specialists, or to its newest diagnostic technology, the x-ray.

Home Encounters

If the office is the major site of care today, that was not the case in the 1930s, when about half of all physician-patient contacts were house calls, though they count for but 1–3 percent of all encounters today. Some idea of what those home visits were like comes from the reminiscences of older physicians[18] who recall prescribing for the kids with the "croup," diarrhea, and earaches, delivering babies, performing kitchen surgery by removing tonsils, sewing up cuts, and draining abscesses, even sometimes treating the pneumonias (as "sulfa drugs" became available) and the heart attacks and failing hearts of aging grandparents, or simply attending to the dying old folks whose deaths had not yet been institutionalized at hospitals and nursing homes. Despite the high volume of home visits (15–20 house calls to 8–10 office visits) compared to today's medical practice, by the 1940s more and more of the doctor's encounters were beginning to shift to the office as patients had the transportation to get there. In addition, the doctor's hospital work was just starting to grow. This latter shift was promoted by the provision of hospital insurance to workers in exchange for wages on the job. Patients could now be hospitalized for "all those tests" without paying out of pocket. That financing made diagnosis and treatment in the hospital a modern patient-doctor convenience, if not a clinical necessity. Thus, by the end of the 1940s, much of the medical practice once performed in the patient's home had moved into the doctor's office, and some of it had moved into the hospital. The site of care changed not only in the United States but also (to a lesser extent) in Great Britain. Even though the British general practitioner (GP) and the British public continue a shared tradition of "domiciliary visits" (and they remain part of the daily GP schedule), such visits are down from a high of 50 percent to 20–25 percent today.

The shift to office care has gained the doctor not only technical efficiency (as so often is claimed and observed from the equipment) but also higher fees and more power. More patients can also be seen. And since the territory of the encounter is the doctor's, advantage belongs , as in any exchange, to the owner, in this case the MD, who can organize the speed, complexity, and volume of diagnosis and treatment. In spite of this modern level of gains and losses in the site of care, several have commented on home visits from other perspectives of the relation but with little chance of reversing the office trend back to home visits or of recapturing some of the past relationship at home (Goldsmith 1979; Fry 1978). However, in obstetrical care, it should be noted that "birthing rooms," "rooming in," and "delivery atten-dance" by fathers (Bradley 1962) are recapturing some features of home deliveries in hospital settings (though the setting is still the hospital with the father attending at 79 percent of births). Meanwhile a trickle of demand for real home deliveries, where fathers are sure to be around (Sagov et al. 1984), continue. Moreover, the family makes the hospital more like home. Just as families attend the patient for bedside care in the hospitals of undeveloped countries, it even happens in the developed ones. An average of 20 percent of the parents of children hospitalized at Massachusetts General Hospital sleep in the adjacent waiting room or in chairs at the child's bedside (John Truman, MGH Pediatrics Service, 1985).

Home visiting, of course, evokes a nostalgic and romantic vision of the doctor attending the whole family (and the sick one), usually in the surroundings of a comfortable urban residence or a humble rural farmhouse, as in Dr. Arthur E. Hertzler's (1938) *The House and Buggy Doctor*, seldom in a city tenement, as in William Carlos Williams's (1984) stories. But even that pleasant old image of the family doctor has been tarnished by recent historical interpretations. Home visiting reportedly became dominant just as home crafts moved out of the family workshop to the factory for the increased productivity pro-vided by machines, an event that increased the number of middle-class mothers who stayed at home with their children. In this context, Christopher Lasch (1977), Barbara and John Ehrenreich (1974), and others view the doctor as one of the new class of "experts" that emerged in the nineteenth century. His visits *invaded* the family at home, bringing bourgeois values on medical care and child rearing that tied mothers to their houses and children rather than liberating them by encouraging work outside the home.

It is widely assumed that patients left their homes to visit doctors' offices in search of more scientific diagnostic technology to look at and in their bodies for more accurate diagnoses than they could get from the doctor's bag he brought to the house. But did the office x-ray for bones and chests, its electocardiogram (EKG) for the heart, and its microscope for blood and urine tests really increase the volume of office visits? Certainly not by themselves. Even before these office technologies were firmly in place, easy transportation by the private car and public trams increased medical visiting at the office. In an essay on these themes, Paul Starr (1979) observes that when the doctor's car replaced the horse and buggy in the early 1900s, he could easily see more patients at home and increase his income, although not through visit fees alone but also through added charges for driving out to the house. Moreover, the automobile was cheaper than the horse (Flink 1970). But later experience has shown that the doctors could handle even more visits when patients could take the city streetcars or drive their own car to the office or get medical advice on the telephone that might have previously been only given at home. Indeed, much of the increase in office visiting preceded the availability of EKGs, chest x-rays, and blood tests in the office as more of the public, with rising personal incomes, sought professional medical advice over their self, lay, or mothers' home treatment. Quite in advance of the medical technology was the larger search for the professional relationship—and the promise of the healthy body.

Viewed as special relationships, home visits no longer evoke the image depicted in Sir Luke Fildes's famous 1890s painting *The Doctor*, in which the doctor waits with the family, sitting at the bedside of a dying child (Gifford 1973). Here the doctor continues to "attend" the patient at home without "doing anything," but nonetheless providing what John Berger and J. Mohr (1967) call the "fraternal comfort" of one who had witnessed others' death, acting out that older idea of medicine as a religious "calling." For these seemingly antique functions of *comfort* and *witness*, patients may still be taken to the doctor at the hospital today; however, their unstated requests may go unacknowledged by the staff members as doctors try to "cure" the patient at all costs or, at least, to maintain a semblance of treatment, e.g., by "giving IV fluids," while avoiding behaviours that might be viewed

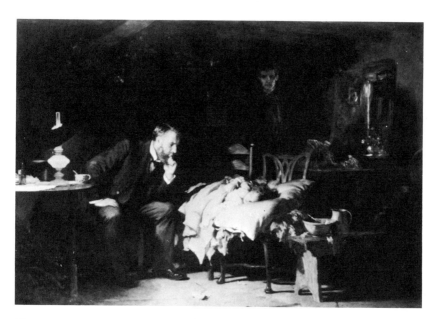

The Doctor, by Sir Luke Fildes (1891).

as merely pastoral. Today the doctor's technical interventions for the dying may themselves seem excessive—certainly in comparison with "bearing witness"—and, in the opinion of some critics, may be (costly) self-serving professional acts that deny a "death with dignity." However, such "all-out" medical intervention in the hospital away from home is strongly supported by an activist public and profession that view illness and dying as things that can be and ought to be controlled, not as matters to be left to fate or nature or (least of all in this uncertain modern world) unattended at home.

Nowadays, popular belief would hold that there is but one life to lead, and the doctors are no longer gatekeepers to the "better life," only guardians of the precious present which is one's only reality. The older religious view, "He that loseth his life shall save it," is uncommon. Thus, the stakes in medical treatment today are different. In the hospital, these modern expectations, along with the technical imperative of medical treatment, may press the doctor to interventions at any cost—literally—and certainly to interventions that would and could not be acted out in the home. Even if medical treatment might seem inappropriate and excessive, the public may respond gratefully, perceiving any technical intervention as only more devoted care: "The doctors were wonderful. They did everything." Yet gratitude is not universal. The perceived entitlement to eternal life (Andrew

Bodnar, MGH Medical Service, personal communication, 1980) that today's medical treatment is supposed to produce may fail, and when those expectations are not fulfilled the doctor is then the victim of often considerable family wrath.

With the dying, as in so many other medical matters, activist intervention is not a persistently or universally held ideology— witness the growth of the hospice movement, which revives relationships that were once part of home care (Sampson 1977). Hospice care, whether in small facilities or in home programs for the terminally ill, promises patients the prevention of chronic pain and bodily discomforts, readily available support personnel (to use the jargon of modern management), care organized for personal wants and needs, and the participation of patients and their families in care (Lack and Buckingham 1978). These goals are gaining acceptance with the public, the medical profession, and even hospitals, some of which now set aside a section for hospice care. Whether in special treatment facilities or in homes, hospice care attracts staff members with particular orientations; as a result, terminal care is made a divided but common enterprise among nursing, social work, medicine, the patient, and the family, with the relationships less dominated by the doctor or by technique alone.

In trying to come up with a modern rationale for the home as a better site of care than the office, Gibson and Kramer (1965) rediscovered the old adage that the doctor who saw a patient at home would see and hear more than just the patient's strictly medical problems. The relationship is altered by more participants, the setting reveals more. Whether today's doctor would respond to the patient's other problems or to the family's concerns is another matter, about which, unfortunately, there are too few facts. Other commentators, indifferent to the reality of relationships developed by house calls, have simply been concerned with whether home visiting is *medically* necessary. From 7 to 12 percent of visits are considered frivolous, and 60 percent a "nurse" might handle.[19] In up to 25 percent of home visits, patients were calling for something other than medical help.[20] The ideal of continuing contact with the same personal doctor for off-hour house calls as for office visits is not always viewed as essential (Hall 1972).[21] Not only does the home visit expand the observed problems of the patient, it also expands the dyadic relation, for now family members often confront the doctor in the territory of the home. As with the Greek physician in the public square, the native witch doctor in ritual healing ceremonies, or the American Indian medicine man in a tribal residence, a lay audience assembles for the medical consultation and examination, which may be held in the kitchen, the living room, or the bedroom. I and my Boston colleagues who have made home visits can report that up to ten friends and family members may surround the consultation, particularly when death is near.[22] More leisure time seems also to have increased the number of "visitors" to the hospitalized patient, too—witness the size of hospitals' parking lots and garages, the night and day movement of people in and out during "visiting hours," and the growth of food, gift, automatic banking, flower shop, and drug store services for visitors and staff.[23] Numbers alone press the doctor to communicate with some, if not all, of the family; so do the visitors themselves, nowadays better informed by longer contacts with the chronic illness and informally educated by relatives working somewhere in the health care industry,[24] if not full of questions about diagnosis and treatment from the media.

Some of these old home relations are being transferred to or re-created in the office or the hospital, although with difficulty. In the case of obstetrics, for example, more home-like treatment comes with birthing rooms and fathers in assistance at the hospital or at free-standing birthing centers (Sagov et al. 1984). To make consultations in the office setting more like home encounters is problematic. The need for a family audience may be hard to gauge, and a family encounter may be difficult to schedule and conduct—especially when the office is small and is separated from the waiting room by a wall of secretaries and receptionists, so that the doctor and the encounter remain unseen, backstage. Despite architectural drawbacks to visibility and space, group consultations with the family are, as David Schmidt (1983) notes, coming back into the office and the hospital for selected purposes, such as deciding on renal transplants, making plans for organ donations, or organizing the discharge of a patient to his or her home, to a nursing home, or to a son's or daughter's resi-dence—negotiating, in effect, who will take care of the patient. To this list should be added the support groups organized for the families of cancer and heart patients during their hospital stays. Like technical treatment, home and family visits are no longer a convenience service but have their clinical indications and rationale which the doctor decides (Billings et al. 1986; Siwek 1985).

Telephone Encounters
Still omitted from this territorial and organizational account are the telephone calls so much a part of modern medical practice. One might think the phone call to be a neutral "territory" for both participants. Hardly the case, since the doctor is harder to reach.

Nonetheless, 20 percent of patients with acute conditions get their medical advice by calling the doctor (Verbrugge 1979). Surveys report that telephone calls make up 10–15 percent of all MD-patient contacts, while clinical observers have reported 30–50 percent. Neither of these figures is surprising in a society in which 94 percent of households have a phone and pay phones are ubiquitous. Pediatricians average 20 office visits per day and 20 phone calls per day, and the calls take 10–15 percent of the doctor's time (Greenlick et al.1973; Bergman et al. 1966; Riley et al. 1969; Heagarty et al. 1968; Lawrence and Fuchsberg 1964).

There are other phone calls that are not recorded in surveys of office practices: those to the doctor's home.[25] Today, the doctor's home phone number has become a privilege, given only to a few long-term patients or (more often) not divulged to patients at all. Doctors can avoid that draining 24-hour availability by exchanging coverage with colleagues through a protective answering service, thus clearly separating their home lives from their professional lives: "to have some real life of my own away from work."

Of patients who phone the doctor, more of those in the upper and middle income groups do so primarily to first and foremost request, "I want to be seen," an appointment (Kedward 1962). This is usually negotiated indirectly with a secretary. Other telephone calls concern prescription refills, medical advice on old and new complaints (and whether they deserve attention or examination), referrals on where to go, reassurance about the patient's current illness, or even "counseling." The average conversation lasts 4.5 minutes (Diseker et al. 1980). The telephone voice exchange lacks the added emotional tone that face-to-face encounters with looking and speaking provide as patients remind us when they insist "You must *see* me" or "I want you to have a *look at me*."

Because the doctor's phone is a source of quick advice, referral, and ventilation, it is really the oldest "hot line." It precedes all those emergency phone contacts for help that proliferated in the expansive 1960s with free clinics and that were later developed by self-help and voluntary groups: the Samaritans, the special-disease associations such as the local branch of the cancer society (Cancer Information Service with their toll-free number from whom referrals on where to go and tape-recorded dial-advice can be had on nearly every ailment), along with suicide-prevention, drug-treatment, poison-control centers, and, not to forget, hospital emergency rooms (Westbury 1974; Lester 1981).[26] The increased use of phone calls to the office along with the "beeper" to locate "the doctor" has made the affiliation of doctor and patient even closer than would be feasible through more and more home and office visits (Weingarten 1982). Indeed, the telephone, as much as the car, accounts for the decline in home visits, though initially doctors thought it would increase them as patients would call to have the doctor come to the house. Often considered an effective substitute for an office visit, telephone advice or "telephone medicine" provides home care and also substitutes for home visits. Answering calls may now be delegated to nurses on the view that they, working under advice protocols or on their own, can handle them as well as doctors (and perhaps better), thus saving the doctor's time for "something else" (Katz et al. 1978; Strain and Miller 1971; Talbot et al. 1984), presumably something more important.

From this account it may seem that phone calls are the patient's guaranteed access to the doctor: "Doctor, please come." But that exchange from patient to doctor is not always the direction of calls. Phone calls may now be initiated by the doctor. Today phone "visits," like operations and home visits, also have professional "indications" as to when they should be done. Typically, doctors make phone calls to report on tests or to supervise the treatment of handicapped and elderly patients who cannot come to the office. Some practitioners have suggested that phone calls from doctors or nurses are a useful way of following the patient's treatment (blood pressure or responses to a new drug) without the necessity of office visits (Bertera and Bertera 1981). Despite physicians' reports that they do phone (for which they are rewarded with gratitude for such faithful, extra attention), the number of such calls they make remains unknown (though sometimes a specific charge for time spent on the phone is noted on a doctor's bill or calculated into the charge for a later office visit).

The Participants: Doctor and Patient

In going to see the doctor outside the hospital, patients are most likely to visit general practitioners, family physicians, internists, or pediatricians—those medical doctors who provide primary or general care, care that provides first-contact treatment, personal continuity, and coordination of services. According to data from the National Ambulatory Medical Care Survey (1975, 1980), visits to these physicians accounted for nearly 60 percent of all office contacts between doctors and patients, although such doctors make up but 44 percent of all physicians. The remaining office visits were to surgeons (20 percent), psychiatrists (3 percent), and a host of other medical specialists and subspecialists.

Overlap in the practice of primary-care doctors and specialists is considerable. Some patients go directly to specialists, who provide some primary care. Specialists have been so overproduced by specialty societies and university medical schools that some cannot keep busy and earn a living practicing their speciality care alone. In dealing with patients seeking general medical aid, they are confronted with, as old and new surveys show, a large segment of patients with undifferentiated complaints and psychological distress, if not psychiatric illness (Regier et al. 1978).

As a result of the discrepancy between patients' needs for specialized technique and patients' illnesses, subspecialists in medicine (cardiologists, nephrologists, hematologists, and rheumatologists) spend 28–53 percent of their time on the general care of patients (Aiken et al. 1979), in which they may have little training or even less interest. Similarly, many surgeons, rather than being completely engaged in their technical area of high expertise, may also maintain general practices because their low rate of operations will not sustain an active surgical practice (though it may still provide much of their income). At present, this national mismatch of patient needs and professional skills is rationalized as inconsequential for the patient and for the quality and costs of care, since the postgraduate training and preparation of doctors in university medical schools and hospitals serve other interests than the appropriate preparation for practice—namely, the economic and status interests of senior specialists who require less expensive junior staff members to whom they can delegate clinical work and the prestige that such training programs bring to the schools and hospitals that the everyday clinical care of patients does not.

Inside hospitals, patients' encounters with medical doctors almost equal those with surgeons—a distinct shift, for until very recently 80 percent of hospital beds were surgical. Now that so many older medical patients are hospitalized for treatment, medical discharges have nearly doubled, going from 7,704,000 (1960) to 14,173,000 (1978) when they surpassed the 12,749,000 general surgical discharges as they have ever since (Commission on Professional and Hospital Activities 1968, 1973, 1978).

Besides these changes in specialists seeing patients, still other shifts in the gender, race, ethnicity and age of doctors and patients make the encounter far more a mixed affair than ever before. Currently, patients are more likely to be female (60 percent) than male (40 percent)

(U.S. Department of Health, Education and Welfare 1980), while the doctor is, with *few* exceptions, male (92 percent). In fact the percentage of women as patients is even higher. Even though pediatric visits are listed by the sex of the child, wise pediatricians, family physicians, and mothers know that the mother is as much the patient as her son or daughter. If half the visits for children under 15 are boys coming with their mothers, the female-to-male ratio of office patients is more likely 70:30, and it would be even higher if we made note of all the daughters who bring their aged parents into the doctor's office or the wives who bring their ailing husbands, as the numbers of elderly grow. Surveys do not count these extras as women patients.

The typical office encounter in the United States is between a male doctor and a female patient (and female escorts). Some commentators, e.g. Ruzek (1978), have seen those gender differences as a built-in source of conflict or domination. Such gender differences are quite different from other countries. Elsewhere, many more women are doctors, for example, 75 percent in the USSR, 35 percent in France, 25 percent in Great Britain, and 20 percent in the Federal Republic of Germany (Josiah Macy Foundation 1970). These differences in physician gender will be coming to the United States, though slowly. The increasing numbers of women recently admitted to American medical schools, a number that is now approaching 30 percent of all classes (Braslow and Heins 1981), as yet has done little to change the male-to-female ratio among American doctors. In 1976 Mark Field estimated that it would be after 1985 before the United States had a significant number of women doctors. The U.S. Department of Health, Education and Welfare (1980a) predicted that by 1990 women will constitute at least 16 percent of all MDs. By 1985 the number of practicing women physicians was already 13 percent (AMA 1985).

This historical male dominance, not the sick role itself, the Ehrenreichs (1974) have argued, has promoted the dependency of women who seek medical help and the control of doctors over them. Despite such assertions, there is surprisingly little in the way of data from the United States or from abroad to indicate whether modern encounters with female doctors make a difference in caring, or whether the doctor is seen to be a good "mama" or "papa" because of or regardless of gender. Marie Haug (1976), as one observer, suggests that the relationship in the USSR is compounded of solicitous "mothering" by female doctors rather than the aristocratic paternalism that presumably typifies (or once typified) male doctoring in the United States.

Kirshner (1978), reviewing the evidence for effects of gender on psychotherapy, found no "systematic influence of gender stereotypes" or that male therapists might, more often or regularly, victimize female patients, but did note studies in which female patients reported greater satisfaction and improvement with female therapists (a preference that may not extend to all types of doctors). Mogul's review "The Sex of the Therapist" (1982) suggests that gender may facilitate the course of therapy, for example when adolescents with identity problems work with therapists of their own gender. Recording medical encounters, Wallen et al. (1979) found that the sex of patients affected the amount of information they recieved from male doctors. Female patients recieved the same number of spontaneous explanations as male patients, but women asked more questions and, in turn, received more explanations, though at a lower level of technicality. Other data also suggest that gender certainly has importance. In some 75 nonclinical studies of dyadic communication reviewed by Judith Hall (1978), more studies showed that female gender was an advantage in decoding nonverbal clues. In a family-practice setting, Candace West (1984) studied the distribution of interruptions in the medical interview, finding that patients interrupted female doctors as much as or more than the doctors interrupted them, whereas male doctors interrupted their patients far more than they were interrupted by them. Such differences in the effect of gender will need further clinical study, but they already suggest a therapeutic advantage to the female doctor for some patients while others write on how to improve communication for females (Borisoff and Merill 1985), hoping that gender inequalities can be reduced. Analyzing more than the interview exchange, namely, female-male differences in treatment, using the National Ambulatory Care Survey, Verbrugge and Steiner (1981) noted that female patients underwent more tests and more blood-pressure checks, had more medication prescribed, and made more return visits than men. Whether more female doctors will alter these differences is a question.

Whatever the answer the entry of greater numbers of women into the profession should make it easier for both women and men who prefer female physicians to seek them out. Some women, whether or not they are involved in feminist movements, prefer female doctors— perhaps because today they are younger and do not behave with the authoritarian style of many older male doctors, and perhaps because they are preferentially selected for gynecological checkups, which are of special concern to women (Armitage et al. 1979; Shapiro 1979). The expectation that the caring behaviors of the profession will improve with more female doctors is an ideological notion; it is difficult to prove (despite the assertion) and as yet there are few empirical descriptions of the purported differences in care. Since women are reportedly less interested in power than men, presumably female doctors would, at least, be less dominating in relationships with patients (Symonds 1980; Heins et al. 1979). Whether male doctors have some of the attributes of the "female" (for example, mothering) has not been tested, but personal observation would certainly suggest they do but do not admit it; it should also be added that some male doctors claim to "do my own social work"—an oblique suggestion that such personal care need not be delegated to female social workers.

Quite apart from the expectation of more humane treatment from female doctors is another transition that their increasing number is likely to bring: a decline in the professional status of the doctor. As Vincente Navarro (1975) and others (Ehrenreich and English 1979) have argued, this may result from structural constraints against women in the organization of health services where their position is or has been subordinate to men in charge of organized services (Schwartz 1980; Rinke 1981). Diminished status accompanied the feminization of schoolteaching, and this may occur in medicine (Field 1975)—not solely, of course, because of the entrance of women, but also because of a large surplus of doctors, cultural factors, and the public's diminished view of the profession in general.

The changing racial and ethnic makeup of the medical profession, too, is bringing promises of new choices for patients, though new problems for both doctors and patients. In the case of race, the 8,000 black MDs now constitute so small a percentage (2.2 percent) of practicing doctors that very few encounters occur between black MDs and white patients (U.S. Department of Health, Education and Welfare 1979). In actual fact, only 13 percent (5.8 million) of all visits to black doctors (most of whom are in solo practice) were by white patients; on the other hand, 41 million (8 percent) of all visits to white doctors were by black patients. Mixed encounters, particularly of white patients with black doctors, may become a bit more frequent as more blacks enter the profession, at least in proportion to their percentage of the population (10 percent), and as black doctors choose to practice in medical groups, where they may more readily build up a panel of white as well as black patients. Mixed practices are beginning. In a 1984 survey of 175 minority graduates from 1975, black physicians had 56.4 percent of patients who were black but also 32.9

percent white patients, the remainder from other minorities (Keith et al. 1985). And yet, these long-range prospects remain uncertain.[27]

The encounter today is more likely to be "mixed" by age and ethnicity, as well as by gender and race. While the population is getting older, doctors are getting younger. A large cohort of younger doctors is entering practice as a result of the expansion of the medical schools from the 1950s to the 1970s. Ethnicity has also changed on both sides of the encounter. To help meet the "doctor shortage" between 1950 and 1975, a large number of doctors immigrated from the Philippines, India, Pakistan, Iran, and Korea. As a result, foreign-born physicians, most from these homelands, now make up some 20 percent of all MDs in the United States (Margulies and Block 1969; Mejia et al. 1980; AMA Center for Health Policy 1984). During this same period, a large popular immigration from Hispanic America and Mexico has made a new ethnic minority, producing still more diversity in doctor-patient backgrounds, promising not only novelty in doctor-patient encounters but perhaps more dissonance in communication that is linguistic, cultural, and related to social class (Harwood 1981; Weitzman and Egeland 1973).

On the subject of communication, still other changes in the participants should also be noted. Some patients (and perhaps some doctors) now seek therapeutic alliances not on the basis of gender, ethnicity, race, or age, but on the basis of sexual preference. That is, some homosexual patients seek out homosexual doctors or go to special medical clinics organized by gay doctors and the gay community. New arrangements to match doctor and patient are in the tradition of organizing special practices and clinics to serve particular segments of the population, rather than to treat particular diseases, a recognized need because some people are often handicapped in access to care in mainstream institutions.[28]

Elements of the Consultation

In the office encounter, several actions take place: the wait; the reception; the interview before, during, or after the physical examination; and sometimes "lab tests," x-rays, electrocardiograms, prescriptions, referrals, discharges, and return visits.

A medical sociology text describes the initial consultation of the patient with the doctor as follows:

The physician is trained, when seeing a patient for the first time, to interview the patient in order to complete a history of the patient's present and past illnesses. This history which the physician learned in medical school has a rather stylized format—beginning with the patient's chief complaint, that is, what is causing the patient to see him on that day and progressing through the patient's history of the present illness, the past medical history, family and social history. Once the physician has taken this history, he examines the patient physically, looking for physical signs of illness. The examination is also stylized and comprehensive, beginning at the head and ending at the feet.

On the basis of the information gained through his history and physical examination, the physician formulates a hypothesis of what is wrong with the patient which he calls the diagnosis. Based on this diagnosis, he formulates a plan of action. (Robertson and Heagarty 1975)

While this stereotyped account from the doctor's perspective may describe the logic and the order of a medical encounter, it does not begin to describe the action that goes on.

Practice is different!

Waiting for the Encounter
Much has been written about the patient's decision to seek medical aid and the choice of pathways to the doctor (Zola 1966, 1972c; Stoeckle et al. 1963) but little about the fact that in order for that decision to lead to an encounter with the doctor a visit must be organized—and waited for, a wait often negotiated with a secretary viewed as "a dragon behind the desk" (Arber and Sawyer 1985). In 1977, the National Health Care Expenditures Study found that the average waiting period for an appointment with a doctor was 7.0 days. The waiting period was somewhat longer for visits to hospital outpatient departments (10.1 days) than for those to doctors' offices (6.9 days) and longer (14.1 days) for visits involving preventive services (e.g., general examinations, immunizations, prenatal and postnatal care) than for visits not involving such services (4.4 days) (National Center for Health Services Research 1981). Adults waited longer for their appointments than children, women longer than men (7.8 versus 5.9 days), and blacks longer than whites (7.2 versus 5.3 days). In a 1980 American Medical Association survey, marginal differences were noted in those same overall waiting times (Goldfarb 1981). New patients waited 8.1 days, old ones 4.5; by 1983 the wait for a new patient was down to 6.3 days (Reynolds and Ohsfeldt 1984).

Once at the doctor's office there was yet another wait for the doctor, with a mean of 27.9 minutes.[29] The longest waits were at emergency wards (39.1 minutes). Differential waiting by race occurs in the same practice setting and in the same treatment institution;

whites waited 28.4 minutes versus 39.4 minutes for other groups in doctors' offices, and 40.9 minutes versus 61.4 for blacks in outpatient departments. Such differentials not only illustrate the duration of the waiting experience but also show how the relationship often begins and continues to differ with the perceived importance and status of some patients over others, even in and between institutions that presumably have a single standard of care and when nearly everyone is a paying patient of equal status (or was until the 1980s' cuts in health-care funding). Capitalizing—literally—on that waiting disparity, today's commercial walk-in clinics advertise "no waiting."

To wait is usually to sit; at least that is the usual image in calculating the number of waiting room chairs. That positional passivity is hard for some to maintain, as standing up to wait not only occurs with a fully occupied room but as a break in the irritating tedium of waiting and the monotony of sitting—a familiar scene not only at emergency rooms and crowded clinics but occasionally outside the offices of private doctors.

In his book *Queuing and Waiting*, Barry Schwartz (1975) discusses the dynamics and the meaning of waiting in treatment organizations and professional relationships. He notes that more waiting can be used to insult and devalue patients (as doctors and their staff members well know from conscious and unconscious practice) and that when waiting is imposed, consciously or not, its origin lies not only in the adminstrative design or misdesign of the office schedule by operational researchers trying to cut the queues (Luck et al. 1971) but also in the doctor's power to run the schedule. A reduction in waiting times may not only bring a gain in efficiency; it may also signal a more egalitarian relationship or even a shift in relative status (as when the doctor "waits on" and "waits for" a celebrity patient, in the ancient tradition of the attending court physician). Schwartz, however, omits consideration of some benefits of extra waiting in medical practices. To those who are not searching for instant services or quick cures (for example, leisured indigents, retirees, or unemployed handicapped persons), the waiting room can serve as a temporary "hangout"—a reality that has been formally organized in day care centers but that can also be observed every day in the informal life of hospitals and clinics.[30] Neither is Schwartz aware of the field observations of Francis Powell (1975), who found that the waiting room in a diabetes clinic was also used by nurses and doctors for social conversation with patients' families or for history-taking from families outside of emergency wards.

To get into the office, the patient may be greeted and escorted into the doctor's office by a nurse, a receptionist, or the doctor. The traditional greeting, "Mr.," "Ms.," or "Mrs.," has sometimes been omitted and patients demeaned of late by calling them by their first names (presumably to appear nonauthoritarian) or by a fake chumminess, particularly to older persons, who are called "dearie" and "honey," names that hardly shore up the patient's already diminished sense of status and self-esteem (Conant 1983), or remove any of the hidden shame that may still accompany seeking help in a society where everyone is presumed to be self-reliant and nervous about dependency of any sort.

The Interview

In the usual picture of medical consultation the doctor and the patient are dressed and seated; the doctor is engaged in "history taking" and the patient in "complaining." While most patients are first interviewed with their clothes on, some are not. In emergency wards and in certain clinics and practices, patients are first undressed and covered with gowns; they then wait on the examining table or stretcher for the interview and physical examination, during which the dressed doctor often stands while the draped patients lies or sits. This positional and sartorial dominance is not uncommon in obstetrical, gynecological, and family-planning clinics, in some arthritis and orthopedic clinics, in visits following surgical operations, and even in the offices of private dermatologists, orthopedists, and gynecologists, where practitioners may quickly inspect incisions and rashes and easily move joints and perform pelvic exams while standing and talking to patients who are sitting or reclining, partially dressed in examination gowns. Of course, by doing two things at one time, these practitioners are being more productive in "processing" patients; they are also, like dentists, standing up much of the day, which is hardly a reflective posture.

Doctors may respond quite differently to patients depending on their position but also on their dress or undress. As a result, some women insist on being interviewed while dressed in order to regain status and respect, and similarly some patients' responses to the doctor may be affected if the doctor is tieless or in sneakers.

The actual garb of patients at encounters has changed less than that of doctors. The doctor's traditional white coat (a symbol of the antiseptic cleanliness of the operating room and the authority of the scientific laboratory) and the business suit for office work have often given way to more informal attire. Some male doctors now wear a shirt and tie but no coat, and both male and female doctors may wear denims and carry the stethoscope as a necklace. Such informal dress is not only for the sake of comfort but also, some feel, to diminish the doctors' authoritarian distance from the patient.

In his essay "The Doctor's White Coat," Blumhagen (1979) attributes to the white coat several symbolic meanings—not only the ones mentioned above but also purity, protection, goodness, and unaroused sexuality. These meanings facilitate the physical examination of patients, especially that of gowned female patients by male doctors. The white coat also serves to separate the professional staff from employees in the bureaucratic stratification of hospital life. That visible stratification is hard to maintain as the doctor's other hospital garb (the casual "OR" shirt) and even the "white coat" popularize into summer clothing. The patient undressed but gowned had still other meanings. The Medical Clinic of Massachusetts General Hospital once put white gowns on both men and women patients before their consultation, while each could wait one to two hours for the doctor. This custom was presumably meant to improve the efficiency of practice, not merely to permit easier physical access to the body. Whether the request is "Please strip to the waist and get up on the table" or "Please get undressed and into this gown," undressing times have always been short, averaging but 1.5 minutes in a study reported by the Scottish Home and Health Services Department (1979) and 1.7 minutes in our own group practice (except for the disabled elderly, who take longer to undress and may need assistance). Perhaps these stripping times seemed worth eliminating when doctors faced 20 patients in two hours, but today, with far fewer patients, these few minutes for advanced undressing now seem a very small gain in a search for office efficiency and serve only to further depersonalize the beginning of the encounter.

Informal dress, less for comfort than purposely to diminish the doctor's authoritarian distance from the patient (Selzer 1960), shades into informal "address," an ideology so prominent in the free-clinic movement of the 1960s, when doctors and patients vied to call each other by first names while dressing informally alike (Stoeckle et al. 1972). Among younger doctors and their younger patients, first-name informality of address persists. Still, many don't like the asymmetry, as Natkins notes in "Hi, Lucille, this is Dr. Gold," especially when the first-name address is not negotiated (Natkins 1982). Harry Senger (1984), who has queried professionals, notes that some give patients the license to use first names more than others. Psychologists (perhaps the newest and youngest of psychotherapists) readily give patients permission to address them by their first names, while social workers are less willing, and psychiatrists even more reluctant, even as more socialized against it. Yet not all first-name greeting is the doctor's; sometimes the patient closes the distance. Examples of calling doctors by their given names come naturally out of the patient's friendship with the doctor outside the office, at the country club, church, lodge, neighborhood, or summer home, where the relationship is a familar one by the time an office consultation occurs. Even without that friendship, patients may initiate informal, first-name address but get no reciprocity from the doctor; this is most common among patients of working-class backgrounds, who may call any doctor by his first name simply because that is how they deal with everyone. A novel and sometimes surprising break in the usual formality of the patient addressing the physician as "Doc" or "Doctor" is "Tell me, John, how do I take those pills?" In general, younger patients are more likely to respond favorably to informal dress and address while older ones appear to like the doctor's formal attire and title, with their symbolic if not actual promise of professionalism, authority, and therapeutic efficacy.[31]

In obtaining a "complete history" of the patient's illness, the doctor traditionally got all the facts in face-to-face communication with the patient, first asking the patient about the "chief complaint," second allowing the patient to tell "the story" (the history or narrative of the illness), and then questioning the patient like a police detective or a reporter in order to get the facts (clues) of "the story" straight. The physical exam followed. With the logic of internal consistency, the doctor, like a detective, could then unravel the clues of symptoms (and signs) to diagnose (detect) the disease, while later testing the body for additional confirmation, thereby completing the search for the diagnosis. This ancient sequence in the search is not always followed today because aides, nurses, and physician assistants intervene and may interview first, then the patient may be asked to pencil in a history questionnaire or take a "computerized medical history" (Slack and Slack 1978). Such information tactics are intended to save the doctor's time in asking questions—and increase the number of patients that can be examined. Little attention has been paid to whether doctors use the information gathered by others and machines, but it appears that they often do not (Grossman et al. 1971).

The use of a computer in taking the patient's history is frequently abandoned, even though it might seem to have several advantages: to divert the patient during the wait, to provide the patient with attention and novelty (if not regularly repeated), to question the patient on more topics than the doctor would (yielding more information than the doctor could use or even write down), to make the record a more legible document (though in uniformly boring type compared to the varied challenging script of doctors), and to make the information easily retrievable for "quality assurance." Those who would romanticize the doctor-patient relation for every service may be surprised when some patients report liking the encounter with the machine better than one with the "Doc." At least they report liking the machine better when they have tried it but once and when they are in the office where they will be seen eventually by the MD (Slack and Slack 1968). Except for the questionnaire on the initial computer interview, liking it better than a "real doctor" is never tested again, but undoubtedly patients can have a brief transference to it just as they may to other high-tech machines, doctors, and institutions (Schwitzgebel and Taugoff 1968).

Time for Communication

It takes time to take the initial complete medical history, perform a complete physical examination, and give medical advice as sketched in the sociology text. However, in a medical practice, only 10–20 percent of office visits are by patients seeking the doctor's aid for the first time (*Advanced Data* 1978). Thus, only a minority of the patients in practice may receive "the one-hour examination" that has been the trademark of the "complete initial workup" by the internist or medical specialist. Judging from the work schedules of these practitioners, even the face-to-face initial visit is now more likely to be 30 minutes (sources: scheduling practices at Internal Medicine Associates, Massachusetts General Hospital; private-practice colleagues, Boston; Kaiser Clinic, Santa Clara, CA; Harvard Community Health Plan, Boston). "Old patients" (those the doctor has asked to come back for treatment and those who are known and who return for "new" or old complaints) get still shorter visits. Return patients constitute 80–90 percent of those attending medical practices, and their agenda with the doctor is usually more treatment than diagnosis. Since visits and patients have both increased, the explanation of limited time for encounters may be that more patients are seen and return more often, but for shorter visits. The average annual number of visits to doctors rose from 2.6 per person in 1930 to 5.0 in the 1970s and the 1980s, and in those same years the percentage of the population going to see the doctor at least once a year rose from 48 to 72 (Peterson 1972). In the 1980s the percentage rose to 80.

The time for a visit with the doctor often seems, and may be, limited, but it greatly depends on national and personal perspectives. In Great Britain, for example, the average time the patient spends in consultation with a general practitioner is reported to be 6 minutes, with the patient having the opportunity to ask about three questions (Royal College of General Practitioners 1973; Eimerl and Pearson 1966). Not surprisingly, patients think it is longer (9 minutes); likewise, doctors invariably give longer estimates of their time with patients (Lister 1974). To some, these minutes seem trivial, too short for any significant interaction even when the patient may be well known to the doctor. However, for Enid Balint and J. S. Norell (1973), even the 6 minutes for the British patient is ample opportunity for psychotherapy, as their little book *Six Minutes for the Patient* attests—particularly if the patient is seen often enough. For similar treatment in the United States, at least 20 minutes has been argued, the so-called "20 minute hour" (Castelnuovo-Tedesco 1962).

The National Ambulatory Care Survey reports the average U.S. office visit to be 12 minutes (Noren et al. 1980), and in 1981 47.1 percent lasted 10 minutes or less (U.S. Dept. of Health and Human Services 1985). Elsewhere, visiting times may still be somewhat briefer. Looking at general-practice workloads in different parts of the world, Yamamoto and others report that in Japan it is not rare for a doctor to see 100 patients a day, having at the most 3 minutes for each contact (Yamamoto 1978; Locke 1980; Lagone and Thorp 1983), a figure similar to that previously noted for Dutch GPs (Querido 1963). In Japan, "three hours [wait] for three minutes [consultation]" is a well-known expression.[32]

From West Germany, two observers, Lise von Feber and Manfred Pflanz, both report that doctors see 60–120 patients per day (10,000 encounters per year), while having responsibility for practices with 2,500–5,500 persons enrolled (von Feber 1975; Pflanz 1970). By contrast, the daily workload of the British GP is somewhat smaller (30–50 patients per day) and the practice list or panel is smaller (2,000–3,000), but the number of face-to-face visits per year is the same (10,000) (Fry 1980). In the United States, where general care is mostly in the hands of family doctors, internists, and pediatricians, their numbers of daily consultations, respectively, average 35, 25, and 28, and their office consultation times are 12.9, 18.8, and 12.9 minutes (National Center for Health Statistics data 1974 and 1980); these figures are not far from those reported by Mendenhall and his physician respondents who filled out time logs of their practices (Mendenhall et al. 1979) or by physicians reporting to the AMA Survey in 1983 (Reynolds and Ohsfeldt 1984).

One might think that more time with the doctor would always correlate with more satisfaction, but it does not. Some of the requests to be satisfied may take hardly any time at all. Commenting on the West German scene, von Feber notes that "seeing 100 patients" per day is possible because at one-third of those visits only a prescription is requested, a ritual that can often be handled by the doctor's office assistant; this makes the actual workload of the doctors she studied 40–60 patients, a number closer to those for U.S. family practice and British general practice. Surveys of American practitioners indicate that only 1 percent of office patients are not seen by the doctor.

Other medical specialists have it easier, at least when it comes to numbers of visits at the office. For example, internists average but 10–15 visits per day in their offices; the rest of their visits are to hospitalized patients. Yet this limited office practice was not always the case for internists. In the 1930s and the 1940s internists had most of their patient encounters at the office or the patient's home. Few surveys are available, but by 1964 internists were spending 26 percent of their time in hospital visits, a percentage that grew to 42.8 percent in 1974 and then to 48.2 percent by 1976 (Mendenhall 1981; Mendenhall et al. 1979) as hospitals expanded and hospital fees became incentives for physicians to admit patients to this setting. Perhaps because there were more doctors, the percentage of internists' hospital time declined to 38.8 in 1983 (Reynolds and Ohsfeldt 1984). The result of these shifts of medical work to the hospital is that the internist's panel of patients is smaller and contains patients with more complex medical conditions. The internist's panel numbers only 468–953, while the family practitioners have 1,004–1,127 (Altman et al. 1965; Girard et al. 1979). In the case of the British GPs and American family doctors, the cross-national differences in patients per day may be due to the fact that the latter have hospital privileges and may spend up to one-third of the day in the hospital, while British GPs work exclusively in community-based offices outside the hospital.[33]

What rationale sets the numbers for these practice panels, particularly those in primary care? Could it be the idea of an optimal size—one that would ensure that doctors "know their patients," like the idea of the "right" class size for a teacher? Or is the rationale merely an economic one, according to which the size equals the necessary number of patients to ensure the doctor's income given the prevailing fee schedule of the payment system, as is suggested by the case of internists? A historical view suggests that panel size is mostly economically determined. The rising demand for home care by middle-class families in the nineteenth century fostered the idea of the family or personal doctor who would "know his patients." Those families became the doctor's panel of patients when the state, as in Great Britain, paid the doctor per capita, rather than by fee for service, thus providing his income for an assessed measure of clinical work that is now some 2,000 to 2,500 patients.

Besides this administrative-economic factor, panel size may be limited by the doctor's capacity to know and remember all his patients. The optimal number by this criterion is problematic. Practitioners, of course, offer testimonials that they do know their panel of patients, but Michael Balint and his colleagues (1966) in seminars with GPs observed that some do not, at least at a level where it might be of some good. In one small study in which doctors were quizzed on knowledge of their patients, only 50 percent of the patients were "well known" (Hull 1972).[34] A doctor's ability to know all of 2,000 or so patients has never been thoroughly tested, but among anthropologists that number is rumored possible to recall. Doctors, as field workers and participant observers (which they are), resemble anthropologists. From their participant observation among primitive peoples, anthropologists are expected to know all members of 800 families (some 2,000 people, like the doctor's practice list). Elsewhere, Michael Gelfand's (1964) account of native African practitioners, *Witch Doctor*, also suggests that the 2,000 figure for a practice panel may not be too far off. He notes that a *nyganga*'s village practice contains 800 families and that he does "know" all the family relationships and presumably each individual's "psychology." Besides this pyschological knowing, there is simply the very important quick recognition of patients, a skill at which some secretaries and receptionists are marvelous—for they are able to greet patients by name, whether they are steady, regular practice attenders or not. Out of similar easy recognition by the doctor, the personal facts about the patient can easily follow.

No matter what view one takes, the encounter time (and it often seems exceedingly brief to outsiders) has, overall, been getting better and longer, while more people use it. In 1879, at St. Bartholomew's Hospital in London, 120 outpatients were seen by the admitting physician and dismissed in an hour and ten minutes—a rate of 35 seconds per patient (Rivington 1879). Also in the late nineteenth century, three casualty officers (MDs) dealt with 500 patients in a morning (Royal College of General Practitioners 1976)! Richard C. Cabot, working in the Medical Clinic of the Massachusetts General Hospital in the 1900s, saw 30–40 patients in a 2-hour session (3 minutes per patient), most without any examination, as did the other physicians to outpatients (Massachusetts General Hospital, Reports of Medical Administrative Committee and Social Service Department, 1905–1920). It was this desperate pressure of clinical work and the neglect of the patients' personal problems that led Cabot to develop medical social service. By 1915 clinical schedules were much better, according to the hospital's annual report: "No physician [in the Medical Department] should see more than six new cases or twenty old ones [requiring little or no physical examination] within three hours" (White 1922). These old statistics are those of public clinics for the sick poor, not those of private practice, where the demand was nowhere near as intense. In their private offices away from the hospital, Cabot and his colleagues would be busy if they saw four or five upper-middle-class patients an afternoon. Today, consultation times are distributed more equally. In Cabot's old clinic, reorganized in the 1970s as a group practice of internal medicine for patients of all incomes, the encounter time for medical patients now averages 20 minutes (a figure close to the national average of 18 minutes for internists) as the doctor now consults with 8–12 patients in a 2–4-hour session.

The data obtained from direct stopwatch observations of the length of office encounters are similar to those reported in questionnaire surveys. These time-and-motion studies, which measure the contact time of doctor and patient among a long list of other office activities, reveal the essential "piecework" nature of doctoring (Brady and Stokes 1970; Parish et al. 1967; Baker 1978; Peterson 1956; Crombie and Cross 1964) whether the encounters studied were in a personal solo practice or in an impersonal clinic. Most of these studies of the workload of practice are designed not to improve the doctor-patient relationship but to boost office efficiency through the delegation of some of the doctor's work to others.[35]

Even when these studies have measured the temporal dimensions of the doctor-patient relation, few have looked at the distribution of what the doctor and patient actually do together; most have only recorded the time in face-to-face encounters while categorizing the other work of the doctor as health counseling, diagnosis, treatment, record-keeping, prescribing, and administration. One exception to this is the study by Waitzkin et al. (1975) in the Medical Clinic at the Massachusetts General Hospital. According to Waitzkin, the doctor's history taking and the patient's complaining took 22.1 percent of the encounter (4 minutes, 36 seconds), social exchange or "gossip" 7.6 percent (1 minute, 8 seconds), explanation and advice 7.6 percent

(1 minute, 8 seconds), and silence 27.4 percent (6 minutes, 9 seconds).[36] Eight years later, a similar survey in the same clinic revealed that explanation and advice might be better, at least longer, now up to 6 minutes (Billings et al. 1983).

In the hospital, the encounter time at the bedside varies, at the most 10 minutes if only visiting (Payson et al. 1961; Foley 1979)—but more when procedures and special examinations are counted which must be the explanation in the longer times that physicians (who overestimate) reported in Mendenhall's 1977 survey (1981). Onco-logists have reported spending 3.62 ± 2.83 minutes in a patient's room on hospital rounds (Blanchard et al. 1983). For the most part, the content of the bedside communication remains unanalyzed, though it is familiar to doctors who do it as they find out how the patient feels and advise on today's tests and treatments. In visits to the patient at home, the contact averages 30 minutes, at its least 15, for it is often hard to leave without being engaged in social conversation or an offer to eat and drink before leaving the house.

Conclusions vary as to how much of a doctor's time should be set aside for doctor-patient interaction. Some would hope to increase time with patients by expanding patient education to facilitate better compliance with treatment; others would be skeptical, doubtful that additional minutes would be used in interaction with patients, and suggest that they might be spent on "irrelevant" office shoptalk, coffee, or gossip. The skeptics also note that doctors, at least those in training, avoid using the working hours that they do have to talk to hospital patients (Payson et al. 1961; Foley 1979). Despite the presence of patients, interns spent more time talking to each other and to senior staff members when they had the chance. When ethnographers stand by to watch and count interactions on a hospital ward, this natural communication preference of medical staff to talk among themselves is also observed on psychiatric wards (McGuire et al. 1977). The ex-planation is probably not that the interns are inadequately super-vised by senior staff members (who might be expected to demonstrate personal attention to patients that should be copied), but simply that the more dominant individuals (the members of the medical staff), meeting in corridors, conference rooms, and nursing stations away from patients' bedsides, will interact more with each other than with the subordinate individuals (the patients). Why should this be? Because doctors have that option, with its more attractive gratifi-cations of doctors talking to doctors. In natural settings, monkeys behave similarly; the strong interact with each other, ignoring the weak (Fairbank 1980). In attempts to promote the personal care of patients, such ethological accounts have important implications as basic science contributions to patient care and to the conduct of medical rounds. When doctors work in groups or teams seeing patients together, as they do today, special effort is needed to maintain the important dyadic communication between one doctor and one patient, or the patient will be ignored. One of the doctors should regularly provide individual attention and personal communication to a given patient, even though the team members continue to talk among themselves. If one staff doctor is not available for a patient to talk to (often the case), the patient will seize any opportunity for personal communication, whether with a dietician, a nurse, a technician, or a cleaning person—as accounts and anecdotes of hospital life so often detail.

To think that the minutes of each encounter are all-important would be to miss other features of visits to doctors and the relationship. Most important for understanding the implications of these stopwatch checks on the schedule of visits to doctors is their distribution and number over the years, both in and out of the hospital, as well as the continuity that the patient has with one or more doctors at these visits. Thus, medical doctors can have long-term relationships with their patients (Ayleff 1976), reasonably up to 40 years if both can stay alive and remain together, meeting from once to several times a year. A recent survey in London revealed some doctors have even practiced into their 90s, or for 50–60 years (Royal College of General Practitioners 1982), taking part in up to 500,000 encounters in a lifetime of practice. In this period of 50 years, one patient might have seen the doctor 200 times or more, not counting those daily hospital visits when "really sick."

These yearly encounters in long professional lives remain a distinctive feature of medical practice despite all the modern separations that so readily disrupt the continuity of doctor-patient encounters— the more common retirement of doctors; their modern shift work that sometimes makes them unavailable; the moves of both doctor and patient; "doctor shopping"; the the demands for "second opinions" by insurers, families, and patients; and the loss of insurance plan to pay for visits to Dr. A but no longer for Dr. B, to mention but a few. A Louis Harris survey (1985) notes 39 percent of Americans dropped their doctors in 1984. But not all the separations are permanent. Even though 50 percent of patients surveyed "doctor shopped" (Kasteler et al. 1976), within a year they often returned to their own doctor after the opinion from the second. From the patient's side, breaking away may also mean the residential moves of patients, estimated to be 25 percent annually; cheaper insurance premiums that pay for a new doctor at an HMO or group practice but will not at another; the "going to another doctor" out of quick dissatisfaction or for a "second opinion" that results in a new attachment rather than coming back (Clyne et al. 1963); the permanent referral to some specialist or to a nursing or a residential home as the severity of illness, handicap, or age might require; as the patient grows up, a transfer from pediatrician to internist or family doctor, and, in the case of aging women patients with multiple disorders from gynecologist to internist who can now "check on everything" (Cabal 1962; Gray and Cartwright 1953). From the doctor's side, splitting up the relation may come from the departure of GPs for specialty training, from their practice moves (up to three per lifetime), or from that medical shift work, developed in group practices (so that everyone has time off) and from specialization around medical technology (so that the doctor's hours are limited in managing those diagnostic treatment machines at the bedside), all of which make the doctor less available. Finally, despite the high value placed on continuity, some patients may not seek it at all, preferring (or accepting) discontinuity and multiple medical contacts as the natural mode of care because that is all they can get.[37] Like marriage, the steady, long-term medical relation is less common today and less searched for by both sides though it continues to be asserted as the best and proper thing.

The continuity of the relation is of course broken by the patient's death, the numbers of which vary among doctors' practices. In Great Britain, 1 percent of patients (25) on a general practitioner's list (2,500) die each year; 40 percent of those deaths (9) will be outside the hospital, where 4 to 5 might be attended by the GP at home (Fry 1980). In contrast, the hospital-based oncologist naturally attends many more deaths, since many of his patients have advanced cancer. Oncologist colleagues report directly attending 30–40 dying patients per year, while hospital-based general internists attend 10–15 and community-based internists more like 1–4, depending on the ages of their patients.[38]

In Great Britain, where more systematic information has been kept on medical practices (Gray and Cartwright 1953), about 7 percent of a practice list of 2,000–2,500, or 140–175 individuals, leave per year. Family practices in the United States report the annual turnover of patients to be 20 percent, which suggests that in the U.S. these mutual attachments are not as strong or that there are more opportunities to break away and more obstacles to sticking together. In America, health-maintenance organizations, which keep track of their enrollees, report 20–30 percent not reenrolling per year, presumably because their jobs and their insurance benefits have changed; moreover, some patients go outside the plan to consult other doctors, a transient separation common to all practices. In the United States, where specialists have constantly expanded compared to generalists, Osler Peterson noted (personal communication, 1970) that every 10 years one-third of American GPs quit general practice (and their patients) for specialization that often takes them into institutional rather than solo practice, or they go into medical administration rather than "burn out" in patient care. In a study by Holden and Levitt (1978), 16 percent of primary-care physicians changed their specialties over a 5-year period from 1971 to 1976. Resident physicians in teaching hospitals leave after 3–5 years, assuring a break in the attachment and the patient's search for or transfer to yet another doctor in the system (Lichstein 1982). Doctors are also observed as making three practice moves before settling down (Steiber 1982).

Like the patients who quit them, doctors occasionally quit patients whom they judge to be too difficult or mean to deal with, sending them formal letters constructed by lawyers so as not to be accused of abandonment:

Dear Mrs. B.:

I find it necessary to inform you that I am withdrawing from further professional attendance upon you for the reason that you have persisted in engaging in abusive and unacceptable behavior. Since your condition requires medical attention, I suggest that you place yourself under the care of another physician without delay. If you so desire, I shall be available to attend you for a reasonable time after you have received this letter, but in no event for more than five days. This should give you ample time to select a physician of your choice from the many competent practitioners in the city. With your approval, I will make available to this physician your case history and information regarding the diagnosis and treatment which you received from me.

Very truly yours,
Dr. A

In terminating a relationship, doctors may use one of the justifiable reasons listed by the Massachusetts Medical Society:

1. Abusive treatment of the physician by the patient.

2. Continued refusal to pay bills when the physician has used all reasonable means to collect the fees and is satisfied that the patient is financially able to pay.

3. When the disease from the patient suffers is foreign to the physician's

expertise. In this situation, names of other physicians should be suggested to the patient.

4. Repeated failure to follow the physician's advice and treatment.

5. Excessive consultations with other physicians without the knowledge and consent of the primary physician, after making certain that the patient understands the hazards in such situations.

6. Incompatibility of personalities that interferes with the proper investigation and treatment of the patient's illness.

Finally, doctors do retire, although much later than people in most other occupations. The working life of New York State physicians in 1980 was 47.0 years for males and 41.3 years for females, with mean age at retirement 68.23 for males and 66.94 for females (Tu 1985). Some work even after age 75, as revealed by a recent survey of primary-care physicians in London, where 10 percent of the doctors were past 75 and still attending patients, although with fewer patients than the usual 2,000–2,500 (Royal College of General Practitioners 1982). When a doctor dies, patients seek a new practitioner by a variety of paths and try-out relationships to a permanent connection (Toms 1977).

Despite these several reasons and tactics for breaks in the continuity of the patient with the doctor, the gains and losses from staying with one doctor or breaking away to another are largely unknown. Clearly, patients get different things from different doctors, but they do not usually write about them and they do not get surveyed by social scientists except about why they quit going to a doctor or what they do not like. A hidden affiliative literature is suggested by patients' comments and hints as to how much they missed Dr. X, "She was wonderful," or how they always felt comfortable with Dr. A but not with Dr. B or "didn't want to give up Dr. C, since he knows me so well"—all relationship experiences that are rarely explored. In the case of the long-term psychoanalytic relation, Harry Guntrip (1975), himself a distinguished psychoanalyst, has written a moving memoir, "My Experience of Analysis with Fairbairn and Winnicott," about two senior British analysts he consulted, reflecting on what he took to be his different relations with each. From Fairbairn came precise intellectual interpretation, while Winnicott provided "imaginative hypotheses," With the latter acknowledging that he, in turn, was stimulated by working with Guntrip, even when the sessions were less frequent than customary practice.

Whereas patients who quit or are left by doctors discuss the relation among friends and family, doctors who "lose" patients seldom discuss it among themselves. Losing a patient who has been in the practice a long time, not one trying out the doctor for the first time, will puzzle the doctor as to what went wrong, and, regardless of the cause, the doctor is likely to take it personally, feel a twinge of "hurt" and shame for "not measuring up to the patient's expectations," though most would deny it and few would discuss with colleagues "why they got fired from that case."

That subset of patients and doctors who have been together from 20 to 50 years deserves note. In the case of visits, the participants may not need a lot of time together because, knowing each other, they can be enormously efficient in the exchange and transmittal of information—a fact that both doctors and patients will verify. Perhaps, as in an old marriage, the two need less time to reach and communicate understanding, and perhaps there is more time for the patient to "speak" and the doctor to "listen." Among aging doctors and their patients, encounters may be shorter (or longer) and the "docs" more alike in their style, as some contend. Despite such assertions, there is little research on this matter. (See, however, Haug and Lawton 1981.) The usual studies of the practice workload are cross-sectional, sampling doctors and patients at one particular time; they do not examine the frequency, site, and contents of encounters over several years, a temporal variable that should be important for an understanding the impact of long-term doctor-patient relations on patients and their illnesses.

The Physical Exam

The National Survey of Health reports that physical exams are performed in 35.9 percent of office visits. Judging from older surveys of general practice (Peterson 1956; Clute 1963), not enough exams were done, and those done were not complete enough. Indeed, the patient may be examined fully clothed (as when only the blood pressure is taken) or not fully disrobed (as when an examination is limited to one part of the body, such as a joint, the abdomen, the heart, or the chest). Such brief "body-part checks" in the office are quite unlike those in the hospital, where the patient lies in bed in a johnny, always ready for the "complete" body exam. Something else about those limited and repeated checks of body parts is important. If they are not really as diagnostic as they are supposed to be, they may not need to be diagnostic. Perhaps what is needed (but unacknowledged) is only a confirmation of previous exams, a measure of expected therapeutic change, or an assessment of normality. In such cases, the check my serve other functions, such as therapeutic "bodily reassurance" (a function not acknowledged by health-care researchers whose performance yardsticks do not measure it).

Amid all the acts of doctors in the relation, the sequence of the exam may vary. As mentioned, the "physical" and some of the interview may be done together, on the basis of an old clinical view that these acts together are more efficient or, as some claim, more revealing, since patients are more willing to talk and to disclose things when being viewed nearly naked and physically touched by the examiner. Less commonly, the "physical" may precede the interview (the reverse of the traditional clinical method of taking the history first and doing the physical second, a sequence that instructional texts always teach). For example, a pelvic exam, preceded at the most by a quick chief-complaint quiz, may be done first and then discussed when the exam is over. The clinical logic is for an efficiency of communication. Patients expect treatment advice about the body that cannot be given until they have been examined. Also, after the examination, barriers to eliciting information disappear, so that the whole encounter produces more information and advice is transmitted in less time. The last assertion, though untested, is the professional rationale for such practice.

On one hand, the literature on the physical exam is meager; on the other, it is vast. That is, countless medical and surgical texts illustrate the body and how to examine it, while even psychiatric texts may also pay attention to the "physical," with special warnings about how to conduct it with "seductive patients." Yet, despite these many texts that instruct the doctor on how to do or "manage" a physical, the literature on the "physical" from the perspective of the patient is scarce. Little information can be found on the patients' accounts of and responses to their "physicals." Even in this age of survey research and self-awareness, the patient's view is missing, though new lay texts on the body (beginning with *Our Bodies, Ourselves*, and including such other titles as *The Well Body Book* and *Man's Body*) now instruct the patient on knowing about and controlling the body, presumably removing any mystery from the professional exam.

For the doctor the physical exam is an important instrumental check for bodily disease or for the confirmation of body normalcy; for the patient there is often much more to it. The examination may be the most important aspect of the relation with the doctor, even though "talk" with the doctor is so commonly thought to be the very essence of the relationship. In the encounter, the doctor often compares the physical examination to the bodily blessing and healing of the "laying on of hands"—a comparison made more in embarrassed

jest than seriously, since modern medical practitioners wish to identify their healing with science, not religion. In the scientific world
view of today, it is medical cure alone that the doctor thinks he is
accomplishing, not religious or psychological healing, by touch. But
now that nonmedical healers have entered the domain of health in
such numbers, touch as treatment is coming back, and possibly a
scientific interest in the effects of this laying on of hands may develop,
as it has for meditation (Grad 1979; Montague 1977; Frank 1957;
Krieger 1979; Bruhn 1978; Borelli and Heidt 1981). Regardless of the
modern perception, a symbolic equivalent of the act of religious
healing is likely reenacted in the modern office and bedside rites of the
complete physical exam.

The "physical" can also be viewed as a quick, sanctioned, and
cheap dyadic encounter therapy—a bodily touching that at once is
systematic, impersonal, and professional; that is easily arranged by
walk-in or or appointment; and that meets a need for human affiliation and personal attention. As people are prone to separate the body
and the self, the physical is a checkup on body functions and parts in the
image of the "body machine." Patients' expectations of and responses
to the physical exam are probably part of their opinions of the
doctor's "technical" versus "personal" attributes—in this instance,
the doctor's technical body check as a fine mechanic in careful search
of hidden trouble.

One who has written about the meaning of the "manual relation"
between the doctor and patient is the Spanish medical historian Lain
Entralgo (1969), who considers four components to the patient's
experience of the physical:

First an experience in self-assertion. More or less consciously a person who
receives an amorous caress reaches an inner conclusion on a Cartesian
model: "I am being caressed, therefore I am not worthless."
  Secondly, a sense of relaxation, a skillful palpation can succeed (as Nacht
says) "in giving a holiday to the adult man who is unconsciously striving so
hard to quiet the little boy crying inside him." . . . Thirdly, a sense of comfort
and company. Skillfully carried out, such contact is consoling and provides
encouragement and companionship, especially when the person touching is
thought by the person touched as outstandingly important and eminent. . . .
Fourthly, an experience of pleasure, generally felt as well-being and specifically moderated according to the area receiving the amorous contact.

Despite Entralgo's analysis, these expectations about the physical
encounter with the doctor remain largely unexplored, and there are
few empirical data. Patients' comments, of course, are quite sugges-

tive: "No one has touched me since my husband died." "That was the best physical ever." "It's not worth it; I didn't get examined." "I want you to check me." "Would you take my pressure?" "I want to come in; I'd feel better if you looked at me." "They didn't even weigh me." "Would you see (feel) what it is?" "Can I show it to you?" These days, that manual relation is also outside the doctor-patient relation. It is being practiced by women patients and young men taught to palpate their breasts or testes in order to discover cancer early, and it is used even more by nurses and physiotherapists, who handle the body far more in treatment than do doctors in diagnosis. Thus, the hospitalized patient gets more bodily contact from nurses who move them when they are infirm and in bed, while the ambulatory patient (if among the 3 percent referred) gets more from physical therapists who move and massage them in treatment for musculoskeletal disorders. Moreover, thanks to "kits" in mail-order brochures or local drug stores, patients do their own uninstructed exams. And videotapes of encounters will reveal that patients even do their own physicals as they frequently demonstrate personal pain and distress by moving, touching, rubbing, holding, and palpating their own bodies for the doctor—acts they have rehearsed before their visit.

The rules for the conduct of the physical exam state that the doctor touches the patient, but sometimes such conduct may be observed in the reverse. Patients may touch the doctor. On occasion, when patients find verbal descriptions of their distress difficult, they will use not only their own bodies (as they demonstrate on themselves while they complain), but the doctor's body, too, in order to show the location of their distress. For example, a patient may poke the doctor's back with his hand and comment, "Here, Doc, it's right below the shoulder blade." Such infrequent events seem most comfortably initiated by patients who are of the same sex as the doctor but of lower status and in situations where the patient cannot easily demonstrate on himself when asked, "Show me where it hurts."

By defining the "physical" as a manual examination, Entralgo omits a most important feature: the looking of the doctor (and patient) that was once the only technique of examination. The doctor scrutinized the countenance of the dressed patient for signs of disease. Before aural and visual examination was extended by the stethoscope and the ophthalmoscope, the doctor's practiced glance or studied gaze could detect not only signs of physical illness, such as the pallor of anemia, but facial expressions and body movements that might be signs of grief, anxiety, hostility, tensions, or seductiveness. The modern list of useful facial signs can, as Paul Ekman reviews them across cultures, be much longer, containing eighteen types of information—if, indeed, the doctor can decode them (Ekman and Friesen 1978; Ekman 1975, 1982).

Complaints about "physicals" also include complaints about not enough examination or about the male doctor's performance of the pelvic examination and his attitude toward the patient. The women's movement, for example, has argued that draping the body excludes the woman's participation in and control of the process, as does failure to let her visualize her cervix (source: Women's Health Center, Cambridge, Massachusetts). In the modern search for the healthy body and to avoid that entrapment of the "professional" exam, the medical profession is pressured to instruct the public in systematic self-diagnosis, monitoring, and self-examination (as with diagnostic decision rules, blood-pressure measurement, and the testing of blood and urine). Yet these and other efforts are not without contradictions; they can, in fact, lead to more (indeed, excessive and unwarranted) medical attention as doubtful signs from self-examination are brought in for the doctor's (unnecessary) "second opinion." Moreover, without instrumentation and training, complete self-examination is technically difficult (at least in looking inside), and the patient may need to visit the doctor in order to be rechecked and reassured.

Complaints about the physicals done by doctors also have another side. One study has reported that 14 percent of recently discharged hospital patients thought they had been examined too often—by more than four doctors on the average (Houston and Pasanem 1972). However, most patients' complaints about "physical exams" concern the *infrequency* of the "P.E." This may be viewed as a sign of too much distance between doctor and patient. At the other extreme, few complained, until recently, of an underdistancing, such as the doctor's voyeurism of the patient's nakedness or of the patient's dressing and undressing, or even sexual liaison. Unconscious, nonverbal "quasi-courtship behavior" by psychotherapists (involving glances, moves, and seating positions)—tactics to engage the patient's participation—have been described by Albert Scheflen (1965). Usually a suppressed topic heard about only through gossip and bits of lawsuits and behind the closed doors of ethics committees, erotic behavior and sexual intercourse between doctor and patient has recently come out in the open and been reported in newspapers, in magazines ("Sexually abusive doctors: How women are betrayed by the men they trust the most," *Ladies Home Journal* June 1979 p. 55), in books (Szasz 1980), and in professional journals ("The ethics of therapist-patient sex," *Medical World News,* July 12, 1976; Dahlberg 1970), and treated in popular stories about women victims, such as *Betrayal* (Freeman and Roy 1976) and *Second Life* (Cook 1981).

In a survey of a random sample of 460 doctors (including psychiatrists), Kardener et al. (1973) noted that 12.8 percent reported nonerotic hugging, kissing, and affectionate touching of patients, 7.2 percent reported erotic behavior (kissing and genital stimulation), and 7.2 percent reported sexual intercourse. (See also Kardener 1974.) Those reporting intercourse stated that it involved experiences with one to five patients, presumably in brief liaisons and "one-night stands." [39] Reports to the ethics committees of state medical societies include not only the usual claims of overcharging and abusive remarks but also claims of sexually inappropriate behavior when watching undressing and of genital stimulation. More recently, a doctor's rapes of hospitalized patients and of patients at home during house calls have been reported by the Boston press ("Doctor convicted of rape gets prison sentence," *Boston Globe,* March 7, 1985).

Kardener and colleagues suggest that an emotional parallel may exist between doctor-patient and parent-child relations. They note that parent-child incest has a similar 5 percent incidence and that, in 19 percent of the doctor-patient liaisons reported, the doctor expressed the belief that sex could be beneficial to the patient. Wagner (1972), on the basis of another study, notes that 25 percent of male medical students surveyed felt that sexual intercourse with a patient could be appropriate under the "right circumstances." Whether female doctors will also engage in sex with patients as it becomes rationalized as part of the "treatment"—when the domain of "medical treatment" expands to include sexual adjustment—is problematic. Such behaviors have already been reported by female psychologists (Holroyd and Brodsky 1977), but not as yet in a survey of 164 women physicians (Perry 1976). Some argue that erotic behavior toward patients is not confined to particular erotic-prone doctors but may be an extension of doctors' usual non-erotic behavior into the encounter (Kardener et al. 1976; Rynearson et al. 1983).

A recent trend in this vein of physical and social closeness is for doctors to get together with patients after office visits to exercise with them (or, rather, to have them exercise with the doctor). This is distinctly different from the doctor's playing golf or tennis at the country club with a member who happens to be his patient. Doctors (and nurses) now report: "We jog in the gym with our patients who are four to six weeks after a heart attack" (Ballou 1982). Similarly, Mollen, in *Run for Your Life,* does so with healthy normals (Mollen

1975). To these new twists to care and treatment we should add older, persisting social contacts where patients invite doctors to wakes, funerals, gypsy feasts, weddings, bar mitzvahs, and anniversaries— and some doctors go (Tolle et al. 1984; Irvine 1985).

Besides these erotic, therapeutic, and social encounters outside the office, there is another extreme: physical violence between patients and practitioners. Schevert Frazier, who has been keeping count of murdered doctors, reports that over 10 years some 250 U.S. doctors were murdered by their patients (personal communication, 1984). As might be expected, more of the doctor victims were psychiatrists treating "mentally disturbed patients" and surgeons who may have operated on similar ones (Revitch 1979), though Thomas Szasz (1982) has argued in "Shooting the Shrink" that the behaviors are not "mental illness" and that some violence may be a response to psychiatric treatment. Threats of physical harm are one of the responses of the dissatisfied, so much so that a registry of "dangerous patients" is kept for the 2,000 doctors in the Canadian province of Alberta (*Medical World News* 1978); and surveys indicate that physicians fear violence against themselves and their families from disgruntled patients (Mawardi 1979). Both practitioners and patients may bring guns into the consultation room, but in different circumstances. In the southwestern states, where carrying handguns is more a custom than elsewhere, a patient may come to the doctor's office wearing a gun in a holster. In big cities, some doctors carry pistols for self-protection when serving as on-call night substitutes for colleagues. Until the advent of security guards in emergency rooms, doctors and nurses remained unprotected from the physical assaults often attempted by disturbed, psychotic, belligerent, intoxicated, and demented patients (and their friends). Marie Haug (1982) reports from China that fistfights between doctors and patients are known to occur, with rudeness and discourtesies on both sides.

Despite enormous professional taboos and the oath to "do no harm," violence and other harmful acts in the other direction, doctor to patient, are not altogether unknown (Boozer 1980). That other long-disturbing chapter of violence against patients is recorded in the annals of World War II[40]; in newspaper accounts of drug-induced deaths, the rape of female patients, and the sexual abuse of children; and in the articles on Nazi death-camp doctors or the "torture doctors" of Third World countries (Keogh 1977). More recently, execution of criminals by drugs is being suggested, legally sanctioned, and performed by prison doctors (or their agents). Contrary to medical tradition and ethics, drugs are injected by or under the direction of doctors ("A 'More Palatable' Way of Killing," *Time*, December 20, 1982, p. 28), rationalized as a presumably more humane alternative to electrocution (Moore 1980; Curran and Casscells 1980).

Laboratory Tests

The physical examination is followed by advice, referrals, and tests. As more laboratory tests are used to monitor disease and treatment, outpatients have more and more tests done at visits (especially blood counts, chemistries, urinalyses, EKGs, and x-rays). Many more tests are done on hospital patients, of course. Some idea of the extent of testing outside hospitals comes from the National Ambulatory Medical Care Surveys (1974, 1980), which report that laboratory blood and urinalysis tests were performed during 22.0, 20.1, 16.5, and 31.7 percent of visits in general practice, family practice, pediatrics, and internal medicine, respectively.

In the future, it seems likely that patients will have even more tests, as old and new diagnostic techniques for looking inside the body or for measuring physiologic functions (exercise tests, blood flow with ultrasound, nuclear magnetic resonance, digital angiograms) are all moved out of the hospital to be done on an ambulatory basis and as the public and the doctors find the physical exam, blood tests, and conventional x-rays inadequate modes for really looking at and inside the patient in the search for the cause and location of bodily disease and distress. Indeed, the patient's requests "I want you to look at me" or "Aren't you going to do any tests?" can be responded to with a vast array of technologically sophisticated measures that really do "look inside" the body. These varied devices (NMR, ultrasound, CAT scans, thallium scans), with their finely detailed and often highly aesthetic images, are gratifying (and rewarding) for the doctor to use. For the patient, they certainly provide more attention to (if not more reassurance about) the body, perhaps with more magical, therapeutic, and diagnostic effects than the doctor's manual exam and inspection alone provide.

In getting tested, the patient meets a technician at the laboratory or the bedside. Their brief encounter is usually not repeated; continuing relationships are unusual. The technician may but introduce herself and provide directions for the test; often the technician's name tag alone suffices for an introduction. The taking of a blood sample has become so routinized that verbal permission is not usually elicited.

Patients now request particular tests, so familiar are they with medical culture and so concerned are they with their own notions of what is causing their illness: "Doc, I want an x-ray." "Don't you think I need a CAT scan?" College-educated patients attending medical practices come in with an average of five test requests. Decision theorists, trying to reduce the number of tests doctors order, claim that most patients do not need such examinations for diagnosis, not recognizing that patients ask for them and may benefit from them as therapy if not for diagnosis (Murphy 1985).

The rarely addressed topic of technician-patient relations might command attention because of the growing volume of testing. For example, technicians from laboratories outside the hospital may make regular home visits to collect blood samples from housebound invalids in order to regulate anticoagulant therapy. Fifty house calls per day are reported by one Boston laboratory, a frequency of home visiting that would be the equivalent to that done by 120 practitioners with home visits of 3 percent per annum. The high job turnover among technicians and the brevity of their encounters (the length of the entire visit is estimated by those technicians who do it as 4 or 5 minutes, from car door to car door) do not lead to long-term relations. Yet still more technicians may be making these house calls as more complicated treatment technologies, including renal dialysis, intravenous alimentation, and chemotherapy, continue to go into the patient's home.

Inside the hospital, special tests on patients are still more numerous. One recent, routine, ordinary example will illustrate. During a four-week hospital stay, a diabetic patient undergoing an uncomplicated coronary bypass graft was attended daily by technicians for the following studies: 8 chest x-rays, 185 blood and urine tests, 213 blood-chemistry determinations, 9 electrocardiograms, and 13 bacteriologic cultures (taken by nurses). And despite the number and regularity of technician-patient encounters in this particular case, the intelligent and conscious patient remembered none, and had few introductions other than the visibility of a name tag.

Given the frequency of such encounters, it is surprising that the subject of relations with patients is rarely discussed in the professional journals of technicians. This reflects the low priority these relations have within the profession. Nearly all the emphasis has been vertical rather than horizontal, on technicians' relations with doctors and supervisors. Such texts as Williams and Lindberg's (1975) *Introduction to the Profession of Medical Technology* and such old articles as Duncan's (1937) "Technicians and Laboratory Relations" illustrate this focus on interprofessional rather than patient relations for reasons that are most likely related to the technician's subordinate position to the doctor.

Prescriptions

When the consultation is completed, a prescription is written in 50–75 percent of U.S. medical visits (Rabin and Bush 1975; Mendenhall 1981; National Center for Health Statistics 1983 and 1984); in Great Britain, prescriptions are written during two-thirds of adults' visits and three-fifths of children's visits (Dunnel and Cartwright 1972). As a result, the doctor is commonly perceived as a medicine-giver and the patient as a medicine-taker. As a result of prescriptions and over-the-counter purchases, in an average man's lifetime no less than 36,000 pills are reported to be consumed (Rossberg 1983).

Regardless of how many are written, prescriptions are not merely a means for patients to obtain drugs for self-treatment away from the office; they are part and parcel of the doctor-patient relation. Encounters often appear incomplete without a prescription to announce the closure. Barbara Pym (1980) comments on this in *A Few Green Leaves*:

Monday was always a busy day at the surgery, a rather stark new building next to the village hall. "They"—the patients—had not on the whole been to church the previous day, but they atoned for this by a devout attendance at the place where they expected not so much to worship, though this did come into it for a few, as to receive advice and consolation. You might TALK to the rector, some would admit doubtfully, but he couldn't give you a prescription. There was nothing in churchgoing to equal that triumphant moment when you came out of the surgery clutching the ritual scrap of paper.

Lennard and his colleagues (1971) observe that the prescribing of drugs serves several functions for both doctor and patient:

The availability of an effective drug legitimizes the physician-patient contact.... Through giving a drug the physican accepts the patient's discomfort as legitimate, as he agrees with the patient's definition of himself as being sick.

Through prescribing a drug, a physician also reduces the patient's anxiety by implying that he has defined the problem and can relieve the complaint.

Prescribing a drug also helps a physician to maintain a sense of accomplishment and to allay his frustration [in dealing with difficult patients].

Administration of drugs may help some physicians retain a sense of mastery in ambiguous situations, such as those associated with mental illness.

To be added to this list is the fact that the doctor plays a significant role in the effectiveness of the drugs he prescribes. Enthusiastic communication of therapeutic intent produces better drug responses than indifferent prescribing (Liberman 1962). This "placebo effect" is not dissimilar to the effect attributed to the native doctor, who, like his modern counterparts, is also a prescriber, though in the practice of primitive and folk medicine. In primitive cultures, patients believe that medications are potent not in, of, and by themselves, but because they have a supernatural origin, revealed only to the native doctor who prescribes them—a view that might explain possible limits to self-treatment and the modern requests for over-the-counter medicine.

In a small clinical study, *Treatment or Diagnosis, A Study of Repeat Prescriptions in General Practice*, Michael Balint and his general-practice colleagues (1970) also looked at the significance of prescriptions for doctor-patient relations. Of 1,000 preselected patients from ten general practices, 25.4 percent received a "repeat prescription—hardly anything else—from their doctors." From reports about the patients' behaviors and the doctors' responses, they concluded that giving "repeats" was a tactic by which doctors avoided their own difficulties in talking with and listening to patients whose real troubles lay beneath the surface of their bodily complaints. A "repeat" avoided the personal problems of patients. As Franz Kafka wrote in *The Country Doctor*, "It is easier to prescribe than come to an understanding of the patient." Balint's basic assumption is that the uncovering of the patient's personal concerns is always possible and invariably more beneficial than a drug. Yet another view is tenable. Not only is the request for a repeat prescription all that some patients want; it may well be that this is the only relation they can tolerate and, therefore, is one of the *uses* of the doctor. In a similarly loaded vein, practitioners have observed that a patient may terminate the relation if his request for medication is refused; on the other hand, patients have noted that a doctor may close the visit by writing out a "script" (Joyce et al. 1968; Tagliacozzo et al. 1973), a tactic also observed by one of Cartwright's survey informants, who replied that his doctor was "too quick with the pen." Whether patients take the prescribed medicine—and 50 percent are said not to—is the subject of a whole other body of literature on "compliance," in which the doctor-patient relation is the central effective variable (Marston 1970; Foye and Chamberlin 1977).

Important Others: Nurses and Pharmacists

After visits with the doctor may come visits with nurses and pharmacists. Both professions have been expanding their roles in out-of-hospital care by taking more direct responsibility for diagnosis and treatment. In demonstration studies, patients' office encounters with nurse-practitioners (NPs) were reported to be longer than their encounters with medical doctors (often some 20–30 minutes, versus 10–15 minutes), and NPs spent 25.6 minutes per visit with well children versus 17.6 for pediatricians (Sultz et al. 1978). Nurse-practitioners are also reported to spend more time than doctors on some of the common topics of encounters, such as health education, and on patients' personal concerns. Whether these therapeutic time gains of demonstration projects will persist in actual practice remains an open issue (Yedidia 1981). Generally, nurse-practitioners do not meet the economic demands of medical practice. Their practice is not always cost-effective, given the present payment schemes. In many instances, visit charges do not support the salary of the practitioner, who sees the patient every 30–45 minutes. As Michael Yedidia (1981) has noted, nurse-practitioners can see more patients in shorter visits to support themselves, but then the patients lose the benefits of expanded contact.

Pharmacists, like nurses, have also tried to move into the treatment of minor illness, but with even less success. Because they no longer compound but only *dispense* drugs, pharmacists might seem to have more time to give their customers advice on medication or information about minor illnesses. But the other side is that patients may perceive their prepackaged dispensing as "unprofessional." They push pills the contents or consequences of which they do not or cannot know. Historically, the "apothecarists" had a medical job, but they split into two groups: the general practitioners, who gave real medical advice (and eventually charged for it) in addition to prescribing drugs, and the apothecarist-pharmacists, who continued dispensing—a job that ever since has carried the "taint of retail trade" rather than the pure accolade of "profession" (Reader 1966). In regard to the likelihood of pharmacists' recapturing the old advisory and therapeutic functions, their situation alone in the drug store puts them at a disadvantage with respect to nurses, who work alongside doctors in offices. Moreover, it must be remembered that the nation's drug stores are used for a great many nonmedication purchases (everything from camera film to garden hoses), and face-to-face encounters with pharmacists for the purpose of obtaining medicines and advice are limited to only 0.3 per person per year. Most of these encounters are for the refilling of prescriptions (Linn and Lawrence 1978). Of the information requests of customers, 17 percent have been reported to be technical (about over-the-counter and pre-scription drugs and about symptoms); 62 percent to be about costs, availability, and location of drugs or products; and 2 percent to be about nondrug, nonmedical products (Knapp et al. 1980). These three topics of pharmacist-patient exchanges are usually discussed across an open (and higher and higher) drugstore counter—often with an audience of other customers, of whom there are over 100 per day coming for all those other purchases. In any event, all contacts with pharmacists, by phone or face to face, are exceedingly brief (Dickson and Rodowskas 1975a,b). In the case of requests for information about drugs, the time is not always used effectively (Ricci et al. 1978). Moreover, the use of the pharmacist as a source of everyday medical advice and informa-tion is heavily influenced by the scheme of health insurance. Before the introduction of national health insurance in Canada, a two-week survey revealed that 3.9 percent of Montreal residents reported hav-ing sought health advice from a pharmacist, making for a pharmacist-consultation rate of 1.25 per person per year. After national health insurance made physicians' services "free," the consultation rate with pharmacists fell to 0.61 per person per year (National Health Care Expenditures Study, U.S. Department of Health and Human Ser-vices, 1981). The notion that the pharmacist should undertake more formal treatment of patients is not likely to be realized, for that would require a reorganization of pharmacy space, time, and staff, along with massive public education. As the trend for the pharmacy to become part of a larger self-service retail store carrying household products and sundries of all sorts continues, the pharmacist's role in consultation is being taken over by a nearby walk-in medical clinic.

Paying for the Visit

Finally, encounters have a cost, and each contains an ancient ritual of giving and receiving that is part of every helping exchange, whether the helper is a modern medical specialist, a holistic MD, an Indian medicine man, or a witch doctor. As always, the public in general and patients in particular have beliefs about how this economic nexus of the relationship influences its quality and use. The political economy of doctoring "the body"—an economy that begins with the decision whether to seek medical aid or to attempt self-treatment (Turner 1984; McKinlay 1984)—is the subject of worldwide debate, even as the particulars of that economy are mystified, distorted, and misunderstood (when available).

For office visits outside the hospital, only 40 percent of Americans have insurance that pays the doctor; the remainder pay out of pocket. Those 40 percent have Blue Shield or commercial insurance, prepaid health plans, Medicaid (welfare), or Medicare to take care of the physician's office fee (or some of it). By contrast, nearly everyone (95 percent) has insurance for hospital care and the doctor's bedside services it requires. Despite the lack of insurance coverage to pay the doctor in the office, only 15–20 percent of office bills are "bad debts" or "delinquent accounts" because patients failed to pay out of pocket for their visits, the mean charge for which was $21.29 in 1977 (National Health Care Expenditures Study 1981) and $41.81 in 1983 (Reynolds and Ohsfeldt 1984) in striking contrast to the $3.00 visit of the 1930s.

And yet this hospital insurance often does pay for tests performed in the office, even if not for the doctor. This former exchange based on a deeply rooted notion that ordering a test is, like the test itself, an objective, always rational necessity in diagnosis that can be identified, authenticated, and confidently paid for, whereas the doctoring encounter is so subjective and intangible that it cannot be validated or paid. This view also presumes that the patient (or the insurer) can be unnecessarily exploited by doctor-initiated return visits, but not by tests that are ordered, which ignores any irrationality of using them.

Insurance payments for tests also may indirectly benefit the doctor. Doctors spend little or no time in doing them, since office assistants and technicians are primarily responsible. However, the doctor's practice is paid for them, and often more than the actual cost. The profit accrues to the doctor, and, as a result of ordering tests done by their staff, doctors may earn nearly as much from tests as they do from their face-to-face encounters with patients (Bailey 1968). Ironically, present insurance schemes that pay amply for tests but less amply for the doctor's services may account for the limited time given to communication with patients. No matter what the public, patients, and doctors assert about the real value of the encounter, in the medical marketplace less cash value is placed on the doctor-patient relation and communication than on tests. "Art" pays less.

There is really nothing new in the discrepancy between the professed and the real value accorded the medical visit. In Revolutionary America, the 1776 fee schedules of the New Jersey State Medical Society, collected by Mark Blumberg (1979), show that even then the office visit was merely a "loss leader"; the doctor gained his income from his fees for the purgatives he administered and the leeches he applied, not from conversing with or examining the patient. In a more detailed study, *Medical Society Regulation of Fees in Boston, 1780–1820*, Blumberg (1984) notes that the visit was not regularly considered a service until the 1780s, when its price was pegged at 6 shillings or one dollar.

The ancient mystique about and reward of technique persist in the prices of procedures performed by specialists. The high prices of procedures produces an inequity in incomes between generalist doctors who do few procedures and specialists who may do many. The situation stratifies doctors by specialty, procedures, pay, and working hours, with specialists getting the most pay for the least working time. Less tolerable today, the differences in professional rewards are being questioned by generalist doctors who, like most working people, seek equal pay for equal work. To accomplish this reform, the American Society of Internal Medicine is promoting charges for "cognitive" as well as "technical" acts (Felch 1981)—a tactic that may now be supported by insurance carriers hoping to limit rising premiums if not the excessive and costly testing of patients.

Quite apart from the low value accorded the relationship, which always seems to have led to limited charges for medical visits, another important impact on the relation is the source and type of payment of the doctor. From a study of national health-care systems, Mark Field (1961) has noted that indirect payment of the doctor through a third party may actually attenuate the bond between the doctor and patient in comparison with direct payments of the fee by the patient. (However, it must be said that comparative information obtained directly from patients and doctors is missing.) Putting the payment mode aside, it should be noted that the sequence and direction of payment may vary. Traditionally, the doctor is usually paid after providing the service; the doctor's bill comes to the patient in the mail and is quite often the last of the household bills to be paid. Yet the variations are many. Cash on the line before or after the visit is often demanded now, as it once was at some practices during the Great Depression, before the advent of insurance. In the prepaid practice, no bill is presented at all. When a third-party insurer pays the doctor directly, only a statement of the services and the paid-up charges goes to the patient.

The conventional direction of payment is from patient to doctor in exchange for services, but there are occasional radical variations on this arrangement in which patients are paid to take treatment. Some difficult patients who are considered likely to discontinue their treatment have been paid to take their medication (for example, anti-tuberculosis chemotherapy) or to come back to the clinic for checkups; although this has been reported to be effective on a short-term trial or an experimental basis, it is difficult to institutionalize into practice, private or public. Fees in Chinese culture are handled rather differently; often none is reported to be paid unless the patient feels that a cure has been effected.

The doctor's pay and income from encounters today may seem high, and the arrangements by which they are paid—fees for service—may seem like profit-making at public expense. Public critiques have some purchase in this area. According to one study, *Physicians, A Study of Physician's Fees* (Dyckman 1978), doctors account for about 20 percent of overall health-care costs. As the costs of care have risen, restricting the growth of professional fees has become an issue of public policy and a source of professional angst (since income, or relative income, is an assurance of professional autonomy). In the 1930s, the doctor's average income was but 1.5 times the national average, while during the medical expansion from the 1950s to the 1980s it rose to 4–5 times the national average.

If the fee constantly reminds us that the doctor-patient relation does not exist in a vacuum, other exchanges between doctors and patients suggest there is a good deal more to it than the cash nexus. Aside from old-fashioned expressions of gratitude, whether written or spoken, patients also bring gifts. In private, elite practices serving the well-to-do, the gifts may be trips, stocks, and bonds, or, if not something given to the doctor personally, the patient's philanthropic contribution to the hospital or clinic for the support of particular medical research or the capital building campaign—a response to the doctor's special relation to the donor-patient.[41] In clinics and office practices, the more ordinary gifts of food, drink, and candy might be seen as tips for extra service. In hospitals, flowers and boxes of chocolates (impermanent items as the illness itself should be) are sometimes left by departing patients and their families for the nurses. In both these situations, patients report that the gifts are their response to the "caring" rather than the "technical" help of the doctors and nurses. Gifts to doctors are by no means universal acts, though, coming from but 5 percent of patients in a practice.

In a study of gift-giving in a medical group practice (Drew et al. 1983), the reasons for gifts to the staff appeared to be of at least five kinds: for personal service, to be remembered before or on returning from trips, to be tolerated when making special demands, as a sacrifice to the doctor, or as a manipulation for perceived favors. At another level, the giving is one more way that patients try to maintain personal and direct reciprocity with doctors, no matter what the payment system and no matter what rules govern the acceptance of gifts. Visitors from Poland, Czechoslovakia, and Hungary report that the giving of gifts as tips or as payment to the doctor is a regularly used means for breaking the bureaucratic queue for services, and that where the gift precedes the service or favor (as it does when placed on the desk at the time of the visit) it might resemble a bribe, though meant as a personal payment to a poorly salaried doctor in a system of state-run health services. That view of gifts is admittedly an old one. Before this present era of paying resident and staff physicians a salary, the restrictions on gifts were spelled out by hospitals in the United States. In these treatment institutions, restrictions on employees' soliciting or accepting gifts continue today, as is detailed, for example, in the 1979 *Employee's Manual* of Massachusetts General Hospital). In office practices outside the hospital, however, doctors usually are not classified as "employees," and even those who are not so classified within a hospital are not restricted when working on the outside. This has not always been the case. During the decades of hospital charity (from 1900 to the 1950s), when a resident doctor, as a hospital employee, was paid a nominal salary or none at all, doctors were traditionally admonished not to accept gifts: "No resident or house officer shall accept a gift, fee, or gratuity for his services during his term of office" (*House Officer's Manual*, Massachusetts General Hospital, 1932). This rule underscored the disinterested impersonality of doctoring; no one considered the therapeutic benefit that gift-giving might have in relieving the patient's sense of indebtedness to the doctor when the gift evened up the asymmetrical exchange. Rather, a gift was perceived to be a bad "influence" in a relation that was expected to be affectively neutral—a bribe paid to the doctor, or a "payoff" for special favors or unequal attention. By contrast, no restriction is stated in today's staff rules. Since resident physicians are now paid, they are presumably immune from incentives to offer differential treatment to those bringing gifts. Moreover, judging from the Japanese experience (Ohnuki-Tierney 1984), paying doctors decreases gift-giving.

In teaching hospitals and practices, perhaps the greatest gift of patients is their permission for medical students to examine them. This gift for the oncoming generation of doctors was largely taken for granted in the past, when the treatment was "free" in exchange for the student's practice at taking the history of the illness and examining the body; this gift exchange is still often unacknowledged today, when everyone is a paying patient. As direct gifts from patients to doctors have become less frequent, the solicitation of gifts by treatment institutions has become more common. Charitable donations are but 15 percent of their income. Their annual and special fund drives for philanthropic support include systematic mailings to all former patients, not, as in the past, to special patrons alone. Still another 1980s twist to gift-giving is the practice of doctors' sending decorative plants to patients after cataract operations, as a "thank you" for business, much as banks offer gift items to people opening accounts. Sending flowers or cards to hospitalized patients is now suggested as a marketing device by which doctors can keep the patients coming back ("Patient Pleasers," *The Internist*, November– December, 1985, p. 14).

After the patient leaves the office or pays the doctor, the encounter is over. Yet the relation may continue and there may be further encounters; some 60–80 percent of patients are asked to return.

The Literature, Its Themes, and Who Writes It

A brief review of the literature on the doctor-patient relation will provide another useful perspective on the readings that follow. Fortunately, not all the literature is confined to academic journals. Along with doctors and social scientists, patients and popular writers have written on the topic, often examining the relationship incidentally or under other guises.

Patients' Accounts

When so much of the public has at some time been ill and been treated by doctors, it is not surprising that patients have produced their own personal literature about their illness experiences—a literature on, as Henry Lederer (1952) originally phrased it, "how the sick view their world." When patients write about their personal struggles with illness, some other themes of satisfactions and dissatisfactions with doctor-patient relations and the various elements of care sometimes ease into the account. These views of patients about their doctors, their illnesses, and their care are published and collected in several official and personal sources. Among the official sources are government documents reporting the complaints against doctors that patients have taken to public authorities (Klein 1973; Yerby 1975); surveys by social scientists (Ley 1972; Cartwright 1967), and official reports of hospitals' complaint offices (such as the Patient Care Representative's Office at Massachusetts General Hospital).

Some of the most interesting personal accounts are those in which patients tell about their experiences with chronic illness; for example, John Vaizey's *Scenes from Institutional Life* (1959), Virginia Woolf's *On Being Ill* (1930), Orme's *My Fight Against Osteo-Arthritis* (1955), *Journey Round My Skull* (brain tumor) (Karinthy 1939), *Take My Hands* (paraplegia) (Wilson 1963), *Coming to Terms with Rheumatoid Arthritis* (Howard 1956), *Fight Against Fear* (Freeman 1951), *Twice a Victim* (Joyce 1977), *Episode* (Hodgins 1971), *Disabilities* (a collection of vignettes from the British medical journal *The Lancet*) (*Lancet* 1952), the collection *Ordinary Lives* (Zola 1982b), *The Missing Pieces* (Zola 1982a) (a medical sociologist's account of living with disability), and *Timetables* (Roth 1963) (an account of life in a sanatorium). Newspaper advice columns, such as that of Ann Landers, contain patients' stories of their struggles with illness and care, and the "experience of illness" is now a popular theme among sociologists.

Ill and disabled doctors have written about their encounters as patients in books such as *When Doctors Are Patients* (Pinner and Miller 1949), *A Physician Faces Cancer Himself* (Sanes 1979), *Stroke* (Dahlberg and Jaffe 1977), *Vital Signs* (Mullan 1983), and *To Provide Safe Passage* (Rabin and Rabin 1984), and in articles such as Vester 1979, Callard 1972, Eliot 1981, and Abram 1977.[42] More recently, when talking publicly about the personal illness experience is no longer taboo,[43] whether it was President Eisenhower in the 1950s or John Wayne in the 1980s, even jointly authored books and articles by both doctor and patient have appeared, such as *A Coronary Event* (Halberstam and Lester 1976) and "An Experience of Cancer, An Honest Dialogue between Doctor and Patient" (Bennet and Sagov 1973), or George A. White's (1980) interview with Dr. Robert Coles, "The Doctor-as-Patient." The stories about "Ike" and "The Duke" perhaps satisfy those yearnings to know (and to watch) celebrities' trials with illness. In the same vein is a much earlier noncelebrity example: an article, "Self Observations and Psychologic Reactions of Medical Student A.S.R. to the Onset and Symptoms of Subacute Bacterial Endocarditis," written in 1933 by an anonymous Harvard Medical School student being treated at the Peter Bent Brigham and Boston City hospitals. Later edited and published by his distinguished physician, Soma Weiss (1942), the account contains a modern interpretation of personality that only became common in the 1950s, a biographical genre that was, by the time of Lord Moran's extraordinary *Churchill* (1966), an expected exposure of the complex, long-term relationship with a celebrity patient. The doctor's relation to the famous is often one of constant if particular attendance where, as Anastasia Kucharski (1984) writes in "On Being Sick and Famous," there are multiple conflicts around information control, clinical responsibility, and interpersonal care (Kucharski 1978).[37,38]

In the autobiographies and biographies of patients' struggles with their illness and their attempts to make personal meaning of it, comments about "the doctor" are scant and seldom flattering when they are available. While the doctor's role may have had importance during the illness, by the time these retrospective accounts get written the focus radically shifts to the everyday coping the patient endures, reflecting the natural "egocentricity" that goes with being "sick," or the reluctance of the patient to settle scores with the doctor. Stewart Alsop's account of his leukemia, *Stay of Execution* (1973), may contain a bit more than the usual deprecatory remarks on the doctor, as does *Heart Sounds* (Lear 1980), a wife's poignant account of her physician-husband's illness with coronary heart disease and their tangled, often oblique relations with doctors. More analytic is Norman Cousins's *Anatomy of an Illness* (1979), which involved the author in successful bargaining with his doctor. The nastiest (and likely most corrosively self-critical) account is probably James Wechsler's *In a Darkness* (1972), the history of his son's treatment for schizophrenia, which involved more than a score of doctors and institutions and which ended in the young man's suicidal leap from the family apartment.

In general, most of the written comments were favorable to doctors until the 1970s, when anger toward the doctor's presumed expertise and asserted authority began to be expressed more openly and when unnecessary subordination of the patient to the doctor received general criticism from consumerists and, in particular, feminists. This phenomenon is not confined to the medical profession but is widespread in society, as Ralph Miliband (1978) notes in his essay "A State of Desubordination", as Lionel Trilling decried as "adversary culture" (Krupnick 1986), though others may view it as participatory democracy.

Surveys reveal that there is a hidden iceberg of complaints. From 60 to 70 percent of dissatisfied patients do not voice their "gripes" because of fear of retribution in the relation or because of a cynical sense of the futility of expecting that any complaint would receive sympathetic attention, much less corrective action. Those survey results come mostly from critical-care hospitals, where the relationship is often short and the illness acute. In such circumstances, it may not seem safe to speak up about the treatment, which is "chancier," or about the relation, which is often unfamiliar and problematic, since the acutely ill patient is often a stranger to the doctor and the hospital. However, in long-term chronic-care institutions this unexpressed discontent is more readily expressed, as practicing clinicians and staff members can attest. Here the patient's condition is more stable, the care is less technical and more certain, and the relation to the institution and the staff is long-term, with a safer, more secure transference. As a result, families can more easily "unload on staff" who might seem, to some families at least, unable to care properly for their sick son, daughter, or parent (Gans 1983).

With the consumer movement supporting the public in its dissatisfactions, more and more of these hidden complaints appear. The expression of "silent" dissatisfactions may produce a larger literature of "anti-doctor" writings, but the testimonials of grateful patients still seem more numerous. For the most part, both complaints and testimonials go unreported and unpublished and remain simply the gossip of everyday life about "going to see the doctor." Patients who have grievances but do not lodge official complaints give such reasons as that they feel the complaint is too trivial, that they are too shy, or that it is inappropriate to complain.

In the office, most complaints are about the doctor's manner and about limited consultation and communication of information; the others are about seemingly more mundane matters, such as waiting too long, no privacy, "office staff gives little respect," or "doctors are more interested in the disease than the patient's health concern" ("Patients Reveal 10 Most Common Complaints," *Physician Management*, February 1978, p. 39). In the Patient Care Representative's Office at Massachusetts General Hospital, the complaint categories are bills, attitudes and behaviors of the staff, and waiting. In this institution, which averages 2,500 admissions and 40,000 ambulatory visits per month, the number of reported complaints averages 100 per month. This number may be low because other complaints are handled elsewhere and because it is hard to complain to the "front office" while under treatment on the premises.

If most of the antagonisms do not get back to the institution or the doctor, they do circulate as gossip in the patient's social network, as Stimpson and Webb (1975) have noted in their study of patients' reports of the general practitioner's consultation process in Great Britain. These tales and experiences of discontent with the doctor may also rationalize several patient behaviors in and out of the encounter: "not going back to see the doctor," "not going to pay the bill," "not taking the medicine or advice," "changing doctors," even "suing him" and "leaving against advice." None of these behaviors is new; they are only much more prevalent and more often articulated.

The increase in lawsuits against doctors has been reported to be at the center of a "malpractice crisis." Like most labels, this is misleading; there is not a single crisis but a mixture of problems in this area.

First, the financing of malpractice insurance has been strained by the bigger fiscal demands that are made on it. Second, claims have tripled since 1975 (no doubt reflecting the alienation of the public from the profession, viewed as vulnerable with its modern affluence). Third, irrational expectations of medical treatment do not admit acknowledgment of "normal" accidents. Finally, in our litigious society, malpractice claims have risen with the encouragement of large numbers of lawyers. In 1983 the chance that a physician in Massachusetts would be accused of malpractice was about one in eleven, with over nine claims per 100 MDs (Massachusetts Medical Society 1985). Karl Singer (1985) observes that, given the current rate, a doctor would experience a malpractice suit from a patient six times in a practice lifetime. Fortunately, the conflict (though not the anger) is usually negotiated; 92 percent of suits are settled out of court. Of those that come to trial, however, 72 percent are won by the doctor (U.S. Department of Health, Education and Welfare 1973; Curran 1983; Holder 1980; Brinkley 1985). The physician's experience of malpractice action is upsetting, as one account illustrates (Charles and Kennedy 1985), and undoubtedly influences other patient relations, if not some instances of withdrawal from practice.

Whether good, bad, or indifferent, patients' responses to the relation have become part of the new administrative literature on medical care that appears in medical management publications (*Medical Care, Health Service Research, Inquiry*) but even more frequently in the free "throwaway" journals of the last decade, in which themes other than those on "hard" medical science can appear for a quick read (*Medical Economics, Patient Care, Psychology Today, Legal Medicine, Private Practice*), in the new social-science journals (*Journal of Health and Human Behavior, Health and Society, Social Science and Medicine*), and in older medical journals devoted to public health or to general practice (*Journal of the Royal College of General Practice, American Journal of Public Health, The Practitioner, Family Practice*). More often than not, the articles explain the behaviors of patients with doctors in terms of the characteristics of patients. Despite the other variables in the exchange (such as the doctor, the organization of the practice, or the dynamics of the relationship), oddly, only the patient is viewed as prone to inappropriate actions in and out of the encounter. As a result, the causative notions of the patient's behavior are "reframed" by being relabeled with new titles indicating what the patient did or did not do, such as "breaking appointments" (Alpert 1964), "defaulting on accounts," "noncompliance" (Caldwell et al. 1970; Finnerty 1973), "changing practice lists" (Givens 1957; Davis and VonderLippe 1967), and "bringing malpractice suits" (Hirsh and

White 1978). Reframing aside, in actual fact, the doctor-patient relation is the latent theme—a dependent variable, but one that is not systematically studied—in such analyses of the actions of patients (Blum 1960). One exception to attributing these behaviors to patients alone is Richard Blum's 1957 and 1958 accounts of doctors' provoking patients to sue for malpractice. His original studies examined aspects of the doctor's character in the same way that is usually applied to the patient only. Blum gave personality tests and interviews not just to patients but to doctors too, thus collecting data on both sides of the encounter.

Some doctors have shaky self-esteem and "paranoid traits" that make them intolerant of patients who appear ungrateful, noncompliant, and questioning. That some of the dissonance in a relationship may be due to some impairment of the doctor is a theme that even doctors are beginning to address as they give themselves a closer look, recognizing that their side of the relationship has been hidden from view. And with good reason—an estimated 5 percent of doctors are mentally ill, drug addicts, or alcoholics, a situation not in itself conducive to the exercise of professional competence or good patient relations (Green 1978). Some of the maladjustments of doctors have, one would suspect, early roots, as in the prospective study of George Vaillant and colleagues (1972); others have argued that the conditions of modern professional training and work promote emotional distress and depression (Shortt 1982; Pfifferling 1980; Muldary 1983), "burnout" (McCue 1982), alienation (Shem 1978) and suicide (Rose and Rosow 1973).

In any event, the literature on doctor-patient relations from the patient's viewpoint is likely to grow, even as medical professionals become more introspective and self-critical about their own development and behavior, and as medical care is viewed as and made a commodity to be delivered to consumers by physician employees, who look less to control their work than to have a life away from it. Like the industrial productivity of blue-collar workers, the satisfactions and dissatisfactions of physicians in their work—indeed, their alienation—may be studied to make the new health-care corporations more "efficient" (and profitable). When health care is no longer a service between mutually respectful partners or a reciprocal relationship with rights and duties but a product, new data about the relation will be sought in order to improve the management of the "distribution and consumption of health services" (as the current rubric goes). Patients, less impressed by professional expertise than in the past and intolerant of old patterns of subordination, will give their opinions more freely by whatever means are necessary.

Even more assertion of the patient's, if not management, control over the relation may therefore be expected.[44] Indeed, we already see some of the public increasing their efforts to avoid visits to the doctor altogether through increased (sometimes compulsively so) self-care (Katz 1975), such as physical checkups, preventive tests (including those BP units marketed by every gasoline company), managing colostomy and rehabilitation devices, self-prescribing for "minor illnesses," and ever more technical monitoring of chronic diseases. Prepaid practices and plans may also support these efforts when, for example, the cost of treating many hypertensives with limited resources from industry or government-financed services makes some self-treatment a practical and profitable alternative to medical attendance.

With so much written on dissatisfaction, it is not surprising that there is a complementary literature giving potential patients advice and warning on controlling the encounter. Popular writings in this genre on how patients could better manage the relation, or "how to be satisfied and get what you want from doctors," have appeared with such titles as *How to Choose and Use Your Doctor* (Belsky and Gross 1975), *The Active Patient's Guide to Better Medical Care* (Sagov and Brodsky 1976), *Managing Your Doctor: How to Get the Best Possible Health Care* (Freeze 1975), *Talk Back to Your Doctor: How to Demand and Recognize High Quality Health Care* (Levin 1975), *Getting the Most from Your Doctor* (May 1978), *Examine Your Doctor: A Patient's Guide to Avoiding Medical Mishaps* (Kra 1982), and *The Energized Family* (Pratt 1976). Now, even in such a staid old popular monthly as *Family Circle*—"the world's largest-selling women's magazine," distributed at every grocery checkout counter—we read: "If you speak up and ask questions, you help establish the open channels of communication that your doctor needs in order to diagnose and treat you properly." Specific questions to ask the doctor are contained in a seven-page pamphlet put out by the Federal Trade Commission (1985), "Healthy Questions, How to Talk To and Select Physicians, Pharmacists, Dentists, Vision Care Specialists." Such popular writings on the relationship rather than disease are truly modern efforts at its improvement, quite different from books like *The Clay Pedestal* (Preston 1981), *The Great Billion Dollar Medical Swindle* (Lasko 1980), or *Confessions of a Medical Heretic* (Mendelsohn 1979), where the exposure and clarification of the relation are provided by critical dissatisfied practitioners from inside the profession.

One reason that there once were few writings on dealing with doctors was the assumption about who needed help in the medical consultation. Only the poor were assumed to be handicapped in encounters, and they were thought to need patient advocates rather than books. In a popular reform tactic in the 1960s and the 1970s, many positions for special health workers to represent the poor in their encounters with doctors were created, only to be abandoned for bureaucratic or ideological reasons. A realistic alternative, namely public education for the patients' own self-advocacy, has not been used, even though anyone can have problems in medical encounters. Lewis (1974) and others began a demonstration project to teach grade-school children to make simple medical decisions, such as whether to see a doctor or a nurse for a given illness and what examinations and therapies to expect and request. Children were found able to learn to make sensible choices, but this educational innovation has not become a wide social reform or been extended through additional instruction in high school, at home, and at work. In another direction, a small movement for consumer rights in the doctor-patient relationship began in the 1970s with a trickle of writings under the title of "patient rights in health care" in the books of G. H. Annas (1974, 1975), in the more radical of the older medical-school newspapers, and in *Street Medical News, Health Politics, Health/ Pac,* and *Health Rights News.* Later, "rights" were brought to the attention of the public in such left-to-liberal weeklies as Boston's *Phoenix* and *Real Paper.* (See "Doctor, No: A Guide to Patients' Rights," *Real Paper,* August 10, 1975.) This genre of books and articles coaching the patient in the doctor-patient relation, once considered less important (or taboo) than instruction about disease, of course, continues (as with the American Association of Retired Persons 1985 pamphlet "Knowing Your Rights: Check Out the Facts Before You Check Into the Hospital"). But these publications are still much less numerous than those (People's Medical Society 1985) that instruct the public on its search for the healthy body or the treatment of the ill one.

Alongside these new writings are the more conventional medical advice books for ill patients, such as *Living with Your Heart Attack* and *How to Cope with Cancer,* and those for well patients, such as *The Well Body Book* (Bennett and Samuels 1973), *How to Be Your Own Doctor (Sometimes)* (Schneff and Eisenberg 1975), *Take Care of Yourself, A Consumer's Guide to Medical Care* (Vickery and Fries 1976), *The Healthy Body Maintenance Manual* (Diagram Group 1981), and *The People's Handbook of Medical Care* (Frank and Frank 1972), which are meant to instruct about illness or about staying well without a relation with the doctor.

Popular Accounts About Doctors

Beside those patients' reports of encounters is another popular literature, including trash novels (read by millions), in which doctors and medical practice have been vastly promoted, romanticized, and criticized. (See, e.g., Knickerbocker 1960; Hopkins 1974; Green 1979.) Then there is television. A recent TV survey notes that during prime time each week a typical viewer will see no less than a dozen doctors (Gerbner et al. 1981), most of them celebrated as heroes (Wilbanks 1972). While purveying modern medical miracles, TV's Drs. Kildare, Ben Casey, and Marcus Welby, the staffs of "Medical Center," "Doctors' Hospital," "St. Elsewhere," and "Medical Story" (and the newspaper comics' Rex Morgan) all demonstrate cool, benign benevolence to patients. "Lifeline," a program of real-life pictures of real hospital doctors and patients, conveys the same image. Strong and virile, the doctors are as at home giving advice on the body as providing moral education on the emotional and social problems of living (which, most of the time, echoes the beliefs and values of the patient). Except for Welby's work as a family practitioner, the scenes of the TV shows are set in the patient's hospital room or the doctor's office in the hospital—locations that give the doctor the aura of the medical scientist, an image more priestly than that of the ordinary "Doc" in a mundane medical office building. That office setting outside the hospital is not on the screen. In all the scenes the doctor is the leading character; the patients, usually female, are members of the supporting cast. Magazines and newspapers publish the authoritative recommendations of "column docs," such as Dr. Steincorn, while Dr. Timothy Johnson appears on TV.[45] In contrast, regular medical-advice newsletters, such as the prestigious *Harvard Medical School Health Letter*, do not often give by-lines to their physician authors.[40]

Although the doctor is praised in much popular literature, this was not always the case in the past. Louis Hamman's essay "As Others See Us" (1938) notes the ridicule that doctors took from ancient writers such as Pliny, Petrarch, Montaigne, Molière, and Securis—a critical debunking tradition that continues today as the public searches for cures of other kinds when medicine fails (Burnham 1982). More modern literary critiques of doctors are found in George Bernard Shaw's *Doctor's Dilemma* (see Shaw 1965 and Boxill 1925), Sinclair Lewis's *Arrowsmith* (1925), and A. J. Cronin's *Citadel* (1937).[46] Shaw attacked the professional dominance of physicians over patients long before it became a modern sociological theme. Lewis's hero, Arrowsmith, addresses the relationship indirectly while struggling with his own career decision between practice and research: Should he do good by providing medical help to a few patients, remaining a mere practitioner, or should he become more powerful and influential by going into medical research and helping society—a more moral endeavor untainted by the commercial nature of private practice?[47] In *The Citadel*, Cronin's Dr. Manson successively fights, joins, and fights the commercialization of the profession and the exploitation of patients. For the most part, these writings are about the social, economic, and political positions of the doctors and about the self-serving, commercial practitioner versus the selfless "doctor-scientist" who emerged as the ideal of academic medical research in the 1900s (Rosenberg 1970). Most books about doctors, including those discussed above, are not actually about personal relations in practice. However, there are exceptions. Solzhenitsyn's *Cancer Ward* (1975) and Orwell's essay "How the Poor Die" (1956) include keen observations of the doctor-patient relation in public charity hospitals of Moscow and Paris and of treatment, issues explored again by social scientists in a university hospital in the United States in the 1970s (Duff and Hollingshead 1968). Solzhenitsyn reveals the restricted nature of the communication between doctor and patient, while both he and Orwell portray the patient's dissatisfaction and discomfort as a consequence of the difference in power and position between the doctor and the patient.

In the popular medium of cartoons, the relation is also a frequent topic. Unlike television's "doctor shows," cartoons illustrate some of the conflicting expectations of patient and doctor; thus, by their unmediated nature, they come closer to reflecting the real rather than the mythical nature of the encounter. Cartoons from *Medical Economics* (1963, 1966) deal with latent sexual attraction as well as lampooning doctors who pompously dispense trivial and irrelevant advice. Bologh (1979) notes the depiction of patients' alienation, even in comic get-well cards. There is also the film *Hospital*, which depicts an absurd, black-comic world where everybody—doctor, patient, nurse, administrator, community—loses. More recently, the camera has focused on the power dynamics and morality of the conflicted relation in *Whose Life Is It, Anyway?*, where Richard Dreyfuss as the patient goes one-up by physically going one-down. The play *The Elephant Man* (Pomerance 1979) contains a similar exposure (Belli 1984).

Doctors' Accounts

Just as patients speak and sometimes write about their relations with doctors, doctors do the same about patients. But there are differences.

Doctors, of course, write vastly more, but in their articles they do not complain about patients directly, explicitly. Rather, they write in a distanced manner, with a distanced diction, about "managing" or "controlling" the relation. While the management of the relation is the subject of scholarly papers, the actual subjects are those chronic medical patients who in conversation are labeled "difficult patients" because of their "unrealistic demands" or "hostile dependency."

The basic assumption in these prescriptive accounts is that a psychological understanding of types of patients can change the doctor's response to them, promoting caring behaviors towards the most undesirable and disliked of patients. Once it was religion that provided the rationale—the management—for the doctor's decent caring acts. From his patrician background, Richard C. Cabot (1912) wrote while treating the urban poor in the 1900s that "to improve practice requires 'more science and more Christianity.' . . . We need for efficient treatment a fund of patience, cheerfulness, of readiness to be interested in each least promising and most unattractive individual in the Clinic that in my experience comes best out of the spirit of Christianity." Today the modern psychology of patient defenses has been substituted for religion, promising that "understanding" will lead to "acceptance" of the patient and that, if understanding does not work, then the doctor's disclosure of personal discomfort in the privacy of peer groups may remove those professional impediments and increase the doctor's concern for the patient.

The doctor's behavior and discomfort in the encounter, rarely written about or examined, are subjects of "backstage" professional gossip (Goffman 1959). They may come up in educational seminars and support groups where five to ten practitioners or students privately examine their encounters with patients in the attempt to learn to tolerate or like the difficult ones who consult them or, at least, to release their hostilities and insecurities about a patient in the safety of a peer group and so be able to face the patient at the next visit (Balint et al. 1966; deBoer et al. 1970; Gustafason 1981). Out of this tactic of peer discussion or "autoagnosis" and out of the encounters themselves have come many pejorative terms for difficult patients, ranging from "crock"—the word of the 1950s for a frequently visiting patient with multiple bodily complaints (Lipsitt 1970)—to more recent denigrating labels such as "shit-ass," "dirt ball," "gomer," "shpos" (subhuman piece of shit), "gork," "douche bag," and "sleaze bag," some of which serve to reduce the person to an oral or anal body part. The modern oral unrecorded literature of physicians about patients and their relations with them is extensive.[48]

While at first glance such demeaning nicknames for irritating patients seem to reflect moral condemnation or a hostility directed entirely at the patients, they may be displacements from other areas of institutional medical life where scorn is taboo. Thus, this language may actually stem from the unpleasant treatment situation that is the exclusive responsibility of residents but not of senior staff, and institution's "scut" or "dirty work," with its excessive hours and demanding pressures without supervision (or support). Regardless of the origins, the labeling presumably serves to help order medical work by indicating who might be seen last, to relieve the doctor of enough suppressed frustration so that the patient's care can continue, or only to signal that the job of doctoring, like factory work, can be tough and dirty, and that it can keep on coming. Relief from hostile tension through communication fits the current cultural practice of letting feelings out in the safety of secret sessions of professionals. However, the process does not end there.

Nowadays, pejorative terms for patients have sometimes gone outside the inner professional circle to become actual forms of address, exchanged in public—particularly in emergency wards, where verbally (and often physically) abusive alcoholic (drunk), psychotic (demented), substance abuser (drugged), and disordered characters "give it" to the staff, while the staff, in turn, might actually give it back in reciprocal nasty name-calling.[49] Like patients, doctors have ways to exit from an unsatisfying encounter, even though the patient is not dissatisfied. A doctor can rid himself of a patient by several tactics: referring the patient to another doctor, limiting his contact to technical treatment alone, being unavailable, delaying consultation, deliberate offensiveness, and pursuing delinquent bills. The fact that patients express liking their doctor even when he or she may not like them indicates that the "sentiments" the patient arouses (to use Henderson's term) may not alter the doctor's caring behaviors (Block and Gerson 1982). About pursuing delinquent accounts, one doctor writes: "Deadbeats are strictly chaff, cluttering up the office and impeding the management of the wheat. Their demands are louder and their complaints more trivial than any other patient category. So exit the deadbeats. They're eased out with three routine monthly statements followed by four weekly statements with collection stickers of graduated severity. Into the hands of the bill collector and good-bye." (Vincent 1975) Not in a professional journal but in a short story, "A Face of Stone," the Passaic, N.J., poet and GP William Carlos Williams (1966) writes about his irritation at examining a seemingly truculent, resistant child. Yet, as Trautman (1975) notes, Williams explores other aspects of the relation, such as his sensitivity to the child's mother and father. Moreover, what Williams records are those quick flashes of mind and emotion that happen during medical acts—a phenomenology of the doctoring encounter, but not enduring sentiments.

Unlike the behaviors of patients, those of doctors are not commonly or systematically studied by themselves or by social scientists. So far, doctors generally will not allow it. What they do and say is often insulated from observers. Since the 1950s, there have been many more exceptions. Patients and doctors have permitted their encounters to be videotaped and analysed for research, education, and treatment (Goroll et al. 1974), or to have anthropologists, social psychologists, and sociologists sit by as direct and participant observers of the office or bedside consultation for purposes of research, while doctors can do the same as self-observers (Shoen 1983).

Despite some of their professional behaviors, which can resemble "cooling the customer out," doctors usually write positive in-house affirmations about the doctor-patient relation, with three major themes: the therapeutic and ethical responsibilities in the relation, the operational use of the relation in patient care, and the management of the relation with "difficult patients."

On Therapeutic and Ethical Responsibilities

Medical writings in the first category stress the norms and manners of professional behavior and the ethical commitment to therapeutic responsibility in the act of caring. Beginning with the Hippocratic Oath (Jones 1923), the doctor is the patient's socially designated agent and protector. The oath, reproduced here, particularly cautions the doctor against the abuse of his power in relations with the sick:

I swear by Apollo Physician, by Aesculapius, by Health, by Panacea, and by all the gods and goddesses, making them my witnesses, that I will carry out, according to my ability and judgment, this oath and this indenture. To hold my teacher in this art equal to my own parents; to make him partner in my livelihood; when he is in need of money to share mine with him; to consider his family as my own brothers, and to teach them this art, if they want to learn it, without fee or indenture; to impart precept, oral instruction and all other instruction to my own sons, the sons of my teacher, and to indentured pupils who have taken the physician's oath, but to nobody else. I will use treatment to help the sick according to my ability and judgment, but never with a view to injury and wrong-doing. Neither will I administer a poison to anybody when asked to do so, nor will I suggest such a course. Similarly, I will not give to a woman a pessary to cause abortion. But I will keep pure and holy both my life and my art. I will not use the knife, not even, verily, of sufferers from stone, but I will give place to such as are craftsmen therein. Into whatsoever houses I enter, I will enter to help the sick, and I will abstain from all intentional wrong-doing and harm, especially from abusing the bodies of man or woman, bound or free. And whatsoever I shall see or hear in the course of my profession, as well as outside my profession in my intercourse with men, if it be what should not be published abroad, I will never divulge, holding such things to be holy secrets. Now if I carry out this oath and break it not, may I gain for every reputation among all men for my life and for my art, but if I transgress it and forswear myself, may the opposite befall me.

Hippocrates recognized the differences in power between doctor and patient. A helping relation demanded the doctor's therapeutic commitment to the patient and the reciprocity of the patient's trust. In the innumerable medical writings about the doctor-patient relation, these themes recur. Doctors continue to retell the nature of therapeutic responsibility as directly as Francis W. Peabody does in his popular essay "Caring for the Patient": "The secret of caring for the patient is to care for him." Physicians' writings also recognize the attributes doctors must bring to the relation to ensure commitment to and care of patients. The conflicts in the relation have changed, but the attributes of doctors remain largely the same.

On Art and Science
In most of its recent and ancient past, medicine has regarded itself as both art and science. If the craft or technique was science, the care of patient and the application of technique for the benefit of the individual were art. The doctor-patient relation, then, was art in action, the expression of human values in the care and medical treatment of patients.

Around the middle of the nineteenth century, when there was far more art than science to medicine and when "unscientific" medical sects such as Thomsonianism (folk remedies), Grahamism (diet), eclecticism ("try anything"), and homeopathy ("like cures like") were popular (Clarke et al. 1876), Oliver Wendell Holmes (1911) and other leaders of the profession complained about unnecessary treatment of self-limited disorders. Holmes argued for more "science" or medical knowledge of the course of disease; otherwise, the patient would be exploited by the medical ignorance of the doctor and the mere ministrations of his art—the doctor's demeanor, the rituals of examination, and the expression of the doctor's personality—his bedside manner.

With the growth of medical specialization from the 1880s into the 1900s (Rosen 1944), the concern about the relation began to shift; it was argued that technique would dominate the relation. Would the specialist then ignore the patient's needs in the application of a narrow technique in what Cabot (1911) called the "absentmindedness of specialization"? The general practitioners complained that the emerging new class of medical specialists would do just that; moreover, in an era of stiff medical competition and limited economic resources, the specialists would, with false promises about tests and techniques, entice away patients—as indeed they gradually did. In the early twentieth century, with the advent of the hospital laboratory for clinical "testing" and of scientific investigation at the bedside, the concern, now even among hospital specialists, was whether the "art of medicine" would be lost in the pursuit of science. Would the patient be ignored in the study of disease as the full-time laboratory physician came to dominate the care of hospital patients, delegating most of it to junior physicians in training? Such are the themes in William Osler's essays (1952) and in those of generations of physicians he represented and many that followed him. Art was seen as the practitioner's "tailoring of treatment" to the individual, the doctor's clinical judgment and personal care. All this attention to the individual patient might be lost with the expansion of hospital technologies if doctors no longer bothered to learn about the personal lives and backgrounds of their patients in the pursuit of medical diagnosis and treatment. The art of medicine was, then, personal care by attention to the needs and *personality* of the patient.

Eventually, some clinicians, stimulated by Sigmund Freud's recognition of the pervasive subjective element in illness and the intrapsychic and interpersonal roots of psychological and somatic distress, became as interested in what the patient felt, thought, and wanted as in what disease the patient had. This new professional knowledge about the patient's views and psychology was expressed by a determination to meet those personal needs of patients, a theme popularized by such phrases as "the patient as a person" (Robinson 1939; Ramsay 1970). The expanding clinical literature produced by doctors, medical social workers, and psychiatrists on the views, experiences, and concerns of patients took the form of largely anecdotal case reports and "psychosomatic studies" relating life experiences to the onset and course of disease. Meanwhile, still other professions (in particular, medical sociology, following Talcott Parsons's oft-cited 1951 essay on the sick role) began to examine the patient and the relation in scientific detail. By the 1950s, illness and the doctor-patient relation from the patient's perspective had become a specialized topic of the social sciences. For the most part, the phenomenology of the patient, not the doctor, became the major focus of the social or behavioral sciences as they viewed this dyadic relation. In any event, the art of medicine was now behavioral science, a systematic study of the patient's perspective, producing knowledge of what the patient is like.

In later writings of clinicians, these older themes of art and science did not continue. Indeed, they could not. Clinicians could no longer speak about "art" and "science," nor can medical academics or practitioners today comfortably allude to these traditional distinctions. The very idea of the art of medicine appears out of vogue in an age when medicine has aspired, above all, to be a scientific form of human engineering and when human relations in medical practice are thought to constitute a behavioral science of interpersonal skills.[50] Now that these scientific reforms are apparently accomplished, the tension in the doctor-patient relation is not whether the doctor has the proper manners, not whether the doctor's "art" modifies "science" in practice for the benefit of patients, and not whether the doctor pays attention to the patients's psychology, personal needs, and concerns; now it is a question of "bioethics." In a medical world that contains so many expensive, complex, diagnostic, and therapeutic technologies, some of which may be hazardous in themselves and of marginal benefit, old ethical questions are being posed again. What are the rights of patients and the responsibilities of doctors in the decisions to use particular technologies? *Primum utilis esse* ("Above all, be useful") (Nelson 1978) is a complicated dictum to apply in a medical world of high-cost, "high-tech" therapies.

The ethical concerns are much broader today than in the 1900s, when Cabot argued only for telling the patient the truth about diagnosis. This communication was then a potential hazard; since few specific therapies were available, in learning the diagnosis the patient might also learn about a bad prognosis and so lose confidence in the doctor. The conflict today is not over the communication of the diagnosis but over the use of technologies in reducing disability and in prolonging life that may hold no "quality." Decisions on these matters are often being settled by groups, such as medical staff committees, rather than by the judgment of the individual doctor. This group decision-making has developed to fill a vaccum, since doctors have not always thought out the logic and ethics of their decisions on behalf of patients as they have thought out the accuracy of technologies in diagnosis and their efficacy in treatment. The doctor's art is now ethics; the old themes of manners, personal care, and behavioral science are now in the background.

Attributes of the Doctor

Recognizing these enduring but shifting conflicts in the relation, doctors have responded by writing about what a caring relation requires from the doctor, retelling the attributes of the good physician in yearly addresses to graduating classes or to annual meetings of professional societies and occasionally considering qualities of personality and character along with grades and achievements when reviewing the applicants to medical schools and residency programs.

When there appeared to be too much "art" and too little "science" in medicine, the important attribute for the doctor was medical knowledge, or at least knowledge about prognosis. It would, repeating Holmes's (1883) argument, prevent the practitioner from exploiting the patient by prescribing useless nostrums for self-limited diseases. As a professional attribute, scientific knowledge has often been exclusively emphasized by medical educators. The reasons are deeply ingrained in the ideology that medicine should, above all, be scientific. First, anything less than undivided attention to the medical science of disease would diminish the doctor's status, power, and projected image as a scientist; second, lessening attention might also increase the doctor's potential to harm the patient should he neglect to uncover the patient's disease while only attending to his distress; third, while science was said to be self-correcting through experiment and validation, art was not, and so the potential of art (as Plato argued) to create harm was far greater. Unlike science, the contribution of art must depend on the uncertain integrity of the practitioner, not on the supposed certainty of proof from experiment; and, as Henderson noted, the contribution of art may die out with the practitioner because there is no applied science of human relations to instruct the oncoming generation of practitioners. Finally, the assumption is that only science and technology improve care, not organization or relationships. For these reasons, far more ideological than not, some would "scientize" all of medicine and leave nothing to art.

Yet that was not the intent of earlier clinicians. Somewhat after Holmes, when the expansion of science in medicine was beginning, F. C. Shattuck (1907), then the physician-in-chief at Massachusetts General Hospital, spoke directly to the old dilemma, "The Science and Art of Medicine in Some of Their Aspects," in an address to the Yale Medical School class of 1907. He noted seven important personal attributes of doctors: knowledge, thoroughness, common sense, character, enthusiasm, sympathy, and honesty. In that same tradition of analyzing the attributes of doctoring are William Osler's "Aequanimatas" (1952), Francis W. Peabody's "Care of the Patient"

(1927), Joseph Pratt's "Personality of the Physician" (1936), James H. Means's advice to medical residents in *The Amenities of Ward Rounds* (1940), Herman Blumgart's "Caring for the Patient" (1964), and "Characteristics of the Helping Relation" (1961),[51] by Carl Rogers (a distinguished psychologist, not a medical practitioner).

More than 50 years after Shattuck, the medical tradition of writing on the doctor's personal qualities was not yet dead; the attributes listed by Sir Robert Pratt in his essay "Doctor and Patient, Ethics, Morale and Government" (1963) are little different from those given by Shattuck: "Scientific thinking is a necessary but not sufficient condition of good doctoring. It needs other qualities: warmth, feeling, compassion, humor, patience, integrity, and understanding." If the titles and writings discussed above have a quaintly antique flavor, it is because they are, indeed, moral strictures in an age when such topics are not part of the idea of the training of the doctor, when only mastery of technique appears central.

To the classic list of physician attributes put forth by Shattuck and Pratt, probably the only addition from modern commentators is that of *empathy*, a quality of understanding distinct from sympathy and pity. If empathy is so emphasized in teaching today, it may be a counterresponse to the great attention given the search for disease with modern technology, to the neglect of personal suffering (Cassell 1982). If empathy is added, an older quality—sacrifice—seems to be missing from the modern lists, however. Daniel Roche, in his essay "Talent, Reason and Sacrifice: The Physician During the Enlightenment" (1980), analyzes published eulogies about French physicians, noting how sacrifice was considered an essential attribute for a French physician. In that period, sacrifice could even mean death, an accepted risk in the care of patients with contagious disease. Today, sacrifice may have a hollow ring as fewer hazards face doctors and fewer demands are now made on them. Of course, training hours remain strenuous (up to 95 per week) and practice hours often long, but pay (as fees or salaries) is generous and schedules are regular, making physicians more and more like employees in business or industry.

Comments about the attributes of doctors might also be expected in modern textbooks on the interview, which introduce the meaning, use, and discourse of the doctor-patient relation to students. Yet these books speak hardly at all about what the doctor should bring to or develop in the relationship. With remarkable consistency, and in contrast with the previous writings, they address only the characteristics of the patient, usually in terms of one-word diagnoses of character types that can easily become reductive jargon: obsessional, narcissistic, hysterical, paranoid, dependent-passive (Kahana and Bibring 1969). Outside of this personality classification, doctors generate their own pragmatic classification of patients with positive attributes. In a survey of doctors' views of ideal patients, Ford et al. (1967) found they are characterized as trusting, cooperative, well-adjusted, responsive to treatment, and believing that their doctor is "best"—features that would certainly provide gratification to the doctor. Doctors in training as residents report that the "good patient" is the one from whom something can be learned about diagnosis and treatment or on whom a difficult procedure can be successfully tried and mastered.

On the Medical Tasks

Doctors also write about the relation when they discuss how they conduct the care of patients. For the practitioner, the relation is essential in the several tasks of care: the diagnosis and treatment of medical and psychological illness; the communication of information about illness (its diagnosis, treatment, prevention, and prognosis); the personal support of patients of all backgrounds in all stages of illness; the optimal maintenance of the chronically ill; and the prevention, when possible, of disease and disability through education, persuasion, and preventive treatment. All these tasks require information from patients, communication with them, and responses to their needs, requests, and expectations. In each task a relation is essential. Yet most medical writings only emphasize the use of the doctor-patient relation to obtain information for diagnosis.

The literature on the doctor-patient relation in diagnosis is found in textbooks on the medical or psychiatric interview, such as Allen J. Enelow and Scott N. Swisher's *Interviewing and Patient Care* (1972, 1985) and George L. Engel and William L. Morgan's *Interviewing the Patient* (1973). In most texts and pedagogical writings, including those mentioned, more attention is paid to the technique of eliciting information from patients for diagnosis than is paid to the doctor's communication with them (Stoeckle and Billings 1986). Two exceptions (not instructional textbooks) are notable and deserve mention. One is Michael Balint's *The Doctor, His Patient and the Illness* (1957). What is so appealing about this book is Balint's attention to the doctor's responses to the patient's complaints. These back-and-forth negotiated responses with the patient are significant in the definition or diagnosis of the patient's illness, what it is called, what caused it, and what should be done. A second exception are psychoanalytic writings. These, too, look at the doctor's response (countertransference) to patients. They note that the doctor's responses may be rooted in the unconscious (Zabarenko et al. 1970; Greenson 1972). This countertransference, with its origins in the doctor's own early experiences with his or her parents, may handicap the doctor's interaction with patients and is the basis of the vital dictum "Doctor, know thyself."

After the routine of questioning for medical diagnosis (the instructional theme that so dominates textbooks) come medical advice and explanation. Though it is seldom acknowledged, the explanatory content or patient education is as important as the diagnostic questioning in this era of multiple high-tech tests and therapies which the patient must choose or consent to (Stoeckle 1985). Explanation is important for the tasks of care other than diagnosis: psychological treatment, personal support, communication of information, and preventive education. Now that medical diagnosis is so often based on tests on patients rather than on information from them, and when medical practice is so much the care of the chronically ill, the elderly, the dependent, and the handicapped, these communicative tasks of care have become crucial in the patient's choices of treatment.

On Managing the Relation

From psychiatric studies of personality or character and of psychotherapy comes a how-to-do-it literature on how to manage the doctor-patient relation, particularly with "difficult" and "problem" patients. Two themes are the patient's personality and the techniques of psychotherapy. The usual advice is to attend to patients' defenses, their habitual responses that are rooted in their personalities. For example, Steiger and Hansen's *Patients Who Trouble You* (1964) contains advice on several patient types: "The Patient Who Doesn't Trust," "The Seductive Patient," and "The Martyr." Textbooks on the medical interview contain much of the same material as this small popular volume written for an audience of young student practitioners. The other common theme is the doctor's use of psychotherapeutic techniques in the care of medical patients. Derived from psychoanalysis, these techniques, consciously or unconsciously used, include abreaction, clarification, suggestion, manipulation, and interpretation (Bibring 1954).

Most of this management literature focuses on patients' personalities, particularly on hostility, as a source of difficulty for the doctor (Lipsitt 1970; Groves 1978; Drossman 1978; Goodwin et al. 1979; Papper 1970; Najmen et al. 1982). Only rarely is difficulty in the relation attributed to the doctor, even though many patients, if asked, would put the blame squarely on the "doc's" shoulders. Except for

Blum's 1960 study, little has been written about the doctor's personality as a variable in the interaction. The other source of strain in the
doctor-patient relation is the illness situation. Doctors have written
about managing dying patients, chronically ill patients (Gans 1983),
handicapped children, patients undergoing highly technical therapies (such as renal dialysis and transplantation), and patients participating in clinical experimentation (Katz 1972).

Even though the management literature consists of commentaries
on the difficulties of and with patients, the accounts are incomplete.
The difficulties of patients need not always end badly, as George
Pickering records in *Creative Malady* (1974) and P. Sandblom in
Creativity and Disease (1982). Patients change, seeking new directions
and accomplishments; there is not invariably regression and dependence, as so much clinical literature would suggest. Moreover,
doctors do not often record their gratification and inspiration from
relations or their successful, satisfying unique encounters, though
they feel good about them (Messner 1976) and even reminisce about
them years later.

Vivid comments on the experience of "doctoring"—on the phenomenology of the doctor—are rarely found in academic writings.
They are more likely to be found in doctors' biographies and autobiographies, as illustrated by Berger and Mohr's *The Fortunate Man*
(1967) or by this excerpt from William Carlos Williams's chapter on
"The Practice" (1948):

It's the humdrum, day-in, day-out, everyday work that is the real satisfaction
of the practice of medicine; the million and a half patients a man has seen on
his daily visits over a forty-year period of weekdays and Sundays that make
up his life. I have never had a money practice; it would have been impossible
for me. But the actual calling on people, at all times and under all conditions,
the coming to grips with the intimate conditions of their lives, when they
were being born, when they were dying, watching them die, watching them
get well when they were ill, has always absorbed me.

I lost myself in the very properties of their minds; for the moment at least I
actually became them, whoever they should be, so that when I detached
myself from them at the end of a half-hour of intense concentration over
some illness which was affecting them, it was as though I were reawakening
from a sleep. For the moment I myself did not exist, nothing of myself affected
me. As a consequence, I came back to myself, as from any other sleep, rested.

Less vivid, humdrum, uninspired reports of patient-doctor encounters can also be found in clinical literature, as in Hollingshead and
Redlich's *Social Class and Mental Illness* (1958):

Seeing him every morning was a chore; I had to put him on my back and carry him for an hour.

He had to get attention in large doses, and this was hard to do.

The patient was not interesting or attractive; I had to repeat, repeat, repeat.

She was a poor, unhappy, miserable woman—we were worlds apart.

Third-Party Accounts of the Relationship

Because patients and doctors are in the relation they write about, they concentrate on its value to them and on how to change it to make it work better in the tasks of care. Social scientists outside the therapeutic relation can examine it from the different perspectives of their disciplines, where they do not experience its gratifications, attachments, affiliations, frustrations, failures, outright defeats, and therapeutic successes. They have described the structure of the relation—the roles and behaviors of the patient and the doctor—as but one example of dyadic relations in general. For reasons not altogether clear, social scientists, as Judith Swazey (1979) notes, have paid more attention to the patients' experiences and behaviors than to those of doctors (though, as noted earlier, some medical anthropologists have begun to look at the everyday experiences of the doctor more closely; see Hahn et al. 1985). One reason for the social scientists' emphasis on the patient's perspective is that it is not systematically or completely described by doctors or that, when it is described, the clinical accounts are biased with the notions practitioners bring to it. Perhaps, too, social scientists are more sympathetic to the patient, choosing that side of the dyadic relation for greater exploration because the patient, as the "underdog" or victim, has more appeal to scholars who are concerned at heart with social issues, or, because the patient's side is richer, more varied, and more interesting than the top side of the relation where professional life seems more uniform—a fact that even doctors will admit, acknowledging their own fascination with the unique lives and illnesses of their patients. Finally, and most important, the social scientists' preference for studying patients made practical sense. By understanding what patients were like, then practitioners might use the information to improve their treatment. Not just theoretical or descriptive, social-psychological knowledge could be applied. The doctor could better persuade patients to take medication and advice, and could better tailor treatment to their individual needs. In effect, helping medical actions would be both effective and personal, in the tradition of good practice. Because such knowledge about what the patient is like might be usefully applied, the social scientists' search for it was rewarding and has been seen as a contribution to the work of practitioners as well as to general knowledge.

Social scientists have also looked at the effects of a variety of social factors on the amount, content, process, quality, and outcome of doctor-patient interaction. These factors include the cultural, class, and ethnic backgrounds of both doctors and patients (though not equally); the organization of practice, whether private, group, or clinic; the modes of communication; and the special treatment situations of acute, chronic, and terminal patients.

Besides these variables in the microstudies of the doctor-patient relation, particular attention has been paid to the theme of power and authority between doctor and patient. This feature has been reexamined, as modern conditions are changing the sources and nature of that power and authority—as the organization of medical practice has shifted from solo to bureaucratic, as the medical knowledge has grown more technical but also more publicly diffused, as authority has come to be expressed through expertise rather than paternalism, and as professional charisma has become more difficult to sustain in the face of the popularized doctor. While the historian Edward Shorter (1985) and social scientists such as Marie Haug, Marvin Sussman, and Bebe Lavin (1969, 1983) have addressed the erosion of professional power from various points of view (along with reference to the advocacy promoting its decline), the medical profession has already accommodated itself in a variety of ways—some of which can be characterized as professional alienation—to a decline in power that is bureaucratic, economic, charismatic, legal, and interpersonal. Doctors grumble but accept more salaried shift work at less pay within the bureaucratic constraints of treatment institutions (Derber 1984); their charisma is diminished as they willingly get advertised, publicized, and popularized, just as their legal dominance is diminished by the increasing but tolerable legal restrictions and liabilities, the cost of which is passed on to the consumer. At the interpersonal level, patients seeking medical aid are less accepting of professional dominance, since subordinate roles are less acceptable, not only in the relation but everywhere else in society. Patients' rights, unfortunately, are often singlemindedly pursued without regard to patients' duties, in disregard of Simone Weil's (1952) clear philosophic formulation that obligations and duties are necessarily reciprocal. In response to this declining authority in the relation, some doctors are enthusiastically redirecting their efforts at communication and patient education, thus transferring power to patients to exercise in their own self-treatment and decision-making. Others, feeling demoralized by external changes, are searching for a closer attachment to patients in the quiet solace of the office; more are leaving the office early, investing less of the professional self in practice life, while a few are leaving altogether.

The readings that follow touch on many of these themes. The several authors examine the structure, dynamics, nature, and conflicts of the doctor-patient relationship, describe the good relation, and discuss the possibilities for research.

Notes

1. Using U. S. Bureau of Census data, Betz and O'Connell (1983) report that people in the professional class increased from 9 to 16 percent of the work force between 1950 and 1980.

2. The 1980 average stay of 8 days was down to 6.6 days in 1984, and is likely to go lower as capitation payments for a diagnosis rather than daily charges give hospitals incentives to move patients out quickly.

3. Nurses account for 50 percent of these contacts, pharmacists for 12 percent.

4. Holistic and alternative practitioners as well as behavioral therapists are not included in conventional surveys. Smoking (and chronic lung disease), drinking (and chronic liver disease), overeating (and obesity), anxiety (and hypertension), and sexual disorders can all be treated by "behavioral modification" outside of strictly medical practice (Mattarazzo et al. 1984), in free-standing or corporate chain clinics, or in medical-specialty boutiques for single disorders only (e.g., Nutrition, Inc.). Recent surveys from Belgium (Foets et al. 1985), the Netherlands (Oijendiijk 1980), and Great Britain (Fulder and Monro 1985) show that 1, 4, and 2.5 percent of their populations respectively see marginal or alternative practitioners. Moreover, these visits are made by the better educated, over one-third of whom also see the doctor. The visit characteristic most valued by British patients is time, 30 minutes compared to the usual 6 from the GP.

5. Indeed, doctor-patient encounters are not always the most important, as patients will readily report liking those with physical therapists and nurses better in some stages of illness (Davis 1963; Robinson 1956).

6. The politics was national, not local—the Hill-Burton Act of 1946. This act for hospital construction was followed by regulations requiring that "the planning of out-patient facilities shall provide for the privacy and dignity of the patient during interview, examination and treatment" (DHEW Human Resource Services 1978).

7. Surprising or not, the U.S. Department of Health, Education and Welfare's 1980 *Practice Management Guide Book* for National Health Service Corps physicians working in underserved and poor communities recommends that exam and treatment rooms be 9 by 11 feet and that the consultation room (the physician's office) be 100 square feet. Presumably space is cheaper away from the cities.

8. Self-disclosure is evident in the photographs of Freud's unoccupied office in *Berggasse 19, Sigmund Freud's Home and Office, Vienna 1930* (University of Chicago Press,

1981), with its display of archaelogical artifacts, pictures, and books; in the office photographs of rural general practitioners and their patients in the 1930s (Stoeckle and White 1980, 1985), showing the utilitarian roll-top desk, shelf of medical texts, hat rack, and papers unfiled; and in the photographs of empty and occupied medical suites from the architectural ads in *Erdman Medical Modules* (Madison: Marshall Erdman and Associates, 1982) with their crisp, modernistic, colorful interiors.

9. Identification pictures were removed not only from medical records but also from school and job applications. Doctors now carry those pictures of patients on color slides for use in lectures. Another photograph exchange is patient-to-doctor. Wallets or pocketbooks hold snapshots of children, grandchildren, weddings, anniversaries, and graduations to show the doctor. Mark Rosenberg's photo essay *Patients: The Experience of Illness* contains office views.

10. In one recent advertising spread, three of twelve doctors depicted were female, one was black, and two were older—media acknowledgement of doctors' changing gender, age, and race.

11. The mother, the father, the wife, the husband, a son, a daughter, a friend, or a home health aide is said to accompany every 2.4–2.6 eye patients. This figure on the number of people who came with the patient seems high, and the term *escort* obscures that fact that this person often has complaints or information about the patient that may also require attention. At the highest, the British report one escort per 3 or 4 patients in medical clinics surveyed (Nuffield Provincial Hospital Trust and University of Bristol 1955; Hockey 1968), a figure consistent with our own local experience with a group-practice population containing fewer visually handicapped patients but more elderly patients and patients with language differences. That makes the doctor in need of linguistic assistance and creates triangular rather than linear dyadic exchanges. The escort-patient ratio is likely to decrease as future medical practice populations contains still more dependent elderly, chronically ill, and physically handicapped patients, so that the encounter with the doctor, more often than not, will be a three-person exchange. This triad has always been the norm in pediatrics, and it is now nearly the norm in adult medical practice as a daughter or sometimes a son is bringing mom or dad to the doctor, the aging wife comes with her ailing husband, and home health aides escort the widowed and childless. Age, not numbers, makes the context of the visit different as the frail elderly parent over 80 comes with daughter (or son) over 60, both of them often drained by a burden of chronic illness and care—and its social costs.

12. The doctor's chair is usually different from the patient's. An executive-style swivel bucket seat or armchair that is movable and larger than the straight-back chair that fixes the patient in one place, it signals the dyadic differences in authority, control, and movement in the office encounter. Swivel chairs reportedly came out in the 1850s (Grant 1976). How soon they were adopted by medical practitioners is not known, but they certainly contributed to the profession's authoritarian position in the office encounter. Sometimes the doctor in American clinic offices sits to interview on a rotating movable stool, yet the patient traditionally remains fixed in a chair (Cambridge Hospital, U.S. Army Outpatient Department). The doctor's chair is usually but not always different. Kopat-Holim clinics in Israel have fixed chairs for both MD and patients, and they are alike.

13. Students of proxemics have yet to examine whether sitting still closer in talking to patients makes a difference in the comfort of the doctor and the patient or in the content of their discourse.

14. Visits to renovated hospitals here and abroad show that this trend toward privacy continues everywhere. In two- and four-bed rooms, current U.S. regulations call for 3 feet of space around each bed. In intensive-care units, beds must be 4 feet from the wall and 8 feet apart, making more room for machines (the monitors and assist devices) at the bedside, as well as for staff and visitors (U.S. Department of Health, Education and Welfare [PHS, HRA] 1978). While ordinary rooms require 3 feet around the bed, even then visitors often stand or visit in shifts, as so many come today. Such amenities of space are not everywhere. In Great Britain, Ann Cartwright (1964) reported that private rooms were less common (4 percent single, 12 percent in 2–4-bed units, 41 percent in 20-bed units, and 12 percent with 30 beds or more), but even in Great Britain the shift to smaller units continues.

15. A patient, recently hospitalized for a myocardial infarction, underwent the placement of a pulmonary-artery "line" (catheter) a balloon assistance, a gated-blood pool scan, a cardiac catherization, and transfer to a convalescent floor, for a total of 10 days of hospitalization. He (or his body) had contract with 55 different hospital staff members (nurses, resident and staff physicians, medical students, technicians, dieticians, clerks, transport aides). Few time motion and content studies are done of the actual interactions with so many different personnel. In one preliminary study by M. Jean Daubenmire and colleagues (1986), a surgical patient during a one-week hospital stay had, 1,902 interactions with various staff in the hospital room alone. While the numbers sound like an applied biological assembly line, in a study of the care of hospitalized patients Strauss et al. (1985) note that the medical work is technical but, more than that, some of it even sentimental.

16. Bedside visits by anesthesiologists began in the 1960s. Such visits and communications became routine when anesthesia was performed by the physician, and by the early 1980s nurse-anesthesiologists were doing the same.

17. Using the language of sports and the psychology of industrial production, doctors, nurses, and social workers began to care for the "sick poor" as "teams" in the early 1900s (Cabot 1907). Quite in contrast to solo practice, he wrote: "Medical organization in a dispensary means not only the team work of peers. It means the stratification and sifting out of jobs, so that the physician never need spend much time on work a less highly trained person can do."

18. Personal communications, Drs. Harriet L. Hardy, Northampton, MA; John Angley, Brockton, MA; John D. Goodson, Sr., Kansas City, MO; Max Pearlstein, Braintree, MA; Lewis Dimsdale, Sioux City, IO; and Salvatore Lima, Boston MA. See also Barnett 1979. The site of care changed not only in the United States but also, to a lesser extent, in Great Britain. Even though the British GP and the British public continue a shared tradition of "domiciliary visits" (and they remain part of the daily GP schedule), such visits are down from a high of 50 percent to 20–25 percent today.

19. However, this is an unlikely task for the nursing profession, which is so deeply invested in hospital work; moreover, nursing services are neither organized nor available in the numbers that would be required for this amount of home care. This comment is made despite the valuable home-practice work of the Visiting Nurse Associations; unfortunately, their efforts are generally limited to day shifts and to lower-income patients. Others will argue that home-care corporations will fill the gap as insurers pay for more technical treatment at home, including chemotherapy, dialysis, and nutritional therapy.

20. The nature of these requests has received much comment though not detailed examination (Wolfe et al. 1968; Elford et al. 1962; Pinsent 1964; Botherston et al. 1959; Scott and McVie 1979; Richman 1965; Bailey 1979; Cauthen 1981). From the case reports in *Night Calls*, Max Clyne (1961) provides some hints with descriptions of family quarrels as one example of the "intermediaries" who call a doctor for the "sick" when they are really the ones in need of attention.

21. Doctors who have their night calls covered by others have reported that the personal doctor might make "a difference" in but 30 percent of those nocturnal visits (and yet 30 percent seems high). When patients in a Danish study were questioned, they welcomed home visits no matter what doctor came, though it should be said that these respondents were mostly old and infirm and had never experienced home visiting (Bentzen et al. 1976). Views from the patients' side, in general, go unrecorded in the literature and are only reported informally by general practitioners abroad. They note that the public continues to want home visits even as such visits are decreasing from a high of 50 percent to a low of 20 percent of the practitioners' work (personal communication, William Sagar, Boston, England).

22. Other observations on families are made in *Night Calls* (Clyne 1961) and by practitioners who have answered house calls. Today the full attention of the family audience and the patient may have to be secured by a quick switch-off of the TV and the visit closure delayed by a cup of coffee on the way out (William Sagar, General Practice Training Unit, Boston, England, personal communication, 1984). In the case of more traditional healers, the African witch doctor, and even today's Indian medicine man (Hawk LittleJohn, Cherokee County, NC, personal communication, 1980), home visiting may be organized as an extended experience for both. The witch doctor and medicine man then live with the family during one or more weeks of healing practice, a residential tactic that would hardly meet today's pressures for cost-effectiveness but one that has been adopted by live-in family psychotherapists determined to alter the "family system" if not the patient. Then there is the hospice movement, with death in the home for which the doctor attends, as carefully described by J. Andrew Billings (1985).

23. Tradition may also make for greater numbers of relatives in the waiting room or surrounding the bedside. Among Gypsies, the numbers from the clan who wait may be 50 or more (Thomas 1985). "Eighty years old, 80 complaints, 80 words of English, and 80 visitors" was once a pejorative, exaggerated claim about Italian-Americans (Peter Rosenberg, Neurology Service, personal communication).

24. The health-care industry is said to be the fifth largest. In 1984, 7,934,000 persons were employed in health service sites—offices, hospitals, convalescent institutions— making for a sizable public informed about health and illness from their work inside these treatment institutions (U.S. DHHS 1986). Add to persons informed by on-the-job medical knowledge the 20 percent high school and college educated public (Hacker 1983).

25. The British National Health Service has considered a yearly stipend of 600 pounds for doctors' wives who answer the home phone.

26. Clinics and hospitals also provide dial-advice. For example, the Tel-Med tape library of the Lahey Clinic, in Burlington, Massachusetts, lists 271 wide-ranging titles, from birth control and development (the teen years) to symptoms of diseases (chronic cough, cancer of the bone) and mental health (When should I see a psychiatrist?).

27. The prospects for more black enrollments is dim. In 1979, only 5.7 percent of those enrolled in medical schools were black (Health/PAC 1980) against the expected 10 percent proportion. In 1986 minority enrollment (blacks, American Indian, Mexican-Americans, and Puerto Ricans) was only 8.5 percent (Iglehart 1986). More certain is a mixed health-care encounter of another kind: the homebound white patient with homemakers and home health aides who, in Eastern cities, are so often black or Hispanic.

28. For example, in the 1980s, clinics for the newly romanticized "homeless" (Brickner et al. 1985) repeated the strategies and tactics of the free-clinic movement of the 1960s and the 1970s (Stoeckle et al. 1972), developing special clinics and facilities, not for diseases but for special people, and now with public and foundation funding rather than volunteer work.

29. This is somewhat longer than the 19.7 (1980) and 18.8 minutes (1983) reported in AMA 1984, and close to the 30 minutes reported in Aday et al. 1984. The wait was 46.6 minutes in hospital outpatient departments—considerably longer than the average wait of 25.0 minutes reported in a 1952 survey of British outpatient departments (Nuffield Provincial Hospitals Trust 1965), even though the British doctors were, on average, 15 minutes late in starting their clinic sessions, like doctors everywhere, even today.

30. In a 1984 survey of persons waiting in the lobby of the Massachusetts General Hospital's Ambulatory Care Center, 8 of 10 persons were neither patients nor employees nor connected with patients coming to the Center.

31. Social psychologist Roger Brown (1965) notes that between persons of unequal status forms of address and names promote status or solidarity (intimacy). We have no surveys of patients' use of the title "Dr." versus doctors' first names or of doctors' use of Mr., Mrs., Ms. versus patients' first names. Everywhere egalitarian pressures for solidarity seem greater than those for status. First names are promoted for face-to-face and voice-to-voice communication in all service encounters between strangers— in restaurants ("I'm Ann, your waitress"), banks ("Thank you, John"), hotels, stores, garages—and even between doctors of different status. Nowadays nurses introduce themselves to patients by their first names, while the appointment card from the physical therapsit indicates the return visit will be with "Rita," and the reminder card for a visit is addressed "Dear Danny." The disappearance of formal nursing uniforms adds to the patient's confusion over identification. As one patient recently remarked, "Can't tell who's who here."

32. The very high number of office visits in Japan is due in part to the dispensing of drugs (rather than the writing of prescriptions) at the doctor's office rather than at the pharmacy, the limited payment for a visit, and the time limits on prescribing and dispensing (2 weeks, compared to 6 months to a year in the U.S.). The average number of visits per year is 20 (Kickai et al. 1977). No matter what the communication, verbal or nonverbal, the Japanese doctor and patient have a visual familarity with each other from these numerous visits greater than that reported from any other country.

33. How many patients can be treated in a day or a week? Cynics will say, "Lots, all quick visits." The answer is also "the doctor's work week is long"—some 50–60 hours (56.8) in 1984, with about 51 hours per week devoted to patient-care contacts alone. Some suggest that working hours are going down a little—3 percent, according to Freeman and Marder (1984). Regardless, the long hours can mean starting the

day early at 7–7:30 A.M., as busy surgeons (and less than 50 percent are) often do with hospital rounds before going to the operating room at 8 A.M. Some psychiatrists begin even earlier, seeing patients at their home office at 7 A.M. before the patients have to report to their own jobs (personal survey, Dr. Doris Held). While psychiatrists may be among the earliest starters, they report working the least—51.1 hours per week, compared to 59.5 for internists (the longest hours reported). Then there are the medical practitioners who hold evening office hours up to 9 P.M. one or two days a week, making physicians one of the few professions among the 12 million "night workers" (Carpentier and Carzamian 1977). Doctors average 47 weeks in practice per year (AMA 1985), taking a longer vacation than most.

34. Rosenberg and Pless (1985) examined the knowledge practitioners had of their patients' personal backgrounds and families and found that the doctors' knowledge of patients was not associated with either high satisfaction or good compliance by patients. Yet such questionnaire inquiries do not tap the affective aspects of the relation.

35. With clinics there has always been a vision of clinical productivity resembling the industrial "assembly line," as reformers since the 1900s have tried to transform medicine from a cottage trade into a modern corporate industry (Davis 1912).

36. The silence may be accounted for, in part, by the physical exam, which is so often conducted with little or no dialogue between doctor and patient. Clearly some minutes are already underutilized for communication, and some might be used differently. Columnist Ann Landers reports that women feel uncomfortable about quiet physical examinations and complain about not hearing the intentions, proce- dures, or findings of the physician as the exam is done ("An interview with Ann Landers on doctors and patients," *Behavioral Medicine*, July 1979, p.29).

37. This sometimes seems to be the case in lower-class life where the options for steady medical relationships are also fewer and, in fact, may not be preferred (Lambert and Freeman 1967). Some would even facilitate all patients changing doctors. David Mechanic (1985) remarks that patients locked into bureaucratic systems of prepaid practices need to have their match with the doctor carefully made, encouraging their choice (and perhaps "tryouts" with MDs), allowing patients to change doctors readily if nothing works in the short or long haul of illness. Among disabled children, Breslau and Mortimer (1981) observe that "seeing the same doctor" is more satisfy- ing, while Ettlinger and Freeman (1981) find a personal doctor (presumably "the same doctor") better for patient compliance.

38. Besides death, the encounter is broken off by other external events—when, for example, divorce breaks up a marriage, and one partner seeks another doctor; when families leave town for the father's job-hunting or his company transfer; when patients are incarcerated because of age, disease, and dementia into distant nursing homes the last eight or ten years of their lives; and even when some are sent to prison, but for shorter average terms of 3.5 years. Fry (1980) notes 4 adults in prison from a practice list of 2,500; the author's practice list contains two.

39. Surprisingly, these survey studies of sexual contacts never include questions on how many doctors marry patients with whom they had an affair or whom they met in the office. I know of four instances (not including the sanitarium encounter of Dr. Dick Diver and Nicole in Fitzgerald's *Tender Is the Night*), and more of nurses marrying their patients, often under circumstances of long-term care and rehabilita- tion. A recent survey ("Psychiatrist-patient sex topic of survey, " *AMA News*, May

23, 1986, p. 3) indicates that 6 percent of psychiatrists, including female therapists, admit to sexual contacts.

40. Experimentation on humans can be included here.

41. A contribution made in gratitude for a certain doctor's care can, of course, increase the doctor's influence, if not power, in the institution. At least it is formally acknowledged:

Dear Dr. X,

The officers and staff of the Massachusetts General Hospital wish you to know that a contribution in your honor has been gratefully received from. . . .

Sincerely,
President of the Corporation

42. Although this list of writings from doctors' pens might be expanded, it is surprisingly short in light of the estimate that some 87,000 practicing MDs (18 percent of the total) are physically disabled (Lewis 1983) and presumably have an illness experience to recount. Also missing from the literature of disabled doctors is their professional relationship with patients when they recover. Do patients get more from disabled doctors who have successfully made it back, as did those TB patients who were taken care of by cured TB doctors who stayed on in the sanitoriums to make a clinical career—inspired that they too can make it back? Or do disabled doctors hide their disability in a specialty such as radiology where patient contact may not be large or hide it by denying it and failing to acknowledge or discuss it in the relationship where the patient expects the doctor not to be or get sick?

43. My search for illness accounts from the 5 percent of physicians impaired by drugs, alcohol, or psychiatric disorders revealed few published accounts, though no doubt their stories are told in group therapy and AA meetings. One recent MD account is Gehring's (1985) *Rx for Addiction*.

44. This new consumer ideology has already appeared in a Canadian government-supported "study" of the prescribing habits of doctors in different practices (Renaud et al. 1980) in which simulated patients were used without informed consent, an undercover investigation of what the doctor did that does not deserve to be labeled "research."

45. Despite the vast popularization of the doctor as a modern folk hero, Myerhoff and Larson (1958) view such exposure and celebrity status as a loss of the profession's charisma and, one could add, of some of the power that goes with that charisma.

46. Readers and bibliographies on "the doctor in literature" provide even more references to (and critiques on) the position and the role of the doctor; see Peschel 1980, Silvette 1967, Cousins 1982, and Trautman and Pollard 1975. Syllabi from the many courses now offered in Medical Humanities also contain reading lists on doctors—and patients.

47. The idea of research as a self-sacrificing career is something of a myth that seems self-serving in retrospect. Even William Osler, who epitomized the early self-sacrificing academic at McGill and Hopkins, reportedly charged very high fees, equivalent to $5,000 for a private consultation (Harrell 1982), in order to support his library, while today modern medical research that has become well-paid has resulted in fraud that has not gone unnoticed by "whistle-blowers" (Swazey and Sober 1982). Meanwhile, academic medical researchers can go to the drug and bio-tech industries for lucrative jobs or become members of their boards of directors.

48. In casualty (accident and emergency) departments of British hospitals an account of what patients are called is similar. From his observational study, Jeffrey (1979) reports that deviant patients are referred to as "normal rubbish," though with variations such as "dross," "dregs," "crumble," and "grot." "Normal rubbish" would include trivial cases (nothing wrong), drunks, overdoses, and tramps. Felicity Stockwell, in her study *The Unpopular Patient* (1984), notes the more genteel term British nurses used for patients they did not like: "hospital birds." Once labeled, however, all disliked patients might be subject to long waits; occasional verbal hostility (from the medical staff!), though fairly restrained compared to comments in discussion with other staff; and, finally, when in desperate need for their physical control, calls to the hospital's security staff, who have been added on to modern treatment institutions, as they are to nearly every institution except the church. While such derogatory language or its equivalent is hard to find in older writings and is quite in contrast to the older religious appeal expressed by Cabot, it can, of course, he heard outside of medicine on the street, in the dialogue of movies, and in novels. Such typification of patients seems to be used more by the medical staff in institutions who are insulated from public view; more by young doctors in training, on front-line duty, than by older staff who are not; and more in those clinical situations of intense work pressures (emergency rather than hospital wards) (Leiderman and Grisso 1985; Mizrahi 1985, 1986).

49. Perhaps these verbal extremes in talking back come out of a culture in which deference and sometimes politeness (Martin 1984) have long since disappeared in all "consumer" areas—banking, schooling, shopping. This trend now seems to have touched medical practice, at least with some of the patient clientele who are at the bottom or who carry high levels of entitlement for services.

50. Even without the rhetoric of "art" and "science," physicians still express these indirectly in how they characterize the good physician. Tinsley Harrison (1980), author of the famous text *Principles of Internal Medicine*, writes: "No greater opportunity or obligation can fall the lot of a human being than to be a physician. In the care of suffering he needs clinical skill, scientific knowledge, and human understanding. He who uses these with courage, humility and wisdom will provide a unique *service* for his fellow man and will build an enduring edifice of character within himself. The physician should ask of his destiny no more than this, and he should be content with no less." Alpha Omega Alpha, the medical fraternity, has the motto "Worthy to serve the suffering."

51. The last-mentioned work is cast not in the rhetoric of professional attributes used in the previously mentioned writings but in the language of therapeutic relationships.

References

Abram, H. S. 1977. Emotional aspects of heart disease: A personal narrative. *Int. J. Psychiat.* 8: 3.

Aday, L. A., Flemming, G. V., and Andersen, R. 1984. *Access to Medical Care in U. S.: Who Has It; Who Doesn't.* Chicago: Pluribus.

Advanced Data. 1978. 1976 summary: National ambulatory medical care survey. *Advanced Data*, no. 30, July 13, 1978.

Aiken, L. H., Lewis, C. F., Craig, J., Modehall, R. C., Blendon, R. J., and Rogers,

D. E. 1979. The contribution of specialists to the delivery of primary care: A new perspective. *New Engl. J. Med.* 300: 1303.

Alpert, J. J. 1964. Broken appointments. *Pediatrics* 34: 127.

Alsop, S. 1973. *Stay of Execution*. Philadelphia: Lippincott.

Altman, I., Kroeger, H. H., Clark, D. A., Johnson, A. C., and Sheps, C. G. 1965. The office practice of internists. II. Patient load. *JAMA* 193: 667.

AMA. 1984. *Center for Health Policy 1984*. Chicago: AMA.

AMA. 1985. *In the Marketplace: Work Patterns, Practice Characteristics, and Incomes of Women Physicians*. Chicago: AMA.

AMA. 1985. *Socioeconomic Characteristics of Medical Practice*. Reynolds, R. A., and Duran, D. J. eds. Chicago: AMA.

American Hospital Association. 1975. Survey of Changes in Community Hospitals as of January 1975. Chicago: AHA.

American Hospital Association. 1985. *Trends*. A Report on Community Hospital Finances, Utilization and Staffing Based on Data from the National Hospital Panel Survey. Chicago: AHA.

Annas, G. H. 1974. The hospital: A human rights wasteland. *Civil Liberties Rev.* 1: 9.

Annas, G. H. 1975. *The Rights of the Hospital Patient: A Basic Guide to a Hospital Patient's Rights*. New York: Avon.

Antonovsky, A. 1972. A model to explain visits to the doctor with special reference to the case of Israel. *J. Health and Soc. Behav.* 13: 446.

Apple, R. A. 1984. *Illustrated Catalogue of the Slide Archives of Historical Medical Photographs at Stony Brook*. Westport, Conn.: Greenwood.

Arber, S., and Sawyer, L. 1985. The role of the receptionist in general practice: A "dragon behind the desk"? *Soc. Sci. Med.* 20: 911.

Armitage, K. L., Schneiderman, L. J., and Bass, P. A. 1979. Response of physicians to medical complaints of men and women. *JAMA* 241: 2186.

Ayleff, M. J. 1976. Seeing the same doctor. *J. Roy. Coll. Gen. Pract.* 26: 47.

Bailey, A. 1979. Home visiting: The part played by the intermediary. *J. Roy. Coll. Gen. Pract.* 29 : 137.

Bailey, R. M. 1968. Economies of scale in outpatient medical practice. *Group Practice*, July, p. 24.

Baker, A. S. 1978. What do family physicians in a prepaid group do in their offices? *J. Fam. Pract.* 6: 335.

Balint, E., and Norell, J. S. 1973. *Six Minutes for the Patient*. London: Tavistock.

Balint, M. 1957. *The Doctor, His Patient and the Illness*. New York: International Universities Press.

Balint, M. E., Balint, E. B., Gosling, R., and Hindebrand, R. 1966. *A Study of Doctors*. New York: Lippincott.

Balint, M. E., Hunt, J., Joyce, D., Marinker, M., and Woodock, J. 1970. *Treatment or Diagnosis, A Study of Repeat Prescriptions in General Practice*. London: Tavistock.

Ballou, A. "MGH cardiac patients learn the joy of exercise." *Boston Globe*, January 8, 1982.

Barnett, S. W. 1979. In *Pure Nostalgia*, ed. C. Hamilton. Ames: Iowa State University Press.

Baron, C. H. 1982. Licensure of health care professionals: The consumer's case for abolition. *Am. J. Law Med.* 9: 335.

Becker, E. M., and Della Penna, R. D. 1975. *Health Care in Correctional Institutions.* Washington, D.C.: National Institute of Law Enforcement and Criminal Justice, U.S. Department of Justice.

Beeson, P. B. 1975. The ways of academic clinical medicine in America since WWII. *Man and Med.* 1: 65.

Belli, A. 1984. Morality and medicine on the modern stage. *Pharos* 47: 11.

Belsky, M. S., and Gross, L. 1975. *How to Choose and Use Your Doctor, The Smart Patient's Way to a Longer, Healthier Life.* New York: Arbor House.

Bennet, J. B., and Sagov, S. E. 1973. An experience of cancer: An honest dialogue between doctor and patient. *Harper's*, November, p. 94.

Bennett, H., and Samuels, M. 1973. *The Well Body Book.* New York: Random House.

Bentzen, N., Russell, I., and Spark, M. G. 1976. Deputizing services in Denmark. *J. Roy. Coll. Gen. Pract.* 26: 37.

Berger, J., and Mohr, J. 1967. *A Fortunate Man, The Story of a Country Doctor.* London: Penguin.

Bergman, A. B., Dassel, S. W., and Wedgewood, B. G. 1966. Time and motion study of practicing pediatricians. *Pediatrics* 38: 254.

Bertera, E. M., and Bertera, R. L. 1981. The cost effectiveness of telephone versus clinic counseling for hypertensive patients: A pilot study. *Am. J. Publ. Health* 71: 626.

Betz, M., and O'Connell, L. 1983. Changing doctor-patient relationships and the rise in concern for accountability. *Social Problems* 31: 84.

Bibring, E. 1954. Psychoanalytic and diagnostic psychotherapy, similarities and differences. *J. Am. Psychoanal. Assoc.* 2: 745.

Bice, T. W., and White, K. L. 1965. Factors related to use of health services: An international comparative study. *Med. Care* 7: 124.

Billings, J. A. 1983. Communication Times in Medical Practices. Unpublished study, Massachusetts General Hospital.

Billings, J. A. 1985. *Outpatient Management of Advanced Cancer.* Philadelphia: Lippincott.

Billings, J. A., Rubin, F., and Stoeckle, J. D. 1986. Home care. In *The Practice of Geriatric Medicine*, ed. E. Calkins. Philadelphia: Saunders.

Blanchard, C. G., Ruckdeschel, J. C., Blanchard, E. B., Arena, J. G., Saunders, N. L., and Molloy, E. D. 1983. Interactions between oncologists and patients during rounds. *Ann. Int. Med.* 9: 694.

Block, S. W., and Gerson, S. 1982. The affective tone of the MD-patient relationship. *Psychosom. Med.* 44: 115.

Bloom, F. 1977. Psychotherapy and moral culture: A psychiatrist's field report. *Yale Rev.* 66: 321.

Blum, R. H. 1957. *The Psychology of Malpractice Suits.* San Francisco: California Medical Association.

Blum, R. H. 1958. *Malpractice Suits: Why and How They Happen.* San Francisco: California Medical Association.

Blum, R. H. 1960. *The Management of the Doctor-Patient Relationship.* New York: McGraw-Hill.

Blumberg, M. S. 1979. Physician Fees as Incentives. Proceedings of the Twenty-First Annual Symposium of Hospital Affairs, Center for Health Administration Studies, Chicago.

Blumberg, M. S. 1984. Medical society regulation of fees in Boston, 1780–1820. *J. Hist. Med. and Allied Sci.* 39: 303.

Blumgart, H. L. 1964. Caring for the patient. *New Engl. J. Med.* 270: 449.

Blumhagen, D. W. 1979. The doctor's white coat: The image of the physician in modern America. *Ann. Int. Med.* 91: 111.

Bologh, R. W. 1979. Alienation in the patient role: Source of ambivalence and humor in comic get-well cards. *Sociol. Health and Illness* 1: 138.

Boozer, J. S. 1980. Children of Hippocrates: Doctors in Nazi Germany. *Ann. Am. Acad. Polit. and Soc. Science* 450: 83.

Borelli, M. D., and Heidt, P. 1981. *Therapeutic Touch.* New York: Springer Publishing.

Borisoff, D., and Merrill, L. 1985. *The Power to Communicate: Gender Differences as Barriers.* Prospect Heights, Ill.: Waveland.

Botherston, J. H. F., Cartwright, A., Cowan, J., Baldwin, J. T., Douglas, E. C. K., and Steele, G. A. 1959. Night calls: Their frequency and nature in one general practice. *Brit. Med. J.* 2: 1169.

Boxill, R. 1925. *Shaw and the Doctors.* New York : Harcourt, Brace.

Bradley, R. A. 1962. Father's presence in delivery rooms. *Psychosomatics* 3: 474.

Brady, B. L., and Stokes, J. 1970. Use of professional time by internists and general practitioners in group and solo practice. *Ann. Int. Med.* 73: 741.

Braslow, J. B., and Heins, M. 1981. Women in medical education: A decline or change? *New Engl. J. Med.* 304: 1129.

Breslau, N., and Mortimer, E. A., Jr. 1981. Seeing the same doctor: Determinants of satisfaction with speciality care for disabled children. *Med. Care* 19: 741.

Brickner, P. W., Scharer, L. K., Conavan, B., Elvy, A., and Savarese, M. 1985. *Health Care of Homeless People.* New York: Springer Publishing.

Brinkley, J. 1985. Physicians have an image problem—It's too good. *New York Times,* February 10.

Brown, R. 1965. The basic dimensions of interpersonal relationship. In *Social Psychology.* New York: Free Press.

Bruhn, J. G. 1978. The doctor's touch: Tactile communication in the doctor-patient relationship. *South. Med. J.* 71: 1469.

Burnham, M. C. 1982. American medicine's golden age: What happened to it? *Science* 215: 1474.

Burns, S. B. 1980. The doctors. *Artforum* 19(3): 10.

Butler, P. W., Bentley, J. D., and Knapp, R. M. 1980. Today's teaching hospitals. *Ann. Int. Med.* 93: 614.

Cabal, M. F. 1962. What the public thinks of the family doctor: Folklore and facts. *GP* 25: 146.

Cabot, R. C. 1907. Suggestions for the reorganization of hospital outpatient departments with special reference to the improvement of treatment. *Maryland Med. J.* 50: 81.

Cabot, R. C. 1911. Humanizing the care of the sick poor. *City Club Bull.* 4: 113.

Cabot, R. C. 1912. Outpatient work, the most important and most neglected part of medical service. *JAMA* 113: 1.

Cabot, R. C. 1927. *Physical Diagnosis*. New York: William Wood.

Caldwell, J. R., Cobb, S., Dowling, M. D., and de Jongh, D. 1970. The drop-out problem in anti-hypertensive therapy. *J. Chron. Dis.* 22: 579.

Callard, C. H. 1972. Iatrogenic problems in end-stage renal failure. *New Engl. J. Med.* 287: 334.

Candib, L. 1982. Personal communication.

Carpentier, J., and Cazamian, P. 1977. *Night Work*. Geneva: International Labor Office.

Cartwright, A. 1964. *Ward Size: Human Relations and Hospital Care*. London: Routledge and Kegan Paul.

Cartwright, A. 1967. *Patients and Their Doctors. A Study of General Practice*. New York: Atherton.

Cassell, E. 1982. The nature of suffering and the goals of medicine. *N. Engl. J. Med.* 306: 458.

Castelnuovo-Tedesco, P. 1962. The twenty minute hour: An experiment in medical education. *New Engl. J. Med.* 266: 283.

Cathell, D. W. 1882. *The Physician Himself and What He Should Add to His Scientific Achievements*. Second edition, revised. Baltimore: Cushings and Gailey.

Cauthen, D. B. 1981. The house call in current medical practice. *J. Fam. Pract.* 13: 209.

Charles, S. C., and Kennedy, E. 1985. *Defendant: A Psychiatrist on Trial for Medical Malpractice*. New York: Free Press.

Clarke, E. H., Bigelow, H. J., Gross, S. D., Thomas, T. G., and Billings, J. S. 1876. *A Century of American Medicine, 1776–1876*. Philadelphia: H. C. Lea.

Clute, K. F. 1963. *The General Practitioner: A Study of Medical Education and Practice in Ontario and Nova Scotia*. University of Toronto Press.

Clyne, M. B. 1961. *Night Calls: A Study in General Practice*. London: Tavistock.

Clyne, M. B., Hawes, A. J., Lask, A., and Saville, P. R. 1963. The discontented patient, leaving by notification. *Roy. Coll. Gen. Pract.* 6: 87.

Coble, R. J., Sinnott, S. K., and Walz, T. H. 1982. The family physician's office: Proposed design criteria for family-centered medical care. *J. Fam. Pract.* 14: 77.

Cochrane, A. 1972. *Effectiveness and Efficiency*. London: McHield.

Commission on Professional and Hospital Activities. 1968, 1973, 1978. *Hospital Resource Study*. Ann Arbor: Commission on Professional and Hospital Activities.

Committee on the Costs of Medical Care. 1932. *Medical Care for the American People*. University of Chicago Press.

Commonwealth of Massachusetts. Department of Public Health. 1975. Long-Term Care Patient Survey.

Commonwealth of Massachusetts. Department of Public Health. 1983. Rules and Regulations for the Licensing of Long-Term Care Facilities, 1977. 105 CMR 150-159.

Conant, E. S. 1983. Addressing patients by their first names. *New Engl. J. Med.* 308: 266.

Cook, S. *Second Life*. 1981. New York: Simon and Schuster.

Cousins, N. 1979. *Anatomy of an Illness as Perceived by the Patient*. New York: Norton.

Cousins, N., ed. 1982. *The Physician in Literature*. Philadelphia: Saunders.

Cowan, P. 1964. Studies in the growth, change and aging of buildings. London: University College. (Trans. Bart. Soc. 1, 1962)

Cox, A., and Groves, P. 1981. *Design for Health Care*. London: Butterworth.

Crombie, D. L., and Cross, K. W. 1964. The workload in general practice. *Lancet* 2: 354.

Cronin, A. J. 1937. *The Citadel*. Boston: Little, Brown.

Curran, W. J., and Casscells, W. 1980. The ethics of medical participation in capital punishment by intravenous drug injection. *New Engl. J. Med.* 302: 226.

Curran, W. J. 1983. Medical malpractice claims since the crisis of 1975: Some good news and some bad. *New Engl. J. Med.* 309: 1107.

Dahlberg, C. C. 1970. Sexual contact between patient and therapist. *Contemp. Psychoanal.* 6(2): 107.

Dahlberg, C. C., and Jaffe, J. 1977. *Stroke, A Doctor's Personal Story of His Recovery*. New York: Norton.

Daubenmire, M. J. School of Nursing, Ohio State University, personal communication.

Davis, F. 1959. The cab driver and the fare: Facets of a fleeting relationship. *Am. J. Sociol.* 65: 158.

Davis, F. 1963. *Passage through Crisis, Polio Victims and their Families*. Indianapolis: Bobbs-Merrill.

Davis, M. M., Jr. 1912. Efficiency tests of out-patient work. *Boston Med. and Surg. J.* 165: 915.

Davis, M. S., and VonderLippe, R. P. 1967. Discharge from hospital against medical advice: A study in reciprocity in the doctor-patient relationship. *Soc. Sci. and Med.* 1: 336.

deBoer, R. A., Jaspars, J. M. F., van Leeuwen, P. van der Meer, F., Radder, J. J., and van Schaik, C. T. H. 1970. An evaluation of long-term seminars in psychiatry for family physicians. *Psychology* 33: 468.

Derber, C. 1984. Physicians and their sponsors: The new medical relations of production. In *The Political Economy of Health Care*. ed. J. B. McKinlay. New York: Tavistock.

Diagram Group. 1981. *The Healthy Body Maintenance Manual*. New York: New American Library.

Dickson, W. M., and Rodowskas, C. A., Jr. 1975a. A comparative study of community pharmacy practice: Chain and prescription oriented pharmacies. *Drugs in Health Care* 2: 153.

Dickson, W. M. and Rodowskas C. A. 1975b. Verbal communication of pharmacists. *Med. Care* 13: 486.

Diseker, R. A., Michielutte, R., and Morris, V. 1980. Use and reported effectiveness of Tel-Med: A telephone health information system. *Am. J. Publ. Health* 70: 229.

Dorsey, J. 1969. Physician distribution in Boston and Brookline, 1940 and 1961. *Med. Care* 7: 429.

Drew, J., Stoeckle, J. D., and Billings, J. A. 1983. Tips, status and sacrifice: Gift giving in the doctor-patient relation. *Soc. Sci. and Med.* 17: 399.

Dreyfuss, J. L. 1971. On evaluating upper gastro-intestinal symptoms by provocative study. *Radiologic Clinics of North America* 9: 15.

Drossman, D. A. 1978. The problem patient. *Ann. Int. Med.* 88: 366.

Duff, R. S., and Hollingshead, A. B. 1968. *Sickness and Society*. New York: Harper & Row.

Duncan, R. E. 1937. Technicians and laboratory relations. *Am. J. Med. Tech.* 3: 81.

Dunnell, K., and Cartwright, A. 1972. *Medicine Takers, Prescribers and Hoarders*. London: Routledge and Kegan Paul.

Dyckman, Z. Y. 1978. Physicians: A Study of Physician Fees. Washington, D.C.: Council on Wage and Price Stability, Executive Office of the President.

Egbert, L. D., Battit, G. E., Welch, C. E., and Bartlett, M. K. 1964. Reduction in post-operative pain by encouragement and instruction of patients: A study of doctor-patient rapport. *New Engl. J. Med.* 270: 825.

Ehrenreich, B., and Ehrenreich, J. 1974. Health care and social control. *Soc. Pol.*, July–August, p. 26.

Ehrenrich, B., and English, D. 1979. *For Her Own Good, 150 Years of the Experts' Advice to Women*. New York: Anchor.

Eimerl, T. S., and Pearson, R. J. C. 1966. Working time in general practice: How GP's use their time. *Brit. Med. J.* 2: 1549.

Ekman, P. 1978. Facial signs: Facts, fantasies and possibilities. In *Sight, Sound and Senses*, ed. T. Sebock. Bloomington: Indiana University Press.

Ekman, P., ed. 1982. *Emotions in the Human Face*. Cambridge University Press.

Ekman, P., and Friesen, W. V. 1975. *Unmasking the Face: A Guide to Recognizing Emotions from Facial Clues*. Englewood Cliffs, N.J.: Prentice-Hall.

Elford, R. W., Whitney Brown, J., Robertson, L., Alpert, J. J., and Kosa, J. 1962. A study of house calls in the practices of general practitioners. *Med. Care* 10: 173

Eliot, R. S. 1981. What I learned from my MI. *Modern Medicine*, June, p. 62.

Enelow, A. J., and Swisher, S. N. 1972, 1985. *Interviewing and Patient Care*. London: Oxford University Press.

Engel, G. L., and Morgan, W. L., Jr. 1973. *Interviewing the Patient*. Philadelphia: Saunders.

Entralgo, P. L. 1969. *Doctor and Patient*. New York: McGraw-Hill.

Ettlinger, P. R. A., and Freeman, G. K. 1981. General practice compliance study: Is it worth being a personal doctor? *Brit. Med. J.* 282: 1192.

Eyles, J., and Woods, K. J. 1983. *The Social Geography of Medicine and Health*. New York: St. Martin's.

Fairbank, L. A. 1980. Relationships among adult females in captive vervet monkeys: Testing a model of rank related attractiveness. *Anim. Behav.* 28: 853.

Falk, I. S., Rorem, C. R., and Ring, M. D. 1933. *The Costs of Medical Care*. University of Chicago Press.

Federal Trade Commission. 1985. *Healthy Questions, How To Talk to and Select Physicians, Pharmacists, Dentists, Vision-Care Specialists*. Washington, D.C.

Felch, W. C. 1981. The internist cognoscenti and cognition. *Internist*, August, p. 12.

Field, M. 1961. The doctor-patient relationship in perspective of "fee-for-service" and "third-party" medicine. *Health and Hum. Behav.* 2: 252.

Field, M. 1975. Feminization of the medical profession, American and Soviet medical manpower: Growth and evolution, 1910–1970. *Int. J. Health Services* 5: 455.

Field, M. G. 1976. Approaches to Correct the Underrepresentation of Women in the Health Professions, A U.S. Response to a Look at the U.S.S.R. In Proceedings of the International Conference on Women in Health. DHEW publication (HRA) 76–51. Washington, D.C.: U.S. Department of Health, Education and Welfare.

Finnerty, P. A., Mattie, E. C., and Finnerty, F. A. 1973. Hypertension in the inner city. *Circulation* 43: 73.

Flink, J. J. 1970. *America Adopts the Automobile, 1895–1910*. Cambridge, Mass.: MIT Press.

Foets, M., Berghmans, F., and Janssens, L. 1985. The primary health care project in Belgium: A survey on the utilization of health services. *Soc. Sci. Med.* 20: 181.

Folev, R., Smilansky, J., and Yonke, A. 1979. Teacher-student interaction in a medical clerkship. *J. Med. Ed.* 54: 622.

Ford, A., Liske, R. E., Ort, R. W., and Denton, J. C. 1967. *The Doctor's Perspective*. Cleveland: Case Western Reserve University Press.

Foye, H., and Chamberlin, R. 1977. Content and emphasis of well-child visits. *Am. J. Dis. Child* 131: 794.

Frank, A., and Frank, S. 1972. *The People's Handbook of Medical Care*. New York: Vintage.

Frank, L. K. 1957. Tactile communication. *Genet. Psych. Monogr.* 56: 209.

Freeman, I., and Roy, T. 1976. *Betrayal: The True Story of the First Woman to Successfully Sue Her Psychiatrist for Using Sex in Guise of Therapy*. New York: Stein and Day.

Freeman, L. 1951. *Fight Against Fear*. New York: Crown.

Freeman, M. P., and Marder, W. D. 1984. Changes in the hours worked by physicians, 1970–80. *Am. J. Pub. Health* 74: 1348.

Freeze, A. S. 1975. *Managing Your Doctor: How to Get the Best Possible Health Care*. New York: Stein and Day.

Fry, G., and Roy, G. I. 1972. Twenty-one years of general practice—Changing patterns. *J. Gen. Pract.* 22: 521.

Fry, J. 1978. Home visiting: How much is necessary? *Update* 16: 1119.

Fry, J., ed. 1980. *Primary Care*. London: Heinemann.

Fuchs, V. R. 1974. *Who Shall Live? Health Economics and Social Choice.* New York: Basic Books.

Fulder, S. J., and Munro, R. E. 1985. Complementary medicine in the United Kingdom: Patients, practitioners, and consultations. *Lancet* 1: 542.

Gammock, R. 1982. *Primary Health Care Buildings, Health Centers, Neighborhood Clinics and Group Practice Surgeries: A Building and Design Guide for Architects and Their Clients.* London: Nichols.

Gans, J. S. 1983. Hate in a rehabilitation setting. *Arch. Phys. Med. Rehab.* 64: 176.

Gartner, A., and Riessman, F., eds. 1984. *The Self-Help Revolution.* New York: Human Sciences Press.

Gehring, W. R. 1985. R_x *for Addiction.* Grand Rapids, Mich.: Zondervan.

Gelfand, M. 1964. *Witch Doctor, Traditional Medicine Man of Rhodesia.* London: Harvill.

Gerbner, G., Gross, L., Morgan, M., and Signorielli, N. 1981. Health and medicine on television. *New Engl. J. Med.* 305: 901.

Gibson, C. D., and Kramer, B. M. 1965. Site of care in medical practice. *Med. Care* 3: 314.

Giffin, M. P., Frazier, S. H., Robinson, D. B., and Johnson, A. M. 1957. The internist's role in the successful treatment of anorexia nervosa. *Proc. Staff Meeting Mayo Clinic* 32: 171.

Gifford, G. E. 1973. Fildes and "The Doctor," *JAMA* 5: 61.

Girard, R. A., Mendenhall, R. C., Tarlov, A. R., Radecki, M. A., and Abrahamson, S. 1979. A national study of internal medicine and its specialties. I. An overview of the practice of internal medicine. *Ann. Int. Med.* 90: 965.

Givens, J. T. 1957. Thirteen reasons why patients change doctors. *Nat. Med. Assoc.* 49: 174.

Goffman, E. 1959. *The Presentation of Self in Everyday Life.* New York: Anchor.

Goldfarb, D. L., ed. 1981. *Profile of Medical Practice, 1981.* Chicago: Center for Health Services Research and Development, American Medical Association.

Goldsmith, S. B. 1979. Housecalls: Anachronism or advent? *Pub. Health Rep.* 94: 299.

Goodman, P. 1959. Meaning of functionalism. *J. Arch. Ed.* 14: 32.

Goodwin, J. M., Goodwin, J. S., and Kellner, R. 1979. Psychiatric symptoms in disliked medical patients. *JAMA* 241: 117.

Goroll, A. H., Stoeckle, J. D., and Lazare, A. 1974. Teaching the clinical method in walk-in clinics. *J. Med. Ed.* 49: 957.

Grad, G. 1979. Healing by the laying on of hands: A review of experiments in ways of health. In *Holistic Approach to Ancient and Contemporary Medicine,* ed. D. Sobel. New York: Harcourt Brace Jovanovich.

Grant, I. 1976. The machine age. In *The History of Furniture.* New York: William Morrow.

Gray, P. G., and Cartwright, A. 1953. Choosing and changing doctors. *Lancet* 2: 1308.

Green, G. 1979. *The Healers.* New York: Putnam.

Green, R. C., Carrol, G. J., and Buxton, W. D. 1978. *The Care and Management of the Sick and Incompetent Physician.* Springfield, Ill.: Thomas.

Greenlick, M. R., Freeborn, D. K., Gambill, G. L., and Pope, C. P. 1973. Determinants of medical care utilization: The role of the telephone in total medical care. *Med. Care* 11: 121.

Greenson, R. P. 1972. *Technique and Practice of Psychoanalysis*. New York: International Universities Press.

Grossman, J. H., Barnett, G. O., McGuire, M. T., and Shedlow, D. B. 1971. Evaluation of computer-acquired histories. *JAMA* 215: 1286.

Groves, J. 1978. Taking care of the hateful patient. *New Engl. J. Med.* 298: 883.

Guntrip, H. 1975. My experience of analysis with Fairbairn and Winnicott. *Int. Rev. Psychoanal.* 2: 145.

Gustafson, J. P. 1981. The control and mastery of aggression by doctors: A focal problem for the Balint group with medical residents. In *Group and Family Therapy*, ed. L. R. Wolberg and M. L. Aronson. New York: Brunner/Mazel.

Hacker, A. 1983. *US: A Statistical Portrait of American People*. New York: Viking.

Haggerty, R. G., Roghmann, K. J., and Pless, I. B. 1975. In *Child Health and the Community*. New York: Wiley-Interscience.

Hahn, R. A., and Gaines, A., eds. 1985. *Physicians of Western Medicine, Anthropological Approaches to Theory and Practice*. Boston: Reidel.

Halberstam, M., and Lester, S. 1976. *A Coronary Event*. New York: Lippincott.

Hall, D. W. 1972. The off-duty arrangements of general practitioners. *Med. Care* 10: 173.

Hall, E. T. 1968. Proxemics. *Curr. Anthropol.* 9: 83.

Hall, J. A. 1978. Gender effects in decoding nonverbal clues. *Psycho. Bull.* 83: 845.

Hamman, L. 1938. As others see us. *Trans. Assoc. Am. Phys.* 53: 22.

Hannay, D. R. 1979. *The Symptom Iceberg: A Study of Community Health*. London: Routledge and Kegan Paul.

Harrell, G. T. 1982. The Osler family. *JAMA* 248: 203.

Harrison, T. 1980. *Harrison's Principles of Internal Medicine*. New York: McGraw-Hill.

Harwood, A. 1981. *Ethnicity and Medical Care*. Cambridge, Mass.: Harvard University Press.

Haug, M. 1976. Erosion of professional authority: Cross-cultural inquiry in case of physicians. *Health and Soc.* 54: 83.

Haug, M. 1982. Doctor-Patient Relations in Different Societies. Unpublished.

Haug, M., and Lavin, B. 1983. *Consumerism in Medicine: Challenging Physician Authority*. Beverly Hills, Calif.: Sage.

Haug, M., and Lawton, M. P., eds. 1981. *Elderly Patients and Their Doctors*. New York: Springer.

Haug, M. R., and Sussman, M. B. 1969. Professional autonomy and the revolt of the client. *Social Problems* 17: 153.

Haupt, B. 1983. 1982 Summary National Hospital Discharge Survey, National Center for Health Statistics. *Advance Data* 95: 1.

Havens, L. 1976. *Participant Observation*. New York: Aronson.

Heagarty, M. C., Robertson, L., Kosa, J., and Alpert, J. J. 1968. Use of telephone by low-income families. *J. Pediatr.* 73: 730.

Health/PAC. 1980 *Double Indemnity*. New York: Health/PAC.

Health Policy Institute. 1982. *The Physician Resource: A Profile of Supply*. Health Policy Institute, University of Pittsburgh.

Heins, M., Hendricks, J., Martindale, L., Smock, S., Stein, M., and Jacobs, B. 1979. Attitudes of women and men physicians. *Am. J. Publ. Health* 69: 1132.

Hertzler, A. E. 1938. *The Horse and Buggy Doctor*. New York: Harper Brothers.

Hirsh, H. L., and White, E. T. 1978. The pathologic anatomy of medical malpractice claims. *Legal Med.*, January, p. 25.

H. J. Kaiser Foundation. 1981. *Medical Practice in the 1980s: Physicians Look at Their Changing Profession*. Prepared by Louis Harris and Associates.

Hockey, L. 1968. *Care in the Balance. A Study of Collaboration Between Hospital and Community Services*. Cambridge: Queen's Institute of Nursing.

Hodgins, E. 1971. *Episode*. New York: Simon and Schuster.

Hoggart, R. 1961. *The Uses of Literacy: Changing Patterns in English Mass Culture*. Boston: Beacon.

Holden, W. D., and Levitt, E. J. 1978. Migration of physicians from one specialty to another. *JAMA* 239: 205.

Holder, A. R. 1978. Trends in malpractice litigation. *Yale J. Biol. and Med.* 53: 333.

Hollingshead, A. B., and Redlich, F. C. 1958. *Social Class and Mental Illness: A Community Study*. New York: Wiley.

Holmes, O. W. 1883. The young practitioner. In *Medical Essays, 1842–1882*. Boston: Houghton Mifflin.

Holmes, O. W. 1911. *Currents and Counter Currents in Medicine. Medical Essays*. Volume 9 in *The Writings of O. W. Holmes*. Boston: Houghton Mifflin.

Holroyd, J. C., and Brodsky, A. M. 1977. Psychologists' attitudes and practices regarding erotic and non-erotic physical contact with patients. *Am. Psychologist* 32: 843.

Hopkins, H. 1974. *Grand Rounds*. Boston: Little, Brown.

Houston, C. S., and Pasanem, W. E. 1972. Patients' perceptions of hospital care. *Hospitals* 46: 70.

Houston, W. R. 1936. *The Art of Treatment*. New York: Macmillan.

Howard, M. 1956. *Coming to Terms with Rheumatoid Arthritis*. London: Faber and Faber.

Hull, F. M. 1972. How well does the general practitioner know his patients? *Practitioner* 208: 688.

Iglehart, J. K. 1986. Health Policy Report: Federal support of health manpower education. *New Engl. J. Med.* 314: 324.

Illich, I. 1976. *Medical Nemesis*. New York: Pantheon.

Irvine, P. 1985. The attending at the funeral. *New Engl. J. Med.* 312: 1704.

Janzen, J. M., and Ackinstall, W. 1978. *The Quest for Therapy in Lower Zaire*. Berkeley: University of California Press.

Jeffery, R. 1979. Normal rubbish: Deviant patients in casualty departments. *Sociol. of Health and Illness* 1: 90.

Jones, W. H. S. 1923. *Hippocrates.* London: Heinemann.

Josiah Macy Foundation. 1970. Annual Report for the Year 1970. New York.

Joyce, C. 1977. *Twice a Victim.* London: Robert Hale.

Joyce, C. R. B., Last, J. M., and Weatherall, M. 1968. Personal factors as a cause of differences in prescribing by general practitioners. *Brit. J. Prev. Soc. Med.* 22: 170.

Insights: Foreign Medical Graduates. *JAMA* 252: 2402, 1984.

Kahana, R. J., and Bibring, G. L. 1969. Personality types in medical management. In *Psychiatry and Medical Practice in a General Hospital*, ed. N. E. Zinberg. New York: International Universities Press.

Kaplan, R. S., and Leinhardt, S. 1975. Determinants of physician office location. *Med. Care* 11: 406.

Kardener, S. H. 1974. Sex and the physician-patient relation. *Am. J. Psychiat.* 131: 1134.

Kardener, S. H., Fuller, M., and Mensh, I. N. 1973. A survey of physicians' attitudes and practices regarding erotic and non-erotic contact with patients. *Am. J. Psychiat.* 130: 1077.

Kardener, S. H., Fuller, M., and Mensh, I. N. 1976. Characteristics of "erotic" practitioners. *Am. J. Psychiat.* 133: 11.

Karinthy, F. 1939. *Journey Round My Skull.* London: Faber and Faber.

Kasteler, J., Kane, R. L., Olsen, D. M., and Thetford, C. 1976. Issues underlying prevalence of "doctor shopping" behavior. *J. Health and Soc. Behav.* 17: 328.

Katz, A. H. 1975. Some Thoughts on Self-Help Groups and the Professional Community. Talk, mimeo. National Conference on Social Welfare, San Francisco, May.

Katz, H. D., Pozen, R., and Mushlin, A. I. 1978. Quality assessment of a telephone care system utilizing non-physician personnel. *Am. J. Publ. Health* 68: 31.

Katz, J. 1972. *Experimentation with Human Beings.* New York: Russell Sage Foundation.

Kedward, H. B. 1962. Social class habits of consulting. *Brit. J. Prevent. and Social Med.* 16: 147.

Keith, S. N., Bell, R. M., Swanson, A. G., and Williams, A. P. 1985. Effects of affirmative action in medical schools: A Study of the class of 1975. *New Engl. J. Med.* 313: 1519.

Keogh, J. P. 1977. Physicians and torture. *New Engl. J. Med.* 297: 178.

Kessel, N., and Sheppard, M. 1969. The health and attitudes of people who seldom consult a doctor. *Med. Care* 7: 124.

Kickai, K., Kimata, S., Kurata, M., Hashimoto, M., Hashimoto, S., and Ichijyo, K., eds. 1977. *Health Services in Japan.* International Hospital Congress, Tokyo.

Kirk, P. T., and Sternberg, E. D. 1955. *Doctors' Offices and Clinics.* New York: Reinhold.

Kirshner, L. A. 1978. Effects of gender on psychotherapy. *Comp. Psych.* 19: 79.

Klein, R. 1973. *Complaints Against Doctors.* London: Charles Knight.

Kleinman, A. 1973. Toward a comparative study of medical systems: An integrated approach to the study of the relationship of medicine to culture. *Sci. Med. and Man* 1: 55.

Kleinman, A. 1980. *Patients and Healers in the Context of Culture.* Berkeley: University of California Press.

Knapp, D. A., Wolf, H. H., Knapp, D. E., and Rudy, T. A. 1969. An experimental analysis. The pharmacist as drug advisor. *Am. Pharm. Assoc.* 10: 502.

Knaus, W. A. 1972. *Inside Russian Medicine: An American Doctor's First-Hand Report.* New York: Everest House.

Knickerbocker, C. H. 1960. *The Hospital War: A Novel of Medical Intrigue.* Garden City, N.Y. : Doubleday.

Kohn, R., and White, K. L. 1976. *Health Care, An International Study.* London: Oxford University Press.

Kra, S. J. 1982. *Examine Your Doctor: A Patient's Guide to Avoiding Medical Mishaps.* New Haven, Conn.: Ticknor and Fields.

Krieger, D. 1979. *The Therapeutic Touch: How to Use Your Hands to Help or Heal.* Englewood Cliffs, N.J.: Prentice-Hall.

Krupnick, M. 1966. *Lionel Trilling and the Fate of Cultural Criticism.* Evanston, Ill.: Northwestern University Press.

Kucharski, A. 1978. Medical management of political patients. *Perspect. Biol. and Med.* 22: 115.

Kucharski, A. 1984. On being sick and famous. *Political Psychol.* 5: 69.

Lack, S., and Buckingham, P. W. 1978. *First American Hospice.* New Haven, Conn.: Hospice.

Lagone, J., and Thorp, D. 1983. Japanese medicine. *Medical Month,* December: 22.

Lambert, C. J. R., and Freeman, H. E. 1967. *The Clinic Habit.* New Haven: College and University Press.

Lancet. 1952. *Disabilities and How to Live with Them.* London: The Lancet.

Lasch, C. 1977. *Haven in a Heartless World, The Family Besieged.* New York: Basic Books.

Lasko, K. A. 1980. *The Great Billion Dollar Medical Swindle.* New York: Bobbs-Merrill.

Lawrence, P. S., and Fuchsberg, R. R. 1964. Medical care, health status, and family income. *Vital Health Statistics* (U.S. DHEW), series 10, no. 9.

Lear, M. W. 1980. *Heart Sounds, The Story of Love and Loss.* New York: Simon and Schuster.

Lederer, H. D. 1952. How the sick view their world. *Soc. Issues* 8: 4.

Leiderman, D. B., and Grisso, J. A. 1985. The gomer phenomenon. *J. Health and Soc. Behav.* 26: 222.

Lennard, H. L., Epstein, L. J., Bernstein, A., and Ransom, D. C. 1971. Mystification by the medical profession. In *Mystification and Drug Misuse.* San Francisco: Jossey-Bass.

Lester, D. 1981. The use of the telephone in counseling and crisis intervention. In *The Social Impact of the Telephone,* ed. I. de Sola Pool. Cambridge, Mass.: MIT Press.

Levin, A. 1975. *Talk Back to Your Doctor: How to Demand and Recognize High Quality Health Care.* Garden City, N.Y.: Doubleday.

Lewis, M. A. 1974. Child-initiated care. *Am. J. Nurs.* 74: 652.

Lewis, S. 1925. *Arrowsmith.* New York: Harcourt, Brace.

Lewis, S. B. 1983. The physically handicapped physician. In *The Physician, a Professional under Stress,* ed. J. P. Callahan. New York: Appleton-Century-Crofts.

Ley, P. 1972. Complaints made by hospital staff and patients: A review of the literature. *Bull. Brit. Psycho. Soc.* 25: 115.

Liberman, R. 1962. Analysis of the placebo phenomenon. *J. Chron. Dis.* 15: 761.

Lichstein, P. R. 1982. The resident leaves the patient: Another look at the doctor-patient relationship. *Ann. Int. Med.* 96: 762.

Linn, L. S., and Lawrence, G. D. 1978. Requests made in community pharmacies. *Am. J. Publ. Health* 68: 492.

Lipsitt, D. 1970. Medical and psychological characteristics of "crocks." *Psychiatry in Medicine* 293: 15.

Lister, J. 1974. By the London Post: Complaints in medicine. The miner's health. Postscript. *New Engl. J. Med.* 290: 827.

Locke, M. M. 1980. Doctor-patient relationships in cosmopolitan medicine. In *East Asian Medicine in Urban Japan, Varieties of Medical Experience.* Berkeley: University of California Press.

Loudell, F. S. 1974. Folk medical beliefs and their implications for care of patients. *Ann. Int. Med.* 81: 82.

Louis Harris & Associates. 1985. Americans and Their Doctors.

Luck, G. M., Luckman, J., Smith, B. W., and Stringer, J. 1971. Waiting for attention. In *Patients, Hospitals and Operational Research.* London: Tavistock.

McCue, J. D. 1982. The effects of stress on physicians and their medical practice. *New Engl. J. Med.* 306: 458.

McGuire, M. T., Fairbanks, L. A., Cole, S. R., Sabardone, R., Silvers, R. M., Richards, M., and Akers, J. 1977. Study of four psychiatric wards: Patient, staff and systems behavior. *J. Psychiat. Res.* 13: 146.

McKeown, T. 1971. A Historical Appraisal of the Medical Task. In *Medical History and Medical Care.* London: Oxford University Press.

McKinlay, J. B., ed. 1984. *Issues in the Political Economy of Health Care.* London: Tavistock.

McKinlay, J. B., and McKinlay, S. M. 1977. The questionable contribution of medical measures to the decline of mortality in the United States in the twentieth century. *Health and Society* 55: 405.

Malkin, J. 1982. *The Design of Medical and Dental Facilities.* New York: Van Nostrand–Reinhold.

Margulies, H., and Block, L. S. 1969. *Foreign Medical Graduates in the United States.* Cambridge, Mass.: Harvard University Press.

Marsh, G. N. 1968. Visiting—falling workload in general practice. *Brit. Med. J.* 1: 633.

Marston, M. V. 1970. Compliance with medical regimens: A review of the literature. *Nursing Res.* 19: 312.

Martin, J. 1984. The pursuit of politeness. *New Republic,* August 6.

Massachusetts Medical Society. 1985. *Malpractice Law Reform: Everybody's Business.*

Mattarazzo, J. D., Weiss, S. M., Herd, J. A., and Miller, N. E., eds. 1984. *Behavioral Health: A Handbook of Health Enhancement and Disease Prevention.* New York: Wiley.

Mawardi, B. 1979. Satisfactions, dissatisfactions, and causes of stress in medical practice. *JAMA* 241: 1483.

May, L. 1978. *Getting the Most from Your Doctor.* New York: Basic Books.

Means, J. H. 1940. *The Amenities of Ward Rounds.* Massachusetts General Hospital (privately printed).

Mechanic, D. 1985. Public perceptions of medicine. *New Engl. J. Med.* 312: 181.

Medical Economics. 1963, 1966. *Cartoon Classics* and *More Cartoon Classics.* Ordwell, N.J.: *Medical Economics* Book Divison.

Mejia, A., Pizurki, H., and Royston, E. 1980. *Foreign Medical Graduates: The Case of the United States.* Lexington, Mass.: Lexington Books.

Mendelsohn, R. S. 1979. *Confessions of a Medical Heretic.* Chicago: Contemporary Books.

Mendenhall, R. C., principal investigator. 1981. *Medical Practice in the United States.* Princeton, N. J.: Robert Wood Johnson Foundation.

Mendenhall, R. C., Tarlov, A. R., Girard, R. A., Michel, J. K., and Radecki, S. E. 1979. A national survey of internal medicine and its specialties. II. Primary care internal medicine. *Ann. Int. Med.* 291: 295.

Messner, E. 1976. Inspiration of psychotherapists by patients. *Am. J. Psychiat.* 133: 12.

Miliband, R. 1978. A state of de-subordination. *Brit. J. Sociol.* 29: 399.

Mizrahi, T. 1985. Getting rid of patients: Contradictions in the socialization of internists to the doctor-patient relationship. *Sociol. Health and Illness.* 7: 214.

Mizrahi, T. 1986. *Getting Rid of Patients.* New Brunswick: Rutgers University Press.

Mogul, K. M. 1982. Overview: The sex of the therapist. *Am J. Psychiat.* 139: 1.

Mollen, A. 1975. *Run For Your Life.* New York: Doubleday.

Montague, A. 1977. *Touching: The Human Significance of the Skin.* New York: Harper and Row.

Moore, R. 1980. Doctor as executioner: The argument over death by injection. *New Physician,* September, p. 21.

Moran, L. 1966. *Churchill Taken from the Diaries of Lord Moran.* Boston: Houghton Mifflin.

Muldary, T. W. 1983. *Burnout and Health Professionals.* Norwalk, Conn.: Appleton-Century-Crofts.

Mullan, F. 1983. *Vital Signs: A Young Doctor's Struggle with Cancer.* New York: Farrar, Straus and Giroux.

Murphy, E. G. 1985. Patient Demand for Diagnostic Tests in Primary Care Medicine Setting. Honors thesis, Harvard Medical School.

Myerhoff, B. H., and Larson, W. R. 1958. The doctor as culture hero: The routinization of charisma. *Human Organization* 17: 189.

Najman, J. M., Klein, O., and Munro, C. 1982. Patient characteristics negatively stereotyped by doctors. *Soc. Sci. and Med.* 16: 1781.

National Ambulatory Medical Care Survey, May 1973–April 1974. Vital Statistics Report 214, no. 4, Supplement, 1975.

National Ambulatory Medical Care Survey, 1980 Summary. In *Advance Data*, no. 77, February 22, 1982. From Vital and Health Statistics of National Center for Health Statistics.

National Ambulatory Medical Care Survey of Visits to General and Family Physicians. 1974, 1980. Washington, D.C.: National Center for Health Statistics.

National Center for Health Services Research. 1981. National Health Care Expenditures Study. *Waiting Times in Different Medical Settings: Appointment Waits and Office Waits*. Data Preview 6. Washington, D.C.: U.S. Department of Health and Human Services.

National Center for Health Statistics, 1984. Cypress, B. K. Patterns of Ambulatory Care in Internal Medicine, The National Ambulatory Medical Care Survey, United States, January 1980–December 1981. *Vital and Health Statistics*. Series 13, no. 80. Publ. no. (PHS)84–1741. Washington D.C.: U.S. Department of Health and Human Services.

National Center for Health Statistics, Vital and Health Statistics. Drug Utilization in General and Family Practice by Characteristics of Physicians and Office Visits. National Ambulatory Medical Survey, 1980. Cypress, B. K., *Advanced Data*, no. 87, March 28, 1983.

Natkins, L. G. 1982. Hi, Lucille, I'm Dr. Gold. *JAMA* 247: 2415.

Navarro, V. 1975. Women in health care. *New Engl. J. Med.* 202: 398.

Nelson, L. J. 1978. Primum utilis esse: The primacy of usefulness in medicine. *Yale J. Biol. and Med.* 51: 655.

Noren, J., Frazier, T., Altman, I., and DeLozier, J. 1980. Ambulatory medical care: A comparison of internists and family general practitioners. *New Engl. J. Med.* 302: 11.

Nuffield Provincial Hospitals Trust and University of Bristol. 1955. *Studies in the Function and Design of Hospitals: A Report of an Investigation*. London: Oxford University Press.

Nuffield Provincial Hospitals Trust. 1965. *Waiting in Outpatient Departments, A Survey of Outpatient Appointment Systems*. London: Oxford University Press.

Ohnuki-Tierney, E. 1984. *Illness and Culture in Contemporary Japan: An Anthropological View*. Cambridge University Press.

Oijendijk, W. T. M., Makenbach, J. P., and Limberger, H. H. B. 1980. What is better? An investigation into the use of and satisfaction with complementary and official medicine in the Netherlands. Netherlands Institute of Preventive Medicine and Technical Industrial Organization.

Orme, E. 1955. *My Fight Against Osteoarthritis*. London: Faber and Faber.

Orwell, G. 1956. How the poor die. In *Orwell Reader*. New York: Harcourt, Brace.

Osler, W. 1952. *Aequanimitas with Other Addresses*. Philadelphia: Blakiston.

Paaswell, F. E., and Recker, W. W. 1970. *Problems of the Carless*. New York: Praeger.

Papper, S. 1970. The undesirable patient. *J. Chron. Dis.* 22: 777.

Parish, H. M., Bishop, F. M., and Baker, A. S. 1967. Time study of general practitioners' office hours. *Arch. Envir. Health* 14: 892.

Parsons, T. 1951. Illness and the role of the physician: A sociological perspective. *Am. J. Orthopsych.* 21: 452.

Payson, H. E., Ganselar, E. C., and Stargarder, F. L. 1961. Time study of an internship on a university medical service. *New Engl. J. Med.* 264: 439.

Peabody, F. W. 1927. The care of the patient. *JAMA* 88: 877.

Perry, J. A. 1976. Physicians' erotic and non-erotic physical involvement with patients. *Am. J. Psychiat.* 133: 838.

Peschel, E. R., ed. 1980. *Medicine and Literature.* New York: Neale Watson.

Peterson, O. 1956. An analytic study of North Carolina general practice, 1953–54. *J. Med. Ed.* 31: 1.

Peterson, O. L. 1972. Vanishing physicians. *Ann. Int. Med.* 76: 141.

Pfifferling, J. H. 1980. The problem of physician impairment. *Conn. Med.* 44: 587.

Pflanz, M. 1970. Two faces of the doctor-patient relationship in a changing welfare state: The Federal Republic of Germany. In *The Doctor-Patient Relationship in the Changing Health Scene*, ed. E. B. Gallagher (Washington, D.C.: U.S. Department of Health, Education and Welfare).

Pickering, G. 1974. *Creative Malady.* London: Oxford University Press.

Pinner, M., and Miller, B. F., eds. 1949. *When Doctors Are Patients.* New York: Norton.

Pinsent, R. J. F. 1964. "Send for the doctor...." *Lancet* 2: 464.

Pomerance, B. 1979. *The Elephant Man.* New York: Grove.

Powell, F. D. 1975. The Diabetic Clinic: A Family-Based Improvising Organization. In *Theory of Coping Systems.* Cambridge, Mass.: Schenkman.

Powles, J. 1973. On the limitations of modern medicine. *Sci. Med. and Man* 1: 1.

Pratt, J. H. 1936. The personality of the physician. *New Engl. J. Med.* 214: 264.

Pratt, L. 1976. *The Energized Family.* Boston: Houghton Mifflin.

Pratt, R. 1963. *Doctor and Patient.* London: Nuffield Provincial Hospitals Trust.

Preston, T. 1981. *The Clay Pedestal: A Re-examination of the Doctor-Patient Relationship.* Seattle: Madrona.

Pym, B. 1980. *A Few Green Leaves.* New York: Dutton.

Querido, A. 1963. *The Efficiency of Medical Care.* Leiden: Stenfert-Kraese.

Rabin, D., and Bush, P. J. 1975. Who's using medicine? *J. Comm. Health* 1: 106.

Rabin, D., and Rabin, P. L. 1984. *To Provide Safe Passage: The Humanistic Aspects of Medicine.* New York: Philosophical Library.

Ramsay, J. A., McKenzie, J. K., and Fish, D. G. 1982. Physicians and nurse practitioners: Do they provide equivalent health care? *Am. J. Publ. Health* 72: 55.

Ramsey, P. 1970. *The Patient as a Person.* New Haven, Conn.: Yale University Press.

Reader, W. J. 1966. *Professional Men: The Rise of the Professional Classes in 19th Century England.* New York: Basic Books.

Regier, D. A., Goldberg, I. D., and Taube, C. A. 1978. The de facto U.S. mental health services system. *Arch. Gen. Psychiat.* 35: 685.

Reiser, S. J. 1977. *Medicine and the Reign of Technology.* Cambridge University Press.

Renaud, M., Beauchemin, C. L., Poirier, H., and Berthiaume, S. 1980. Different practice settings and prescribing profiles, Montreal. *Am. J. Publ. Health* 70: 1068.

Revitch, E. 1979. Patients who kill their physicians. *J. Med. Soc. New Jersey* 76: 429.

Reynolds, R. A., and Ohsfeldt, R. L., eds. 1984. *Socioeconomic Characteristics of Medical Practice*. Chicago: Center for Health Policy Research, American Medical Association.

Ricci, E. M., Enterline, P., and Henderson, V. 1978. Contacts with pharmacists before and after free medical care. The Quebec experience. *Med. Care* 16: 256.

Richman, G. 1965. Late call, emergency or anxiety? *J. Roy. Coll. Gen. Pract.* 9: 241.

Riley, G. H., Willie, C. R., and Haggerty, R. J. 1969. A study of family medicine in upstate New York. *JAMA* 208: 2307.

Rinke, C. 1981. The economic and academic status of women physicians. *JAMA* 245: 2305.

Rivington, W. 1879. *The Medical Profession*. Being the essay to which was rewarded the first Carmichael Prize by the Committee of the Royal College of Surgeons. Dublin: Fannin.

Robertson, L. S., and Heagarty, M. C. 1975. *Medical Sociology, A General Systems Approach*. Chicago: Nelson-Hall.

Robinson, G. C. 1939. *The Patient as a Person*. New York: Commonwealth Fund.

Robinson, H. A., Finesinger, J. E., and Bierman, J. S. 1956. Psychiatric considerations in the adjustment of patients with poliomyelitis. *New Engl. J. Med.* 254: 975.

Roche, D. 1980. Talent, reason and sacrifice: The physicians during the Enlightenment, In *Medicine and Society in France*, ed. R. Forster and O. Ranuan. Baltimore: Johns Hopkins University Press.

Roemer, M. I. 1981. *Ambulatory Health Services in America*. Rockville, Maryland: Aspen Systems.

Rogers, C. R. 1961. Characteristics of the helping relation. In *On Becoming a Person*. Boston: Houghton Mifflin.

Rose, K. D., and Rosow, I. 1973. Psychiatrists who kill themselves. *Arch. Gen. Psychiat.* 29: 800.

Rosen, G. 1944. *The Specialization of Medicine*. New York: Froben.

Rosenbaum, J. 1975. What your consultation room furniture reveals. *Practical Psychology for Physicians*, November, p. 46.

Rosenberg, C. E. 1970. *No Other Gods: On Science and American Social Thought*. Baltimore: Johns Hopkins University Press.

Rosenberg, M. L. *Patients: The Experience of Illness*. Philadelphia: Saunders.

Rosenberg, E. E., and Pless, I. B. 1985. Clinicians' knowledge about the families of their patients. *Family Practice* 2: 23.

Rossberg, E. 1983. They all want the best. *Scala Magazine*, February, p. 18.

Roth, J. A. 1963. *Timetables*. New York: Bobbs-Merrill.

Royal College of General Practitioners. 1973. *Present Status and Future Needs: Reports from General Practice, No. 2*. London.

Royal College of General Practitioners. 1976. Editorial: Outpatient follow-up. *J. Roy. Coll. Gen. Pract.* 26: 792.

Royal College of General Practitioners. 1982. *A Survey of Primary Care in London*, Occasional paper 16. London.

Ruzek, S. B. 1978. *The Women's Health Movement. Feminist Alternatives to Medical Control.* New York: Praeger.

Rynearson, R. R., Stewart, W. L., and Bachman, B. A. 1983. Physician-patient sexual relationships. *Patient and Physician*, March, p. 13.

Sachs, B. J. 1975. The opthalmologist's office: Planning and practice. *International Ophthalmology Clinic* 15: 47.

Sacks, O. 1984. *One Leg To Stand On.* New York: Simon & Schuster.

Sagov, S. E., and Brodsky, A. 1976. *The Active Patient's Guide to Better Medical Care.* New York: McKay.

Sagov, S. F., Feinbloom, R. I., Spindel, R., and Brodsky, A. 1984. *Home Birth: A Practitioner's Guide to Birth Outside the Hospital.* Rockville, Maryland: Aspen Systems.

Sampson, W. I. 1977. Dying at home. *JAMA* 238: 2405.

Sandblom, P. 1982. *Creativity and Disease: How Illness Affects Literature, Art and Music.* Philadelphia: Stickley.

Sanes, S. 1979. *A Physician Faces Cancer Himself.* Albany: State University of New York Press.

Scheflen, A. E. 1965. Quasi-courtship behavior in psychotherapy. *Psychiatry* 28: 245.

Schmidt, D. D. 1983. When is it helpful to convene the family? *J. Fam. Pract.* 16: 967.

Schneff, K. W., and Eisenberg, H. 1975. *How to Be Your Own Doctor (Sometimes).* New York: Grosset and Dunlap.

Schwartz, B. 1975. *Queuing and Waiting: Studies in the Social Organization of Access and Delay.* University of Chicago Press.

Schwartz, H. 1980. American medical women's associates: Still rebelling, making few inroads. *Private Pract.*, January, p. 35.

Schwartz, M. 1981. *Designing and Building Your Own Professional Office.* Oradell, N.J.: Medical Economics.

Schwitzgebel, R. I. L., and Taugoff, M. 1968. Initial note on the placebo effect of machines. *Behav. Sci.* 13: 527.

Scott, R., and McVie, D. H. 1979. Doctor in the house and analysis of home visits in general practice. *J. Roy. Coll. Gen. Pract.* 29: 137.

Scottish Home and Health Services. 1979. *Time Study of Consultations in General Practice.* Edinburgh.

Selwyn, P. 1980. Medicine behind bars: Health care inside a maximum security prison. *Present Illness*, Harvard Medical School February–March, p. 3.

Selwyn, P. 1984. Personal communication.

Selzer, M. L. 1960. The use of first names in psychotherapy. *Arch. Gen. Psych.* 3: 215.

Senger, H. L. 1984. First name or last? Addressing the patient in psychotherapy. *Comp. Psych.* 25: 38.

Shannon, G. W. 1980. Space and time in medical geography. In *Conceptuual and Methodological Issues in Medical Geography*, ed. M. S. Meade. Chapel Hill, Department of Medical Geography, University of North Carolina.

Shapiro, E. T. 1979. The gender factor in medical practice: Does the sex of the physician matter? *Behav. Med.*, May, p. 17.

Shattuck, F. C. 1907. The science and art of medicine in some of their aspects. *Boston Med. and Surg. J.* 157: 63.

Shaw, G. B. 1965. *The Doctor's Dilemma.* London: Penguin.

Shem, S. 1978. *The House of God.* New York: Richard Marek.

Shoen, E. 1983. *The Reflective Practitioner.* New York: Basic Books.

Short, P. W. 1980. Why not discard the desk? *J. Roy. Coll. Gen. Pract.* 30: 687.

Shorter, E. 1985. *Bedside Manners.* New York: Simon and Schuster.

Shortt, S. E. D., ed. 1982. *Psychiatric Illness in Physicians.* Springfield, Ill. : Thomas.

Shuval, J., Antonovsky, A., and Davis, M. 1970. *The Social Functions of Medical Practice.* San Francisco: Jossey-Bass.

Silver, G. A. 1980. Chiropractice: Professional controversy and public policy. *Am. J. Pub. Health* 70: 348.

Silvette, H. 1967. *The Doctor on the Stage.* Knoxville: University of Tennessee Press.

Singer, K. 1985. No wonder liability issue is frustrating, MD says. *AMA News,* January 18, p. 5.

Singleton, A. 1982. Sicking out: An ill excuse. *Harvard Independent,* January 7, p. 6.

Sissman, L. E. 1978. Homage to Clotho: A hospital suite. In *Hello, Darkness. The Collected Poems of L. E. Sissman.* Boston: Little, Brown.

Siwek, J. 1985. House calls: Current status and rationale. *J. Am. Fam. Pract.* 31: 169.

Slack, W. V., and Slack, C. W. 1968. Patient reaction to computer-based medical interviewing. *Comput. Biomed. Res.* 13: 267.

Slack, W. V., and Slack, C. W. 1978. Patient-computer dialogue. *New Engl. J. Med.* 286: 1304.

Smith, W. E. 1986. *Let the Truth Be the Prejudice.* Philadelphia Museum of Art.

Solon, J. A., and Greenwalt, L. F. 1974. Physicians' participation in nursing homes. *Med. Care* 12: 486.

Solzhenitsyn, A. 1975. *The Cancer Ward.* New York: Farrar, Straus and Giroux.

Sommer, R. 1969. *Personal Space: The Behavioral Basis of Design.* Englewood Cliffs, N.J.: Prentice-Hall.

Stambler, H. V. 1979. Health manpower for the nation: A look ahead at the supply and requirements. *Publ. Health Reports* 94: 5.

Starr, P. 1979. Medicine, economy and society in nineteenth century America. In *The Medicine Show,* ed. P. Branco. Now York: Neale Watson.

Steiber, S. 1982. Physicians who move and why they move. *JAMA* 248: 1490.

Steiger, W. A., and Hansen, A. V. 1964. *Patients Who Trouble You.* Boston: Little, Brown.

Stimpson, J., and Webb, B. 1975. *Going to See the Doctor: The Consultation Process in General Practice.* London: Routledge and Kegan Paul.

Stockwell, F. 1984. *The Unpopular Patient.* London: Croom Helm.

Stoeckle, J. D. 1975. The reorganization of care in the community. In *Poverty and Health.,* ed. J. Kosa and I. K. Zola, second edition. Cambridge, Mass.: Harvard University Press.

Stoeckle, J. D. 1979. Tasks of care: Humanistic aspects of medical education. In *Nourishing the Humanistic in Medicine*, ed. W. E. Rogers and D. Barnard. University of Pittsburgh Press.

Stoeckle, J. D. 1984. Medical advice books: The search for the healthy body. *Soc. Sci. and Med.* 19: 1.

Stoeckle, J. D. 1985. The role of the academician as a teacher of patient care. *Bull. N.Y. Acad. Med.* 61: 144.

Stoeckle, J. D., and Billings, J. A. 1987. On questioning, listening and talking: A history of the medical interview and its instruction. *J. Gen. Med.* (to appear).

Stoeckle, J. D., and Grossman, J. H. 1977. The out-patient department: Ambulatory care at the hospital. *New Engl. J. Med.* 52: 834.

Stoeckle, J. D., and White, G. A. 1980. *Primary Care in the 1930s: Working People Consulting the Doctor. An Exhibit of FSA Photographs.* Boston: Primary Care Program, Massachusetts General Hospital.

Stoeckle, J. D., and White, G. A. 1985. *Plain Pictures of Plain Doctoring: Vernacular Expression in New Deal Medicine and Photography.* Cambridge, Mass.: MIT Press.

Stoeckle, J. D., and Zola, I. K. 1964. Views, problems and potentialities of the clinic. *Medicine* 43: 413.

Stoeckle, J. D., Zola, I. K., and Davidson, G. E. 1963. On going to see the doctor: The contributions of the patient to the decision to seek medical aid. *J. Chronic Dis.* 16: 975.

Stoeckle, J. D., Anderson, W. H., Page, J., and Brenner, J. 1972. The free clinics. *JAMA* 219: 603.

Stoeckle, J. D., Dineen, J. J., Follayttar, S., Wood, L. C., and Jones, F. 1981. Report of the Board of Managers, Medical Clinics Complex, Massachusetts General Hospital Annual Report, 1975: A Survey Report of the Ambulatory Practices of, at, or Affiliated with the Massachusetts General Hospital.

Stone, D. A. 1979a. Diagnosis and the dole: The function of illness in American distributive politics. *J. Health Politics, Policy, and Law* 4: 507.

Stone, D. A. 1979b. Physicians as gatekeepers: Illness certification as a rationing device. *Public Policy* 27: 227.

Stone, D. A. 1984. *The Disabled State.* Philadelphia: Temple University Press.

Strain, J. F., and Miller, J. D. 1971. The preparation, utilization and evaluation of a registered nurse trained to give telephone advice in a private pediatric office. *Pediatrics* 74: 1051.

Strauss, A., Fagerhaugh, S., Suczek, B., and Weiner, C. L. 1985. *Social Organization of Medical Work.* University of Chicago Press.

Sultz, H. A., Zielezny, M., Gentry, J. M., and Kinyon, L. 1978. *Longitudinal Study of Nurse Practitioners.* DHEW publ. 78–92. Washington, D.C.: U.S. Department of Health, Education and Welfare.

Swazey, J. P. 1979. Health Professionals and the Public: Toward a New Social Contract. Annual oration, Society for Health and Human Values, November 4.

Swazey, J. P., and Sober, S. P., eds. 1982. *Whistle Blowing in Biomedical Research: Policies and Procedures for Responding to Reports of Misconduct.* Washington, D.C.: Superintendent of Documents.

Symonds, A. 1980. Women's liberation, effect on physician-patient relation. *N.Y. State J. Med.* 80: 211.

Szasz, T. H. 1980. *Sex by Prescription.* London: Penguin.

Szasz, T. 1982. Shooting the shrink. *New Republic,* June 16, p. 11.

Tagliacozzo, D., Ima, K., and Lashof, J. 1973. Influencing the chronically ill: The role of prescriptions in premature terminations of outpatient care. *Med. Care* 11: 21.

Talbot, A. A. III, Curtis, P., MacLaren, L., Sanchez, A. F., Jr., and Bissonette, R. 1984. Telephone medicine: A training need in a technological society. *Fam. Med.* 16: 141.

Tanner, R. 1982. Doc in the box: Medical care, fast-food style. *Venture,* October, p. 54.

Taylor, A. D. 1981. Set your sails to doctor at sea. *Physician Management,* November, p. 108.

Thibault, G. E., Mulley, A. G., Barnett, G. O., Goldstein, R. C. H., Reder, V. A., Sherman, E. L., and Skinner, E. R. 1980. Medical intensive care: Indicators, interventions and outcomes. *New Engl. J. Med.* 32: 938.

Thomas, J. 1985. Gypsies and American medical care. *Ann. Int. Med.* 102: 842.

Thompson, J. D., and Golden, G., eds. 1975. *The Hospital: A Social and Architectural History.* New Haven, Conn.: Yale University Press.

Tolle, S. S., Elliot, D. L., and Hickham, D. H. 1984. Physician attitudes and practices at the time of patient death. *Arch. Int. Med.* 144: 2389.

Toms, W. 1977. Analysis of the impact of the loss of a primary care physician on a patient population. *J. Fam. Pract.* 4: 115.

Trautman, J. 1975. William Carlos Williams and the poetry of medicine. *Ethics in Sci. and Med.* 2: 105.

Trautman, J., and Pollard, C. 1975. *Literature and Medicine.* Philadelphia: Society for Health and Human Values.

Tu, J.-C. E. 1985. Working life of New York state physicians, 1980. *Am. J. Pub. Health* 75: 553.

Turner, B. S. 1984. *The Body and Society.* Oxford: Blackwell.

Twaddle, A. C. 1976. Utilization of medical services by a captive population: An analysis of sick-call in a state prison. *J. Health and Soc. Behav.* 17: 236.

U.S. Department of Health, Education and Welfare. 1973. Report of the Secretary's Commission on Medical Malpractice. Publication no. 73–89.

U.S. Department of Health, Education and Welfare. 1978. Report to the President and Congress on the Status of the Health Professions. Publication no. (HRA)78–93.

U.S. Department of Health, Education and Welfare. 1978. Minimal Requirement of Construction and Equipment for Hospitals and Medical Facilities. Publication no. (HRA)79-14500.

U.S. Department of Health, Education and Welfare. 1979. The Treatment Practices of Black Physicians. Publication no. (HRA)80-628.

U.S. Department of Health, Education and Welfare. 1980a. *The Current and Future supply of Physicians and Physician Specialists.* Publication no. (HRA)80-60.

U.S. Department of Health, Education and Welfare. 1980b. The National Ambulatory Medical Survey, 1977 Summary, series 13, no. 44. Publication no. (PHS)80-1795.

U.S. Department of Health, Education and Welfare. 1980c. *The National Health Service Corps Practice Management Guide Book*. Publication no. 77-6008.

U.S. Department of Health and Human Services. 1981a. Charges and Sources of Payment for Visits to Physicians Offices. Data Previews, National Health Care Expenditures Study.

U.S. Department of Health and Human Services. 1981b. *Health U.S. 1981*.

U.S. Department of Health and Human Services. 1981c. Persons Receiving Care from Selected Health Care Practitioners, U.S. 1980. Series B, Descriptive Report no. 6. National Medical Care Utilization and Expenditure Survey.

U.S. Department of Health and Human Services. 1985. *Health United States 1985*.

U.S. Department of Health and Human Services. 1985. *Nonphysician Health Providers: Use of Ambulatory Services, Expenditures, and Sources of Payment*.

University of Pennsylvania Law School. 1973. *Health Care in Pennsylvania Prisons Health Law Project*. Philadelphia.

Vaillant, G. E., Sobowale, N. C., and McArthur, C. 1972. Some psychological vulnerabilities of physicians. *New Engl. J. Med.* 287: 372.

Vaizey, J. 1959. *Scenes from Institutional Life*. London: Faber and Faber.

Van der Berg, J. H. 1967. *The Psychology of the Sick Bed*. Pittsburg: Duquesne University Press.

Verbrugge, L. M. 1979. *Medical Care of Acute Conditions, United States, 1973-1974*. National Center for Health Statistics, series 10, no. 179. Washington, D.C.: U.S. Department of Health, Education and Welfare.

Verbrugge, L. M., and Steiner, R. P. 1981. Physician treatment of men and women patients: Sex bias or appropriate care? *Med. Care* 19: 609.

Vester, J. W. 1979. Lonesome valley: Hospitalization after severe injury. *Forum on Medicine*, March, p. 159.

Vickery, D. M., and Fries, J. F. 1976. *Take Care of Yourself: A Consumer's Guide to Medical Care*. Reading, Mass.: Addison-Wesley.

Vincent, T. S. 1975. So I appall the academicians, I provide necessary medication. *Med. Econ.*, July, p. 53.

von Feber, L. 1975. The doctor's consulting room: Or do doctor and patient communicate? *Hexagon-Roche* 3: 1.

Wagner, N. 1973. Ethical Concerns of Medical Students, 1972. Western Workshop of Center for Study of Sex Education in Medicine, Santa Barbara, Calif. Quoted in Kardener et al. 1973.

Waitzkin, H., and Waterman, B. 1974. *The Penal Institution in the Exploitation of Illness in Capitalist Society*. Indianapolis: Bobbs-Merrill.

Waitzkin, H., Beller, E., and Mons, C. 1975. Information Process in Medical Care: Preliminary Statistical Results. Working Paper no. 10, Department of Medicine, Stanford University.

Wallen, J., Waitzkin, H., and Stoeckle, J. D. 1979. Physician stereotypes about female health and illness: A study of patient's sex and informative process during medical interviews. *Women and Health* 4: 135.

Wardwell, W. I. 1976. Orthodox and unorthodox practitioners. In *Marginal Medicine*, ed. R. Wallis and P. Morley. New York: Free Press.

Wechsler, J. A. 1972. *In a Darkness*. New York: Norton.

Weil, S. 1952. *The Need for Roots: A Prelude to a Declaration of Duties Toward Mankind*. New York: Putnam.

Weingarten, M. A. 1982. Telephone consultations with patients: A brief study and review of the literature. *J. Roy. Coll. Gen. Pract.* 32: 766.

Weiss, J. E., and Greenlick, M. R. 1970. Determinants of medical care utilization: The effect of social class and distance on contacts with the medical care system. *Med. Care* 8: 456.

Weiss, S. 1942. Self-observations and psychologic reactions of medical student A.S.R. to the onset and symptoms of subacute bacterial endocarditis. *Mt. Sinai Hosp.* 8: 1079.

Weitzman, H. H., and Egeland, J. A. 1973. A behavioral science perspective in the comparative approach to the delivery of health care. *Soc. Science and Med.* 7: 845.

West, C. 1984. When the doctor is a "lady": Power, status and gender in physician-patient dialogues. In *Women, Health and Medicine*, ed. A. Stromberg. Palo Alto: Mayfield.

Westbury, R. C. 1974. The electric speaking practice, A telephone workload study. *Canad. Fam. Phys.*, February, p. 68.

White, G. A. 1980. The doctor-as-patient. *Harvard Medical Alumni Bull.* 54: 18.

White, K. L., Williams, T. F., and Greenberg, R. C. 1961. The ecology of medical care. *New Engl. J. Med.* 265: 885.

White, P. D. 1922. Dispensary development, with special reference to the outpatient department of the Massachusetts General Hospital. *Boston Med. and Surg. J.* 56: 693.

Wilbanks, E. 1972. The doctor as romantic hero. *JAMA* 220: 54.

Williams, M. R., and Lindberg, D. S. 1975. *An Introduction to the Profession of Medical Technology*. Philadelphia: Lea and Febiger.

Williams, W. C. 1948. *The Autobiography of William Carlos Williams*. New York: New Directions.

Williams, W. C. 1984. *William Carlos Williams: The Doctor Stories*. New York: New Directions.

Williams, W. C. 1966. A face of stone. In *The William Carlos Williams Reader*, ed. M. L. Rosenthal. New York: New Directions.

Wilson, D. C. 1963. *Take My Hands*. New York: McGraw-Hill.

Wilson, F. A., and Newhauser, D. 1974. *Health Services in the U.S.* Cambridge, Mass.: Ballinger.

Winnicott, D. W. 1978. *The Child, the Family and the Outside World*. New York: Penguin.

Wolfe, S., Badgley, R. F., Kasius, P. V., Garson, J. Z., and Gold, R. J. M. 1968. The work of a group of doctors in Saskatchewan. *Milbank Mem. Fund Quart.* 46: 103.

Woolf, V. 1930. *On Being Ill*. London: Hogarth.

Yamamoto, M. 1978. Health Care and Health Systems in Japan. In Japan and United States: Health Care and Medical Systems, Disease and Health Patterns. Mimeo. New York Academy of Medicine.

Yankauer, A., and Sullivan, J. 1982. The new professionals: Three examples. *Ann. Rev. Publ. Health* 3: 249.

Yedidia, M. 1981. *Delivering Primary Health Care*. Boston: Auburn House.

Yerby, A. 1975. *British National Health Service Complaints Procedure*. Publication no. 76–988. Washington, D.C.: Department of Health, Education and Welfare.

Zabarenko, R. N., Zabarenko, L., and Hengea, R. A. 1970. The psychodynamics of physicianhood. *Psychiatry* 33: 102.

Zola, I. K. 1966. Culture and symptoms. *Am. Sociol. Rev.* 31: 615.

Zola, I. K. 1972a. The concept of trouble and sources of medical assistance: To whom can one turn, with what, and why. *Soc. Sci. and Med.* 6: 673.

Zola, I. K. 1972b. Medicine as an institution of social control. *Sociol. Rev.* 20: 487.

Zola, I. K. 1972c. Studying the decision to see a doctor, review, critique and corrective. In *Advances in Psychosomatic Medicine*, ed. Z. J. Lipowski. Basel: Karger.

Zola, I. K. 1982a. *The Missing Pieces: A Chronical of Living with a Disability*. Philadelphia: Temple University Press.

Zola, I. K. 1982b. *Ordinary Lives*. Cambridge, Mass.: Apple-Wood.

I

The Structure: Ground Rules for the Doctor-Patient Relation

In the history of medical practice, the doctor traditionally acted on the patient with advice and medical treatment. Modern ideas about the relation began with the recognition that the patient might, in turn, influence the doctor. Freud noted this is some detail; simply put, transference explained the effect of the doctor on the patient, counter-transference the patient's effect on the doctor. But it is L. J. Henderson, not Freud, who is credited in America with defining the doctor-patient relation as a reciprocal social system. A physician and professor of chemistry at Harvard University, Henderson was aware of psychoanalytic thought, though, in the main, he derived his ideas about the doctor-patient relation from the physiochemical systems of Willard Gibbs and the social systems analysis of Victor Pareto, an early-twentieth-century Italian sociologist. He did not use Freud's intrapsychic idea of transference to explain the interaction but argued that the patient influences the doctor directly through "sentiments," his or her values and emotions. Henderson's important 1935 paper "Physician and Patient as a Social System," therefore, begins these readings.

Henderson was not widely read by doctors, even though his initial presentation was at the grand rounds of the medical staff at Massachusetts General Hospital. Sociologists, however, were quick to examine his ideas, most notably Talcott Parsons and George Homans, members of the department at Harvard University where Henderson also taught (B. Barber, ed., *L. J. Henderson on the Social System* [University of Chicago Press, 1970]). If Parsons read Henderson, both men also drew their ideas from direct observation of medical practitioners. Henderson did not practice, but he was aware of clinical work through that of his physician colleagues, just as Parsons, who made empirical observations of the medical staff in practice at Massachusetts General Hospital during the 1930s and 1940s.

Parsons's reciprocal role model of the relation is widely known from two contributions: a lengthy statement, "The Case of Modern Medical Practice in the Social System" (in *The Social System*, ed. T. Parsons [Free Press, 1951]), and a shorter exposition, "Illness and the Role of the Physician" (1951), reprinted here. His descriptive role takes a classically functionalist perspective: the rights and obligations of the doctor and the patient complement each other in the common task of returning the patient to normal. The doctor's role is held to be limited to the health problems presented to the doctor. An expert in medicine and affectively "neutral," the doctor is obligated to treat the patient whether he likes him or not. The patient, in turn, has the "obligation" of seeking medical help, bringing appropriate medical complaints, cooperating with the doctor, and working to get well. These were the ground rules by which the self-contained, static, doctor-patient "game" was to be played out.

Revisions and critiques of Parsons's model of the sick role and the doctor-patient relation are now numerous, but no similar distinctive analysis has appeared since this 1951 work. The various critiques of the Parsonian theory have been summarized by Andrew Twaddle in "The Concepts of the Sick Role and Illness Behavior" (in *Advances in Psychosomatic Medicine*, volume 8, ed. Z. Lipowski [Prager, 1972]). Twaddle focuses not on the doctor-patient relation per se but on the sick role (the obverse of the doctor's role in the model of Parsons), noting that the definition of the sick role is limited to industrial societies, applies to a narrow range of illnesses, contains "management bias," and does not even account for variability within modern societies. Omitted from Twaddle's account are the more Marxian critique of Howard Waitzkin and Barbara Waterman (*Exploitation of Illness in Capitalistic Society* [Bobbs-Merrill, 1974]; see also Waitzkin, *The Second Sickness: Contradictions of Capitalist Health Care* [Free Press, 1983]), the interactionist criticism of Michael Bloom and George Horobin ("Conflict and Conflict Resolution in Doctor-Patient Interactions," in *Sociology of Medical Practice*, ed. C. Cox and A. Mead [Collier-Macmillan, 1975]), and the modern elaboration of Samuel Bloom (*The Doctor and His Patient* [Russell Sage Foundation, 1963]). Waitzkin and Waterman argue that the doctor's legitimization of sickness is a conservative form of social control. Since the deviant behavior of being sick is a response to oppressive social conditions, permitting the sick role reduces, then, the potential political opposition to the status quo. The doctor is, thus, an agent in such control. From a less political analysis, Bloom and Horobin observe that the relation is fundamentally conflicted and is neither reciprocal nor consensual (as Parsons argued). In the interactionist definition, the doctors' expectations that patients should use their judgment in seeking help and then defer to the doctor's judgment when consulting place patients in a double bind: an intensely conflicted situation at the outset.

Today, the doctor-patient relation is no longer viewed as a functional consensus, but as a relation that involves conflict, competition, and negotiation from the very beginning.

1

Physician and Patient as a Social System
L. J. Henderson

Medicine is today in part an applied science. Mathematics, physics, chemistry, and many departments of biology find applications in this hospital and in the practice of all skillful physicians. Meanwhile, the personal relations between the physician and the patient remain nearly what they have always been. To these relations, as yet, science has been little applied, and it is unlikely that the men in this room are upon the whole as much concerned about their personal relations with patients as a similar group of Boston doctors must have been in the days of James Jackson. A multitude of important new facts and theories, of new methods and routines, so far absorb the physician's attention and arouse his interest that the personal relations seem to have become less important, if not absolutely, at least relatively to the new and powerful technology of medical practice. This condition, for which nobody is to blame, might perhaps be modified if it were possible to apply to practice a science of human relations. But such a science is barely growing into the stage where applications are possible.

The psychologists and sociologists are the professional custodians of what little scientific knowledge we possess that is conversant with personal relations. But from them we have, as yet, little to learn, for they are in general little aware of the problem of practicing what they know in the affairs of everyday life. Indeed, skill in managing one's relations with others is probably less common among professional psychologists and sociologists than among the ablest men of affairs or the wisest physicians. So the personal relations of the physician with his patients and with their families are still understood, when they are understood, at the empirical level, as they were in the days of Hippocrates. Such skill is not only empirical but it is also, as we vaguely say,

Reprinted, with permission, from *New England Journal of Medicine* 212 (1935): 819–823.

intuitive. Sometimes in those favored persons whose perceptions and sensibilities are well suited to the task, it results in patterns of behavior that are among the most interesting and, if I may use the word, beautiful that I know. As I came into this room, I was saying that if Dr. Frederick Shattuck could only be here he, who knew so much more about my subject than I shall ever know, would have been able after I had finished to say many things to you and to me. Doctors like him have always existed and will always exist, but their skill dies with them except when their apprentices have learned in some measure to imitate them.

The necessary condition for the effective transmission of acquired knowledge seems to be scientific formulation, and for this purpose some kind of theory, working hypothesis, or conceptual scheme is necessary. In this way the natural sciences are preserved and transmitted, and the role of scientific laws and generalizations is seen to be not merely economy of thought, as Mach said, but also the effective remembering of the successful and economical thought of the past. A well learned theory is remembered in the right place at the right time, and this is a necessary condition for its use. Accordingly my first subject is the theory of the relation between physician and patient.

Four centuries ago, Machiavelli was thinking of certain great problems of human society and writing two famous books. In so doing, he reached scientific generalizations about the influence of the sentiments upon the actions of men and, through these actions, upon the fate of human societies. As a whole, these conclusions stand; but from this great and ingenious work of Machiavelli's almost no developments have followed. The science of statecraft and of the influence of the sentiments upon human behavior is little different today from what it was in Florence in the 16th century.

In the following century, another Florentine, Galileo, published his "Dialogues on Two New Sciences." From this work a great part of modern science has grown out. The two men were perhaps equal in ability and in originality. Why has the influence of one been small and that of the other inestimably great?

In seeking a partial answer to this question, I ask you to consider the names of the subjects that are taught in modern universities, and to divide them, so far as may be, into two classes: first, history, politics, economics, sociology, law, literature, etc.; secondly, logic, mathematics, physics, chemistry, biology, grammar, harmony, etc. Most subjects will fall well enough into one or the other of these two classes. Next I ask you to consider the behavior of the professors who cultivate the two classes of subjects. Those who are adepts of subjects of the second class, when they differ, commonly do so at the frontiers of knowledge, where growth occurs. Moreover, their differences are ordinarily settled by observation, experiment, mathematical calculation, and logical analysis. But in the subjects of the first class differences of opinion occur at all points, and frequently they cannot be resolved. The differences and the disputes seem to be interminable, and there is often no accepted method of reaching a conclusion.

Such a contrast between the behavior of the skillful devotees of the two classes of subjects must depend in part upon differences in the nature of the two classes of subjects, for we cannot admit that a natural selection of professors so nearly perfect as to produce this striking result should occur. Now there is, in fact, one difference between the two classes of subjects which, as I think, is sufficient in a rough approximation to explain the phenomenon. The subjects of the second class do not, in general, consider the interrelations of two or more persons. The subjects of the first class always consider the interrelations of two or more persons. Thus in history, politics, economics, sociology, law, literature, etc., the interrelations and interactions of people are always concerned, but in logic, mathematics, physics, chemistry, biology, grammar, harmony, etc., except perhaps in certain subjects on the borders of biology, they are ruled out. Perhaps this distinction also goes far to explain the curious condition of psychology in our own time. At any rate I am persuaded that it goes far to explain why we have little more than empirical knowledge about the relations of physician and patient.

Willard Gibbs's generalized physico-chemical system is possibly the most famous piece of scientific work that has been done by an American. According to Gibbs, any arbitrarily isolated portion of the material universe may be regarded as a physico-chemical system. In a first approximation, it may be characterized as follows: A physico-chemical system is made up of components. Components are individual chemical substances such as water, salt, etc. They exist in phases. Phases are physically homogeneous parts of the system, either solid, or liquid, or gaseous such as ice, a salt solution, or air. The system is further distinguished by the concentration of the components in the phases, by its temperature, and by its pressure. For many purposes no other factors need be considered.

The Italian sociologist Pareto, formerly professor at the University of Lausanne, has described a generalized social system which may be usefully compared with Gibbs's physico-chemical system. Pareto's social system is made up of individuals. They are perhaps analogous to the components of Gibbs's system. The individuals are heterogeneous, that is, unequal. They are unequal in size and in age. There are two sexes. They have different educations. They belong to different social and economic classes, to different institutions, to different social structures. They suffer from different pathological conditions, and their mental differences are different far beyond our computation and description. This heterogeneity suggests the heterogeneity of solid, liquid, and gaseous phases in the physico-chemical system.

These individuals possess, or at least manifest, sentiments. I implore you not to ask me to define the word sentiment, but to permit me to use it without definition to include in its meaning a variety of mental states. For example, I desire to solve a problem; that is a sentiment. You have a feeling that the constitution of the United States should be preserved; that is a sentiment. Affection for the members of your family is a sentiment. The feeling of personal integrity is a sentiment. The desire to express your gratitude for a kindness is a sentiment. The sexual complexes of psychoanalysts, even though they may be unconscious, are for my purpose sentiments.

The individuals who make up social systems also have economic interests, and they have and use language. This use of language is sometimes a non-logical manifestation of sentiments. For example, I read the other day the following title of a sermon, posted up in front of a church in a New England town, "One on God's side is a majority." Language is also sometimes used, though less often than we fondly suppose, to perform logical operations and to express their results.

A physician and a patient make up a social system. And that is my first point.

Many of you, I fear, will think this introduction singularly irrelevant to the subject of my discourse, and so vague and general that it can hardly be of any use in the premises. To them I venture to suggest that it is possible that they may be mistaken, and I ask them to try to follow what I now have to say receptively, postponing criticism until they have received my whole statement.

Two persons, if no more are present, make up a social system. These individuals are heterogeneous. They have and are moved by sentiments and interests. They talk and reason. That is a definition. I shall now state a theorem. In any social system the sentiments and the interactions of the sentiments are likely to be the most important phenomena. And that is my second point. Sometimes the interaction of the sentiments of the individuals making up a social system is hardly less important than gravitational attraction in the solar system.

In the eighteenth century, before a wave of sentimentality swept over the Western world, some people saw human relations pretty clearly. They had not been brought up on Rousseau and others whose writings have continued down almost to the present time to influence the intellectual atmosphere in which men have formed this habit of thought. Among the more successful eighteenth-century observers of the mechanism of human behavior was Lord Chesterfield. From one of his letters to his son I venture to quote:

I acquainted you in a former letter, that I had brought a bill into the House of Lords for correcting and reforming our present calendar, which is the Julian; and for adopting the Gregorian. I will now give you a more particular account of that affair; from which reflections will naturally occur to you, that I hope may be useful, and which I fear you have not made. It was notorious, that the Julian calendar was erroneous, and had overcharged the solar year with eleven days. Pope Gregory the Thirteenth corrected this error; his reformed calendar was immediately received by all the Catholic Powers in Europe, and afterwards adopted by all the Protestant ones, except Russia, Sweden, and England. It was not, in my opinion, very honourable for England to remain in a gross and avowed error, especially in such company; the inconveniency of it was likewise felt by all those who had foreign correspondences, whether political or mercantile. I determined, therefore, to attempt the reformation; I consulted the best lawyers and the most skilful astronomers, and we cooked up a bill for that purpose. But then my difficulty began: I was to bring in this bill, which was necessarily composed of law jargon and astronomical calculations, to both which I am an utter stranger. However, it was absolutely necessary to make the House of Lords think that I knew something of the matter; and also to make them believe that they knew something of it themselves, which they do not. For my own part, I could just as soon have talked Celtic or Sclavonian to them as astronomy, and they would have understood me full as well: so I resolved to do better than speak to the purpose, and to please instead of informing them. I gave them, therefore, only an historical account of calendars, from the Egyptian down to the Gregorian, amusing them now and then with little episodes; but I was particularly attentive to the choice of my words, to the harmony and roundness of my periods, to my elocution, to my action. This succeeded, and ever will succeed; they thought I informed, because I pleased them; and many of them said, that I had made the whole very clear to them; when, God knows, I had not even attempted it. Lord Macclesfield, who had the greatest share in forming the bill, and who is one of the greatest mathematicians and astronomers in Europe, spoke afterwards with infinite knowledge, and all the clearness that so intricate a matter would admit of: but as his words, his periods, and his utterance, were not near so good as mine, the preference was most unanimously, though most unjustly, given to me. This will ever be the case; every numerous assembly is *mob*, let the individuals who compose it be what they will. Mere reason and good sense is never to be talked to a mob; their passions, their sentiments, their senses, and their seeming interests, are alone to be appealed to. Understanding they have collectively none, but they have ears and eyes, which must be flattered and seduced; and this can only be done by eloquence, tuneful periods, graceful action, and all the various parts of oratory.

It is not only to a mob that reason and good sense cannot effectively be talked. A patient sitting in your office, facing you, is rarely in a favorable state of mind to appreciate the precise significance of a logical statement, and it is in general not merely difficult but quite impossible for him to perceive the precise meaning of a train of thought. It is also out of the question that the physician should convey what he desires to convey to the patient, if he follows the practice of blurting out just what comes into his mind. The patient is moved by fears and by many other sentiments, and these, together with reason, are being modified by the doctor's words and phrases, by his manner and expression. This generalization appears to me to be as well founded as the generalizations of physical science.

If so far I am right, I think it is fair to set up a precept that follows from all this as a rule of conduct: The physician should see to it that the patient's sentiments do not act upon his sentiments and, above all, do not thereby modify his behavior, and he should endeavor to act upon the patient's sentiments according to a well-considered plan. And that is my third point.

I believe that this assertion may be regarded as an application of science to the practice of medicine, and that as such it will bear comparison with the applications of physics, chemistry, and biology to practice. However, in this case the application of science to practice is peculiarly difficult. If I am to speak about it, I must in the first place beg explicitly to disclaim any skill of my own. It is not my business to deal with patients, nor has it been my business to perform that kind of operation that Chesterfield so well describes in his letter. Accordingly, what I am now to say to you is, in the main, second-hand knowledge that I have cribbed from others.[1] It represents, so far as I can understand what I have seen and heard, the soundest judgment, based upon experience, skillful performance, and clear analysis in this field. In order to be brief and clear, I shall permit myself the luxury of plain assertion.

In talking with the patient, the doctor must not only appear to be, but must be, really interested in what the patient says. He must not suggest or imply judgments of value or of morals concerning the patient's report to him or concerning the patient's behavior. (To this there is one exception: When the patient successfully presents a difficult objective report of his experiences, it is useful to praise him for doing well what it is necessary that he should do in order to help the physician to help him.) In all those matters that concern the psychological aspects of the patient's experience few questions should be asked and, above all, no leading questions. There should be no argument about the prejudices of the patient, for, at any stage, when you are endeavoring to evoke the subjective aspect of the patient's experience or to modify his sentiments, logic will not avail. In order to modify the sentiments of the patients, your logical analysis must somehow be transformed into the appropriate change of the patient's sentiments. But sentiments are resistant to change. For this reason, you must so far as possible utilize some part of the sentiments that the patient has in order to modify his subjective attitude.

When you talk with the patient, you should listen, first, for what he wants to tell, secondly, for what he does not want to tell, thirdly, for what he cannot tell. He does not want to tell things the telling of which is shameful or painful. He cannot tell you his implicit assumptions that are unknown to him, such as the assumption that all action not perfectly good is bad, such as the assumption that everything that is not perfectly successful is failure, such as the assumption that everything that is not perfectly safe is dangerous. We are all of us subject to errors of this kind, to the assumption that quantitative differences are qualitative. Perhaps the commonest false dichotomy of the hypochondriac is the last of those that I have just mentioned: the assumption that everything not perfectly safe is dangerous.

When you listen for what the patient does not want to tell and for what he cannot tell you must take especial note of his omissions, for it is the things that he fails to say that correspond to what he does not want to say plus what he cannot say. In listening for these omissions, which is a difficult task, you must make use of every aid that is available. Among the available aids are the results of psychoanalysis. Many of them are well established; but if you wish to preserve a scientific point of view, you must beware of psychoanalytical theories. Use these theories, if you must use them, with skepticism, but do not believe them, for they are themselves in no small measure rationalizations built up by an eager group of enthusiastic students who are unquestionably seeking new knowledge, but whose attitude is strangely modified by a quasi-religious enthusiasm, and by a devotion to the corresponding quasi-theological dogmas. As a useful corrective for undue confidence in the importance of such theories, it is well to recall Henri Poincaré's judicious and skeptical remark: "These two propositions, 'the external world exists,' or, 'it is more convenient to suppose that it exists,' have one and the same meaning." In truth, all theories, but above all others those that refer to the sentiments of men, must be used with care and skepticism.

Therefore, beware of your own arbitrary assumptions. Beware of the expression of your own feelings. In general, both are likely to be harmful, or at least irrelevant, except as they are used to encourage and to cheer the patient. Beware of the expression of moral judgments. Beware of bare statements of bare truth or bare logic. Remember especially that the principal effect of a sentence of confinement or of death is an emotional effect, and that the patient will eagerly scrutinize and rationalize what you say, that he will carry it away with him, that he will turn your phrases over and over in his mind, seeking persistently for shades of meaning that you never thought of. Try to remember how as a very young man you have similarly scrutinized for non-existent meaning the casual phrases of those whom you have admired, or respected, or loved.

Above all, remember that it is meaningless to speak of telling the truth, the whole truth, and nothing but the truth, to a patient. It is meaningless because it is impossible;—a sheer impossibility. Since this assertion is likely to be subjected to both objective and subjective criticism, it will be well that I should try to explain it. I know of no other way to explain it than by means of an example. Let us scrutinize this example, so far as we may be able, objectively, putting aside all our habits of moralistic thought that we acquired in early years and that arise from the theological and metaphysical traditions of our civilization.

Consider the statement, "This is a carcinoma." Let us assume in the first place that the statement has been made by a skillful and experienced pathologist, that he has found a typical carcinoma—in short, that the diagnosis is as certain as it ever can be. Let us also put aside the consideration that no two carcinomas are alike, that no two patients are alike, and that, at one extreme, death may be rapid and painful or, at another extreme, there may be but a small prospect of death from cancer. In short, let us assume, putting aside all such considerations, that the statement has nearly the same validity as the assertions contained in the nautical almanac. If we now look at things, not from the standpoint of philosophers, moralists, or lawyers, but from the standpoint of biologists, we may regard the statement as a stimulus applied to the patient. This stimulus will produce a response and the response, together with the mechanism that is involved in its production, is an extremely complex one, at least in those cases where a not too vague cognition of the meaning of the four words is involved in the process. For instance, there are likely to be circulatory and respiratory changes accompanying many complex changes in the central and peripheral nervous system. With the cognition there is a correlated fear. There will probably be concern for the economic interests of others, for example, of wife and children. All these intricate processes constitute the response to the stimulus made up of the four words, "This is a carcinoma," in case the statement is addressed by the physician to the patient, and it is obviously impossible to produce in the patient cognition without the accompanying affective phenomena and without concern for the economic interests. I suggest, in view of these obvious facts, that, if you recognize the duty of telling the truth to the patient, you range yourself outside the class of biologists, with lawyers and philosophers. The idea that the truth, the whole truth, and nothing but the truth can be conveyed to the patient is an example of false abstraction, of that fallacy called by Whitehead "the fallacy of misplaced concreteness." It results from neglecting factors that cannot be excluded from the concrete situation and that have an effect that cannot be neglected. Another fallacy also is involved, the belief that it is not too difficult to know the truth; but of this I shall not speak further.

I beg that you will not suppose that I am recommending, for this reason, that you should always lie to your patients. Such a conclusion from what I have said would correspond roughly to a class of fallacies that I have already referred to above. Since telling the truth is impossible, there can be no sharp distinction between what is true and what is false. But surely that does not relieve the physician of his moral responsibility. On the contrary, the difficulties that arise from the immense complexity of the phenomena do not diminish, but rather increase, the moral responsibility of the physician, and one of my objects has been to describe the facts through which the nature of that moral responsibility is determined.

Far older than the precept, "the truth, the whole truth, and nothing but the truth," is another that originates within our profession, that has always been the guide of the best physicians, and, if I may venture a prophecy, will always remain so: So far as possible, "do no harm." You can do harm by the process that is quaintly called telling the truth. You can do harm by lying. In your relations with your patients you will inevitably do much harm, and this will be by no means confined to your strictly medical blunders. It will arise also from what you say and what you fail to say. But try to do as little harm as possible, not only in treatment with drugs, or with the knife, but also in treatment with words, with the expression of your sentiments and emotions. Try at all times to act upon the patient so as to modify his sentiments to his own advantage, and remember that, to this end, nothing is more effective than arousing in him the belief that you are concerned whole-heartedly and exclusively for his welfare.

What I have said does not conform in my manner of saying it to the rules that I have suggested for your relations with patients. I have tried to talk reason and good sense to you, following, so far as I have been able, the habits of a lecturer upon scientific subjects. With some of you I have surely failed to accomplish my object. To them I suggest that this failure is an excellent illustration of the phenomena that I have been describing, for, unless I am mistaken, if you dislike what I have said, it is chiefly because I have failed to appeal to and made use of your sentiments.

This address was delivered at the Harvard Medical School Colloquium, in Vanderbilt Hall, on December 20, 1934, and at a Medical Staff Meeting at Massachusetts General Hospital on January 21, 1935.

Note

1. I owe my information to my colleagues, Professors Elton Mayo, F. J. Roethlisberger, and their associates. The theory and practice of interviewing developed by Mayo were applied and adapted with the advice and collaboration of the Harvard Department of Industrial Research by the Western Electric Company in the course of an elaborate investigation at the Hawthorne Works of the company. A valuable description of these Western Electric methods of interviewing may be found in Bingham and Moore's *How to Interview* (New York, 1931; second edition, 1935). In all this it is possible to discern more than traces of the methods of psychoanalysis, divested however of the usual theoretical and dogmatic accompaniments, and there considerably modified.

2

Illness and the Role of the Physician: A Sociological Perspective
Talcott Parsons

The present paper will attempt to discuss certain features of the phenomena of illness, and of the processes of therapy and the role of the therapist, as aspects of the general social equilibrium of modern Western society. This is what is meant by the use of the term "a sociological perspective" in the title. It is naturally a somewhat different perspective from that usually taken for granted by physicians and others, like clinical psychologists and social workers, who are directly concerned with the care of sick people. They are naturally more likely to think in terms of the simple application of technical knowledge of the etiological factors in ill health and of their own manipulation of the situation in the attempt to control these factors. What the present paper can do is to add something with reference to the social setting in which this more "technological" point of view fits.

Undoubtedly the biological processes of the organism constitute one crucial aspect of the determinants of ill health, and their manipulation one primary focus of the therapeutic process. With this aspect of "organic medicine" we are here only indirectly concerned. However, as the development of psychosomatic medicine has so clearly shown, even where most of the symptomatology is organic, very frequently a critically important psychogenic component is involved. In addition, there are the neuroses and psychoses where the condition itself is defined primarily in "psychological" terms, that is, in terms of the motivated adjustment of the individual in terms of his own personality, and of his relations to others in the social world. It is with this motivated aspect of illness, whether its symptoms be organic or behavioral, that we are concerned. Our fundamental thesis will be that illness to this degree must be considered to be an integral part of

Reprinted, with permission, from *American Journal of Psychiatry* 21 (1951): 452–460. Copyright 1951 by The American Orthopsychiatric Association, FRC.

what may be called the "motivational economy" of the social system and that, correspondingly, the therapeutic process must also be treated as part of that same motivational balance.

Seen in this perspective illness is to be treated as a special type of what sociologists call "deviant" behavior. By this is meant behavior which is defined in sociological terms as failing in some way to fulfill the institutionally defined expectations of one or more of the roles in which the individual is implicated in the society. Whatever the complexities of the motivational factors which may be involved, the dimension of conformity with versus deviance or alienation from the fulfillment of role expectations is always one crucial dimension of the process. The sick person is, by definition, in some respect disabled from fulfilling normal social obligations, and the motivation of the sick person in being or staying sick has some reference to this fact. Conversely, since being a normally satisfactory member of social groups is always one aspect of health, mental or physical, the therapeutic process must always have as one dimension the restoration of capacity to play social roles in a normal way.

We will deal with these problems under four headings. First something will have to be said about the processes of genesis of illness insofar as it is motivated and thus can be classed as deviant behavior. Secondly, we will say something about the role of the sick person precisely as a social role, and not only a "condition"; third, we will analyze briefly certain aspects of the role of the physician and show their relation to the therapeutic process and finally, fourth, we will say something about the way in which both roles fit into the general equilibrium of the social system.

Insofar as illness is a motivated phenomenon, the sociologist is particularly concerned with the ways in which certain features of the individual's relations to others have played a part in the process of its genesis. These factors are never isolated; there are, of course, the constitutional and organically significant environmental factors (e.g., bacterial agents), and undoubtedly also psychological factors internal to the individual personality. But evidence is overwhelming as to the enormous importance of relations to others in the development and functioning of personality. The sociologist's emphasis, then, is on the factors responsible for "something's going wrong" in a person's relationships to others during the processes of social interaction. Probably the most significant of these processes are those of childhood, and centering in relations to family members, especially, of course, the parents. But the essential phenomena are involved throughout the life cycle.

Something going wrong in this sense may be said in general to consist in the imposition of a strain on the individual, a strain with which, given his resources, he is unable successfully to cope. A combination of contributions from psychopathology, learning theory and sociology makes it possible for us to say a good deal, both about what kinds of circumstances in interpersonal relations are most likely to impose potentially pathogenic strains, and about what the nature of the reactions to such strains is likely to be.

Very briefly we may say that the pathogenic strains center at two main points. The first concerns what psychiatrists often call the "support" a person receives from those surrounding him. Essentially this may be defined as his acceptance as a full-fledged member of the group, in the appropriate role. For the child this means, first of all, acceptance by the family. The individual is emotionally "wanted" and within considerable limits this attitude is not conditional on the details of his behavior. The second aspect concerns the upholding of the value patterns which are constitutive of the group, which may be only a dyadic relationship of two persons, but is usually a more extensive group. Thus rejection, the seducibility of the other, particularly the more responsible, members of the group in contravention of the group norms, the evasion by these members of responsibility for enforcement of norms, and, finally, the compulsive "legalistic" enforcement of them are the primary sources of strain in social relationships. It is unfortunately not possible to take space here to elaborate further on these very important problems.

Reactions to such strains are, in their main outline, relatively familiar to students of mental pathology. The most important may be enumerated as anxiety, production of fantasies, hostile impulses and the resort to special mechanisms of defense. In general we may say that the most serious problem with reference to social relationships concerns the handling of hostile impulses. If the strain is not adequately coped with in such ways as to reduce anxiety to manageable levels, the result will, we believe, be the generating of ambivalent motivational structures. Here, because intrinsically incompatible motivations are involved, there must be resort to special mechanisms of defense and adjustment. Attitudes toward others thereby acquire the special property of compulsiveness because of the need to defend against the repressed element of the motivational structure. The ambivalent structure may work out in either of two main directions: first, by the repression of the hostile side, there develops a compulsive need to conform with expectations and retain the favorable attitudes of the object; second, by dominance of the hostile side, compulsive alienation from expectations of conformity and from the object results.

The presence of such compulsive motivation inevitably distorts the attitudes of an individual in his social relationships. This means that it imposes strains upon those with whom he interacts. In general it may be suggested that most pathological motivation arises out of vicious circles of deepening ambivalence. An individual, say a child, is subjected to such strain by the compulsive motivation of adults. As a defense against this he himself develops a complementary pattern of compulsive motivation, and the two continue, unless the process is checked, to "work on each other." In this connection it may be especially noted that some patterns of what has been called compulsive conformity are not readily defined as deviant in the larger social group. Such people may in a sense be often regarded as "carriers" of mental pathology in that, though themselves not explicitly deviant, either in the form of illness or otherwise, by their effects on others they contribute to the genesis of the kinds of personality structure which are likely to break down into illness or other forms of deviance.

Two important conclusions seem to be justified from these considerations. The first is that the types of strain on persons which we have discussed are disorganizing both to personalities and to social relationships. Personal disorganization and social disorganization are, in a considerable part, two sides of the same concrete process. This obviously has very important implications both for psychiatry and for social science. Secondly, illness as a form of deviant behavior is not a unique phenomenon, but one type in a wider category. It is one of a set of alternatives which are open to the individual. There are, of course, reasons why some persons will have a psychological make-up which is more predisposed toward illness, and others toward one or another of the alternatives; but there is a considerable element of fluidity, and the selection among such alternatives may be a function of a number of variables. This fact is of the greatest importance when it is seen that the role of the sick person is a socially structured and in a sense institutionalized role.

The alternatives to illness may be such as to be open only to the isolated individual, as in the case of the individual criminal or the hobo. They may also involve the formation of deviant groups as in the case of the delinquent gang. Or, finally, they may involve a group formation which includes asserting a claim to legitimacy in terms of the value system of the society, as in joining an exotic religious sect. Thus to be a criminal is in general to be a social outcast, but in general we define religious devoutness as "a good thing" so that the same order of conflict with society that is involved in the criminal case may not be involved in the religious case. There are many complex and important problems concerning the genesis and significance of these various deviant patterns, and their relations to each other, which cannot be gone into here. The most essential point is to see that illness is one pattern among a family of such alternatives, and that the fundamental motivational ingredients of illness are not peculiar to it, but are of more general significance.

We may now turn to our second main topic, that of the sense in which illness is not merely a "condition" but also a social role. The essential criteria of a social role concern the attitudes both of the incumbent and of others with whom he interacts, in relation to a set of social norms defining expectations of appropriate or proper behavior for persons in that role. In this respect we may distinguish four main features of the "sick role" in our society.

The first of these is the exemption of the sick person from the performance of certain of his normal social obligations. Thus, to take a very simple case, "Johnny has a fever, he ought not to go to school today." This exemption and the decision as to when it does and does not apply should not be taken for granted. Psychiatrists are sufficiently familiar with the motivational significance of the "secondary gain" of the mentally ill to realize that conscious malingering is not the only problem of the abuse of the privileges of being sick. In short, the sick person's claim to exemption must be socially defined and validated. Not every case of "just not feeling like working" can be accepted as such a valid claim.

Secondly, the sick person is, in a very specific sense, also exempted from a certain type of responsibility for his own state. This is what is ordinarily meant by saying that he is in a "condition." He will either have to get well spontaneously or to "be cured" by having something done to him. He cannot reasonably be expected to "pull himself together" by a mere act of will, and thus to decide to be all right. He may have been responsible for getting himself into such a state, as by careless exposure to accident or infection, but even then he is not responsible for the process of getting well, except in a peripheral sense.

This exemption from obligations and from a certain kind of responsibility, however, is given at a price. The third aspect of the sick role is the partial character of its legitimation, hence the deprivation of a claim to full legitimacy. To be sick, that is, is to be in a state which is socially defined as undesirable, to be gotten out of as expeditiously as possible. No one is given the privileges of being sick any longer than necessary but only so long as he "can't help it." The sick person is thereby isolated, and by his deviant pattern is deprived of a claim to appeal to others.

Finally, fourth, being sick is also defined, except for the mildest cases, as being "in need of help." Moreover, the type of help which is needed is presumptively defined; it is that of persons specially qualified to care for illness, above all, of physicians. Thus from being defined as the incumbent of a role relative to people who are not sick, the sick person makes the transition to the additional role of patient. He thereby, as in all social roles, incurs certain obligations, especially that of "cooperating" with his physician—or other therapist—in the process of trying to get well. This obviously constitutes an affirmation of the admission of being sick, and therefore in an undesirable state, and also exposes the individual to specific reintegrative influences.

It is important to realize that in all these four respects, the phenomena of mental pathology have been assimilated to a role pattern which was already well established in our society before the development of modern psychopathology. In some respects it is peculiar to modern Western society, particularly perhaps with respect to the kinds of help which a patient is felt to need; in many societies magical manipulations have been the most prominent elements in treatment.

In our society, with reference to the severer cases at any rate, the definition of the mental "case" as sick has had to compete with a somewhat different role definition, namely, that as "insane." The primary difference would seem to center on the concept of responsibility and the mode and extent of its application. The insane person is, we may say, defined as being in a state where not only can he not be held responsible for getting out of his condition by an act of will, but where he is held not to be responsible in his usual dealings with others and therefore not responsible for recognition of his own condition, its disabilities and his need for help. This conception of lack of responsibility leads to the justification of coercion of the insane, as by commitment to a hospital. The relations between the two role definitions raise important problems which cannot be gone into here.

It may be worth while just to mention another complication which is of special interest to members of the Orthopsychiatric Association, namely, the situation involved when the sick person is a child. Here, because of the role of child, certain features of the role of sick adult must be altered, particularly with respect to the levels of responsibility which can be imputed to the child. This brings the role of the mentally sick child in certain respects closer to that of the insane than, particularly, of the neurotic adult. Above all it means that third parties, notably parents, must play a particularly important part in the situation. It is common for pediatricians, when they refer to "my patient," often to mean the mother rather than the sick child. There is a very real sense in which the child psychiatrist must actively treat the parents and not merely the child himself.

We may now turn to our third major problem area, that of the social role of the therapist and its relation to the motivational processes involved in reversing the pathogenic processes. These processes are, it is widely recognized, in a certain sense definable as the obverse of those involved in pathogenesis, with due allowance for certain complicating factors. There seem to be four main conditions of successful psychotherapy which can be briefly discussed.

The first of these is what psychiatrists generally refer to as "support." By this is here meant essentially that acceptance as a member of a social group, the lack of which we argued above played a crucial part in pathogenesis. In this instance it is, above all, the solidary group formed by the therapist and his patient, in which the therapist assumes the obligation to do everything he can within reason to "help" his patient. The strong emphasis in the "ideology" of the medical profession on the "welfare of the patient" as the first obligation of the physician is closely related to this factor. The insistence that the professional role must be immune from "commercialism," with its suggestion that maximizing profits is a legitimate goal, symbolizes the attitude. Support in this sense is, so long as the relationship subsists, to be interpreted as essentially unconditional, in that within wide limits it will not be shaken by what the patient does. As we shall see, this does not, however, mean that it is unlimited, in the sense that the therapist is obligated to "do anything the patient wants."

The second element is a special permissiveness to express wishes and fantasies which would ordinarily not be permitted expression in normal social relationships, as within the family. This permissiveness must mean that the normal sanctions for such expression in the form of disapproval and the like are suspended. There are of course definite limits on "acting out." In general the permissiveness is confined to verbal and gestural levels, but this is nonetheless an essential feature of the therapeutic process.

The obverse of permissiveness, however, is a very important restriction on the therapist's reaction to it. In general, that is, the therapist does not reciprocate the expectations which are expressed, explicitly or implicitly, in the patient's deviant wishes and fantasies. The most fundamental wishes, we may presume, involve reciprocal interaction between the individual and others. The expression of a wish is in fact an invitation to the other to reciprocate in the complementary role, if it is a deviant wish, an attempt to "seduce" him into reciprocation. This is true of negative as well as positive attitudes. The expression of hostility to the therapist in transference is only a partial gratification of the wish; full gratification would require reciprocation by the therapist's becoming angry in return. Sometimes this occurs; it is what is called "countertransference"; but it is quite clear that the therapist is expected to control his countertransference impulses and that such control is in general a condition of successful therapy. By showing the patient the projective character of this transference reaction, this refusal to reciprocate plays an essential part in facilitating the attainment of insight by the patient.

Finally, fourth, over against the unconditional element of support, there is the conditional manipulation of sanctions by the therapist. The therapist's giving and withholding of approval is of critical importance to the patient. This seems to be an essential condition of the effectiveness of interpretations. The acceptance of an interpretation by the patient demonstrates his capacity, to the relevant extent, to discuss matters on a mature plane with the therapist, who shows his approval of this performance. It is probably significant that overt disapproval is seldom used in therapy, but certainly the withholding of positive approval is very significant.

The above four conditions of successful psychotherapy, it is important to observe, are all to some degree "built into" the role which the therapist in our society typically assumes, that of the physician, and all to some degree are aspects of behavior in that role which are at least partially independent of any conscious or explicit theory or technique of psychotherapy.

The relation of support to the definition of the physician's role as primarily oriented to the welfare of the patient has already been noted. The element of permissiveness has its roots in the general social acceptance that "allowances" should be made for sick people, not only in that they may have physical disabilities, but that they are in various ways "emotionally" disturbed. The physician, by virtue of his special responsibility for the care of the sick, has a special obligation to make such allowances. Third, however, the physician is, by the definition of his role, positively enjoined not to enter into certain reciprocities with his patients, or he is protected against the pressures which they exert upon him. Thus giving of confidential information is, in ordinary relationships, a symbol of reciprocal intimacy, but the physician does not tell about his own private affairs. Many features of the physician-patient relationship, such as the physician's access to the body, might arouse erotic reactions, but the role is defined so as to inhibit such developments even if they are initiated by the patient. In general the definition of the physician's role as specifically limited to concern with matters of health, and the injunction to observe an "impersonal," matter-of-fact attitude without personal emotional involvement, serve to justify and legitimize his refusal to reciprocate his patient's deviant expectations. Finally, the prestige of the physician's scientific training, his reputation for technical competence, gives authority to his approval, a basis for the acceptance of his interpretations.

All of these fundamental features of the role of the physician are given independently of the technical operations of psychotherapy; indeed they were institutionalized long before the days of Freud or of psychiatry as an important branch of the medical profession. This fact is of the very first importance.

First, it strongly suggests that in fact deliberate, conscious psychotherapy is only part of the process. Indeed, the effective utilization of these aspects of the physician's role is a prominent part of what has long been called the "art of medicine." It is highly probable that, whether or not the physician knows it or wishes it, in practicing medicine skillfully he is always in fact exerting a psychotherapeutic effect on his patients. Furthermore, there is every reason to believe that, even though the cases are not explicitly "mental" cases, this is necessary. This is, first, because a "psychic factor" is present in a very large proportion of ostensibly somatic cases and, secondly, apart from any psychic factor in the etiology, because illness is always to some degree a situation of strain to the patient, and mechanisms for coping with his reactions to that strain are hence necessary, if the strain is not to have psychopathological consequences. The essential continuity between the art of medicine and deliberate psychotherapy is, therefore, deeply rooted in the nature of the physician's function generally. Modern psychotherapy has been built upon the role of the physician as this was already established in the social structure of Western society. It has utilized the existing role pattern, and extended and refined certain of its features, but the roles of the physician and of the sick person were not created as an application of the theories of psychiatrists.

The second major implication is that, if these features of the role of the physician and of illness are built into the structure of society independent of the application of theories of psychopathology, it would be very strange indeed if they turned out to be isolated phenomena, confined in their significance to this one context. This is particularly true if, as we have given reason to believe, illness is not an isolated phenomenon, but one of a set of alternative modes of expression for a common fund of motivational reaction to strain in the social system. But with proper allowances for very important differences we can show that certain of these same features can also be found in other roles in the social system. Thus to take an example of special interest to you, there are many resemblances between the psychotherapeutic process and that of the normal socialization of the child. The differences are, however, great. They are partly related to the fact that a child apparently needs two parents while a neurotic person can get along with only one psychiatrist. But also in the institutions of leadership, of the settlement of conflicts in society and of many others, many of the same factors are operative.

We therefore suggest that the processes which are visible in the actual technical work of psychotherapy resemble, in their relation to the total balance of forces operating within and upon the individual, the part of the iceberg which protrudes above the surface of the water; what is below the surface is the larger and, in certain respects, probably still the more important part.

It also shows that the phenomena of physical and mental illness and their counteraction are more intimately connected with the general equilibrium of the social system than is generally supposed. We may close with one rather general inference from this generalization. It is rather generally supposed that there has been a considerable increase in the incidence of mental illness within the last generation or so. This is difficult to prove since statistics are notably fragmentary and fashions of diagnosis and treatment have greatly changed. But granting the fact, what would be its meaning? It could be that it was simply an index of generally increasing social disorganization. But this is not necessarily the case. There are certain positive functions in the role of illness from the social point of view. The sick person is isolated from influence upon others. His condition is declared to be undesirable and he is placed in the way of reequilibrating influences. It is altogether possible that an increase in mental illness may constitute a diversion of tendencies to deviance from other channels of expression into the role of illness, with consequences less dangerous to the stability of society than certain alternatives might be. In any case the physician is not merely the person responsible for the care of a special class of "problem cases." He stands at a strategic point in the general balance of forces in the society of which he is a part.

II

The Dynamics: How the Interchange Takes Place

General models of the doctor-patient relation are valued for providing the unstated rules for everyday encounters, but they omit the working dynamics and the many variations of the relation that are met in medical practice. From a review of case studies in the psychoanalytic literature, doctor-patient relations clearly have intrapsychic roots in the early experience between parent and child (W. A. Greene, "Some Perspective for Observing and Interpreting Biophysiologic and Doctor-Patient Relations," *Perspectives in Biol. and Med.*, summer 1959: 453). Accordingly, some writers—and some patients—observe that patients may respond to the medical doctor as a good "mama" or a stern "papa." An aging doctor may even represent a grandparent or, in the case of young medical students caring for the elderly, a son or daughter: "You're just like my son Bill." Still other dynamic factors are directly part of the relation, some of which are illustrated by several writings reprinted here.

Thomas Szasz and Marc Hollender, in "Basic Models of the Doctor-Patient Relationship," note how the physical condition of the individual influences the relation in respect to treatment. That pervasive modern condition is the patient's chronic disease or handicap (e.g., arthritis, heart disease, cancer, stroke), which may be present an entire lifetime; as Alexander Pope wrote, "This long disease, my life." With chronic disorders, the patient is not a passive recipient of treatment, but, in the language of those studies that examine patient behavior, the patient can avoid or adhere to, comply or cooperate with, even participate in or drop out of, treatment. For adherence, the patient must do self-treatment as soon as leaving the medical consultation. As a result, Szasz and Hollender argue, the patient's participation in medical advice and treatment is key. The relation now requires more than authoritarian advice, namely, "mutual participation," accomplished by a negotiated exchange between doctor and patient. Both must agree that the taking of prescribed medicine is important and necessary.

Many examples of chronicity, such as physical impairments, handicaps, and disease, should be mentioned. These include neurological disorders with lingering terminal states as with amyotrophic lateral sclerosis and disabling strokes; kidney failure treated by renal or peritoneal dialysis; long-term experimental drug trials in cancer chemotherapy; genetic disorders such as Mongolism (Down's Syndrome); and being handicapped with blindness, deafness, mental retardation, seizure disorder, arthritis, or post-traumatic spinal-cord injuries. All are special examples of chronicity in which medical cures are not possible, and the patient's participation is essential for any treatment, rehabilitation, or care, and where, despite negotiations, the patient's compliance may not be "all or nothing" but may vary from the ritualistic, retreatist, and innovative to the optimal cooperative response (E. Mumford, "The response of patients to medical advice," in *Understanding Human Behavior in Health and Disease*, ed. R. C. Simons [Williams and Wilkins, 1985]). The special illness situations of the doctor-patient relation are found in numerous writings. In the instance of dying and terminal states, the social features of the relation in hospitals are the contained in David Sudnov's *Passing On: The Social Organization of Dying* (Prentice-Hall, 1967), and the psychological features are covered in Elisabeth Kübler-Ross's *On Death and Dying* (Macmillan, 1969). Renée Fox, in *Experiment Perilous* (Free Press, 1969), writes about the mutual devotion of doctors and patients in experimental trials of new treatments (specifically, renal transplants at the Peter Bent Brigham Hospital in Boston). Charlotte Swartz's article "Strategies and Tactics of Mothers of Mentally Retarded Children," in *Diminished People*, edited by N. Bernstein (Little, Brown, 1970), records mothers' difficulties in getting their requests fulfilled by doctors who took a standard definition of the child's problem rather than the mother's definition. Norman Bernstein (*Emotional Care of the Facially Burned and Disfigured* [Little, Brown, 1976]) notes how patients with facial disfigurement from burns will "disappear" from the relationship because of the shameful necessity of displaying their disfigurement. Robert Goldwyn (*The Patient and the Plastic Surgeon* [Little, Brown, 1981]) discusses the expectations of patients seeking plastic surgery.

Fred Davis discussed another dimension of illness and the relation in "Uncertainty in Prognosis, Clinical and Functional" (*Am. J. Sociol.* 65 [1960]: 41). He noted how uncertainty (especially in the prognosis of poliomyelitis when that disease was prevalent) was employed by the doctor and was a source of tension in the relation. Like guilt in psychotherapy, or in life, such tension about prognosis can be productively used to clarify the goals of treatment, although more commonly it may be used to keep the patient in limbo (or in line), as Davis noted, and may be useful in keeping up patients' hopes about improvement. Thus, systematic attention to the communication of prognostic information might also improve such relations and patient recovery. From an ethnomethodologic view, the physical exam (the pelvic) in the female patient-doctor relationship was examined by Jane Emerson. In "Behavior in Private Places" she discusses the doctor's behavior not only as information transmittal, but also as it defines the nature of the gynecological exam for the patient (and, hence, the dynamics of the interchange).

Looking at the limits of the physician's power, Eliot Freidson, in "Client Control and Medical Practice," notes how the lay referral system, namely, the use of the patients' own social networks and choices of practitioner, provides patients with some control over doctors, limiting doctors' freedom and power to act (or overact). Others, like Thomas J. Scheff, theorize from a variety of empirical studies how doctors actually deal with patients' complaints and requests when they do consult. In "Negotiating Reality," Scheff looks at evidence, from Balint's general-practice seminars to plea bargaining in courts and from the psychiatric interview to fiction, concluding that doctor-patient encounters are in fact negotiations in which the doctor, perhaps, is always one up in influencing the patient in the kind of illness or treatment he thinks is proper. But, as Jay Haley noted in *Strategies of Psychotherapy* (Grune and Stratton, 1963), this does not mean that the patient always loses, as is often implied in analyses of the differences in power between doctors and patients. The actual bargaining that takes place in the encounter, involving both the requests of the patient and the "offers" of the doctor, was discussed in terms of "exchanges" by E. Katz, M. Gurevitch, T. Peled, and B. Danet ("Doctor-Patient Exchanges: A Diagnostic Approach to Organization and the Professions," *Hum. Rel.* 11 [1965]: 309), who noted that the individual faces similar exchanges in everyday life, with police, banks, and workers' committees (E. Katz et al., "Petition and Persuasive Appeals: A Study of Official-Client Relations," *Am. Sociol. Rev.* 31 [1966]: 817). Those who might be interested in measuring the quality of care from an interpersonal rather than a technical viewpoint might examine "good doctoring" in terms of the degree of reciprocity.

In an early essay examining the cash nexus of the contract from comparative studies of the Russian and British medical systems, Mark G. Field ("The Doctor-Patient Relation in the Perspective of 'Fee-for-Service' and 'Third-Party Medicine,'" *J. Health and Hum. Behav.* 2 (1961): 252) wrote on how the payment intervention may alter the interpersonal qualities of the relation. Third parties, whether commercial insurance, the government's Medicare and Medicaid programs, nonprofit Blue Cross–Blue Shield plans, or prepaid HMOs, may depersonalize it, attenuating the bond between the patient and the doctor while diminishing the patient's control as an out-of-pocket payer. This payment transformation of practice is nearly but not quite complete. As previously noted, 92 percent of doctor bills in the hospital are now paid for by third parties, while these payers cover only 35–40 percent of office bills. Even with much indirect payment, some incentive to close involvement with the patient in the office can still be maintained, since the doctor's pay is related to the volume of patients he attracts and the quality of his practice (J. Grossman, J. D. Stoeckle, and J. J. Dineen, "New Organizations Out of Old Ones: Teaching Group Practices Out of OPDs and Private Practice, *Health and Society*, winter 1975: 65). Despite the recent growth of prepayment plans amid fee-of-service medicine, no comparative studies of doctor-patient-relationship differences have been done, even when the reasons why patients go in and out of prepayment and fee-for-service practices are common professional concerns. Unfortunately, the modern issues in health policy are not the quality of therapeutic relations but the cost and what appears to be excessive use of services generated by doctors' decisions and patients' requests.

Influences other than the commercial and cash nexus are examined by Arlene K. Daniels, who looks at the effect of the practice setting. Her paper on medical work in the military services uses psychiatry as an example. Entitled "The Captive Professional," it provides one example of the influence of special institutions on the relation. As previously noted, prisons, colleges, schools, HMOs, factories, and industry may have similar constraints on the doctor working there and on the relation, where, in each situation, if not each consultation, some would argue that the doctor is a double agent serving others besides the patient.

Leo G. Reeder's paper "The Patient-Client as a Consumer: Some Observations of the Changing Professional-Client Relationship" (*J. Health and Social Behav.* 13 [1972]: 406) spoke to cultural influences on the contemporary expert-consumer relation regardless of its setting. In the 1970s he noted the mounting pressures for a more egalitarian relation between "consumers" and "experts," between patients and doctors. Reeder saw a redefinition of the relation: "consumer" patients seeking medical aid of doctors as "providers," an exchange with roots in the consumer movement and the economic model of medical practice. That exchange has become the prevailing view of the competition ideology of the 1980s. The use of the rubric "health-care provider," so common in many treatment institutions, has announced this consumer thinking about, if not actual change in, practitioner-patient relations. Some would extend this idea of the relation beyond the mere influence of a consumer on a professional to a presumably legal notion in which a "contract" is made with the "consumer" over treatment. And yet this seemingly modern idea of the contract is actually not a change (even if accompanied by paperwork), but a metaphor for the relation where agreements are negotiated, not contracted. Writing on the same theme, Marie Haug and Marvin Sussman ("Professional Autonomy and the Revolt of the Client." *Social Problems* 17 [1969]: 153) predicted a restriction of the professional's technical expertise and humanistic action. Yet if many doctors regard such developments as threatening to their future authority, power, and status, many others would observe, or at least feel, that the reduction in physicians' authority, power, and status is already here (P. Starr, *The Social Transformation of Medicine* [Basic Books, 1983]). However, more "equal" relations—and they cannot be altogether equal, despite assertions that they should be—may actually improve the doctor's job by demystifying medical work and reducing irrational expectations. Moreover, those outcomes are not, of necessity, altogether bleak. The shift may also benefit the patient by increasing his rational autonomy in care and treatment and therefore increasing his behavioral compliance.

3

A Contribution to the Philosophy of Medicine: The Basic Models of the Doctor-Patient Relationship
Thomas S. Szasz and Marc H. Hollender

When a person leaves the culture in which he was born and raised and migrates to another, he usually experiences his new social setting as something strange—and in some ways threatening—and he is stimulated to master it by conscious efforts at understanding. To some extent every immigrant to the United States reacts in this manner to the American scene. Similarly, the American tourist in Europe or South America "scrutinizes" the social setting which is taken for granted by the natives. To scrutinize—and criticize—the pattern of other peoples' lives is obviously both common and easy. It also happens, however, that people exposed to cross-cultural experiences turn their attention to the very customs which formed the social matrix of their lives in the past. Lastly, to study the "customs" which shape and govern one's day-to-day life is most difficult of all (Ruesch and Bateson 1951).

In many ways the psychoanalyst is like a person who has migrated from one culture to another. To him the relationship between physician and patient—which is like a custom that is taken for granted in medical practice and which he himself so treated in his early history—has become an object of study. While the precise nature and extent of the influence which psychoanalysis and so-called dynamic psychiatry have had on modern medicine are debatable, it seems to us that the most decisive effect has been that of making physicians explicitly aware of the possible significance of their relationship to patients.

The question naturally arises as to "What is a doctor-patient relationship?" It is our aim to discuss this question and to show that certain philosophical preconceptions associated with the notions of

Reprinted, with permission, from *AMA Archives of Internal Medicine* 97 (1956): 585–592. Copyright 1956 by the American Medical Association.

"disease," "treatment," and "cure" have a profound bearing on both the theory and the practice of medicine.[1]

What Is a Human Relationship?

The concept of a relationship is a novel one in medicine. Traditionally, physicians have been concerned with "things," for example, anatomical structures, lesions, bacteria, and the like. In modern times the scope has been broadened to include the concept of "function." The phenomenon of a human relationship is often viewed as though it were a "thing" or a "function." It is, in fact, neither. Rather it is an abstraction, appropriate for the description and handling of certain observational facts. Moreover, it is an abstraction which presupposes concepts of both structure and function.

The foregoing comments may be clarified by concrete illustrations. Psychiatrists often suggest to their medical colleagues that the physician's relationship with his patient "per se" helps the latter. This creates the impression (whether so intended or not) that the relationship is a thing, which works not unlike the way that vitamins do in a case of vitamin deficiency. Another idea is that the doctor-patient relationship depends mainly on what the physician does (or thinks or feels). Then it is viewed not unlike a function.

When we consider a relationship in which there is joint participation of the two persons involved, "relationship" refers to neither a structure nor a function (such as the "personality" of the physician or patient). It is, rather, an abstraction embodying the activities of two interacting systems (persons) (Dubos 1955).

Three Basic Models of the Doctor-Patient Relationship

The three basic models of the doctor-patient relationship (see table 1), which we will describe, embrace modes of interaction ubiquitous in human relationships and in no way specific for the contact between physician and patient. The specificity of the medical situation probably derives from a combination of these modes of interaction with certain technical procedures and social settings.

1. The Model of Activity-Passivity

Historically, this is the oldest conceptual model. Psychologically, it is not an interaction, because it is based on the effect of one person on another in such a way and under such circumstances that the person acted upon is unable to contribute actively, or is considered to be

Table 1
Three basic models of the physician-patient relationship.

Model	Physician's role	Patient's role	Clinical application of model	Prototype of model
1. Activity-passivity	Does something to patient	Recipient (unable to respond or inert)	Anesthesia, acute trauma, coma, delirium, etc.	Parent-infant
2. Guidance-cooperation	Tells patient what to do	Cooperator (obeys)	Acute infectious processes, etc.	Parent-child (adolescent)
3. Mutual participation	Helps patient to help himself	Participant in "partnership" (uses expert help)	Most chronic illnesses, psychoanalysis, etc.	Adult-adult

inanimate. This frame of reference (in which the physician does something to the patient) underlies the application of some of the outstanding advances of modern medicine (e.g., anesthesia and surgery, antibiotics, etc.). The physician is active; the patient, passive. This orientation has originated in—and is entirely appropriate for—the treatment of emergencies (e.g., for the patient who is severely injured, bleeding, delirious, or in coma). "Treatment" takes place irrespective of the patient's contribution and regardless of the outcome. There is a similarity here between the patient and a helpless infant, on the one hand, and between the physician and a parent, on the other. It may be recalled that psychoanalysis, too, evolved from a procedure (hypnosis) which was based on this model. Various physical measures to which psychotics are subjected today are another example of the activity-passivity frame of reference.

2. The Model of Guidance-Cooperation
This model underlies much of medical practice. It is employed in situations which are less desperate than those previously mentioned (e.g., acute infections). Although the patient is ill, he is conscious and has feelings and aspirations of his own. Since he suffers from pain, anxiety, and other distressing symptoms, he seeks help and is ready and willing to "cooperate." When he turns to a physician, he places the latter (even if only in some limited ways) in a position of power. This is due not only to a "transference reaction" (i.e., his regarding the physician as he did his father when he was a child) but also to the

fact that the physician possesses knowledge of his bodily processes which he does not have. In some ways it may seem that this, like the first model, is an active-passive phenomenon. Actually, this is more apparent than real. Both persons are "active" in that they contribute to the relationship and what ensues from it. The main difference between the two participants pertains to power, and to its actual or potential use. The more powerful of the two (parent, physician, employer, etc.) will speak of guidance or leadership and will expect cooperation of the other member of the pair (child, patient, employee, etc.). The patient is expected to "look up to" and to "obey" his doctor. Moreover, he is neither to question nor to argue or disagree with the orders he receives. This model has its prototype in the relationship of the parent and his (adolescent) child. Often, threats and other undisguised weapons of force are employed, even though presumably these are for the patient's "own good." It should be added that the possibility of the exploitation of the situation—as in any relationship between persons of unequal power—for the sole benefit of the physician, albeit under the guise of altruism, is ever present.

3. The Model of Mutual Participation

Philosophically, this model is predicated on the postulate that equality among human beings is desirable. It is fundamental to the social structure of democracy and has played a crucial role in occidental civilization for more than 200 years. Psychologically, mutuality rests on complex processes of identification—which facilitate conceiving of others in terms of oneself—together with maintaining and tolerating the discrete individuality of the observer and the observed. It is crucial to this type of interaction that the participants (1) have approximately equal power, (2) be mutually interdependent (i.e., need each other), and (3) engage in activity that will be in some ways satisfying to both.

This model is favored by patients who, for various reasons, want to take care of themselves (at least in part). This may be an overcompensatory attempt at mastering anxieties associated with helplessness and passivity. It may also be "realistic" and necessary, as, for example, in the management of most chronic illnesses (e.g., diabetes mellitus, chronic heart disease, etc.). Here the patient's own experiences provide reliable and important clues for therapy. Moreover, the treatment program itself is principally carried out by the patient. Essentially, the physician helps the patient to help himself.

In an evolutionary sense, the pattern of mutual participation is more highly developed than the other two models of the doctor-patient relationship. It requires a more complex psychological and social organization on the part of both participants. Accordingly, it is rarely appropriate for children or for those persons who are mentally deficient, very poorly educated, or profoundly immature. On the other hand, the greater the intellectual, educational, and general experiential similarity between physician and patient the more appropriate and necessary this model of therapy becomes.

The Basic Models and the Psychology of the Physician

Consideration of why physicians seek one or another type of relationship with patients (or seek patients who fit into a particular relationship) would carry us beyond the scope of this essay. Yet, it must be emphasized that as long as this subject is approached with the sentimental viewpoint that a physician is simply motivated by a wish to help others (not that we deny this wish), no scientific study of the subject can be undertaken. Scientific investigation is possible only if value judgment is subrogated, at least temporarily, to a candid scrutiny of the physician's actual behavior with his patients.

The activity-passivity model places the physician in absolute control of the situation. In this way it gratifies needs for mastery and contributes to feelings of superiority (Jones 1951; Marmor 1953). At the same time it requires that the physician disidentify with the patient as a person.

Somewhat similar is the guidance-cooperation model. The disidentification with the patient, however, is less complete. The physician, like the parent of a growing child, could be said to see in the patient a human being potentially (but not yet) like himself (or like he wishes to be). In addition to the gratifications already mentioned, this relationship provides an opportunity to recreate and to gratify the "Pygmalion Complex." Thus, the physician can mold others into his own image, as God is said to have created man (or he may mold them into his own image of what they should be like, as in Shaw's *Pygmalion*). This type of relationship is of importance in education, as the transmission of more or less stable cultural values (and of language itself) shows. It requires that the physician be convinced he is "right" in his notion of what is "best" for the patient. He will then try to induce the patient to accept his aims as the patient's own.

The model of mutual participation, as suggested earlier, is essentially foreign to medicine. This relationship, characterized by a high degree of empathy, has elements often associated with the notions of friendship and partnership and the imparting of expert advice. The physician may be said to help the patient to help himself. The physician's gratification cannot stem from power or from the control over someone else. His satisfactions are derived from more abstract kinds of mastery, which are as yet poorly understood.

It is evident that in each of the categories mentioned the satisfactions of physician and patient complement each other. This makes for stability in a paired system. Such stability, however, must be temporary, since the physician strives to alter the patient's state. The comatose patient, for example, either will recover to a more healthy, conscious condition or he will die. If he improves, the doctor-patient relationship must change. It is at this point that the physician's inner (usually unacknowledged) needs are most likely to interfere with what is "best" for the patient. At this juncture, the physician either changes his "attitude" (not a consciously or deliberately assumed role) to complement the patient's emergent needs or he foists upon the patient the same role of helpless passivity from which he (allegedly) tried to rescue him in the first place. Here we touch on a subject rich in psychological and sociological complexities. The process of change the physician must undergo to have a mutually constructive experience with the patient is similar to a very familiar process: namely, the need for the parent to behave ever differently toward his growing child.

What Is "Good Medicine"?

Let us now consider the problem of "good medicine" from the viewpoint of human relationships. The function of sciences is not to tell us what is good or bad but rather to help us understand how things work. "Good" and "bad" are personal judgments, usually decided on the basis of whether or not the object under consideration satisfies us. In viewing the doctor-patient relationship we cannot conclude, however, that anything which satisfies—irrespective of other considerations—is "good." Further complications arise when the method is questioned by which we ascertain whether or not a particular need has been satisfied. Do we take the patient's word for it? Or do we place ourselves into the traditional parental role of "knowing what is best" for our patients (children)?

The shortcomings and dangers inherent in these and in other attempts to clarify some of the most basic aspects of our daily life are too well known to require documentation. It is this very complexity of the situation which has led, as is the rule in scientific work, to an essentially arbitrary simplification of the structure of our field of observation.[2]

Let us present an example. A patient consults a physician because of pain and other symptoms resulting from a duodenal ulcer. Both physician and patient assume that the latter would be better off without these discomforts. The situation now may be structured as follows: Healing of the ulcer is "good," whereas its persistence is "bad." What we wish to emphasize is the fact that physician and patient agree (explicitly or otherwise) as to what is good and bad. Without such agreement it is meaningless to speak of a therapeutic relationship.

In other words, the notions of "normal," "abnormal," "symptom," "disease," and the like are social conventions. These definitions often are set by the medical world and are usually tacitly accepted by others. The fact that there is agreement renders it difficult to perceive their changing (and relativistic) character. A brief example will clarify this statement. Some years ago—and among the uneducated even today—fever was regarded as something "bad" ("abnormal," a "symptom"), to be combated. The current scientific opinion is that it is the organism's response to certain types of influences (e.g., infection) and that within limits the manifestation itself should not be "treated."

The issue of agreement is of interest because it has direct bearing on the three models of the doctor-patient relationship. In the first two models "agreement" between physician and patient is taken for granted. The comatose patient obviously cannot disagree. According to the second model, the patient does not possess the knowledge to dispute the physician's word. The third category differs in that the physician does not profess to know exactly what is best for the patient. The search for this becomes the essence of the therapeutic interaction. The patient's own experiences furnish indispensable information for eventual agreement, under otherwise favorable circumstances, as to what "health" might be for him.

The characteristics of the different types of doctor-patient relationships are summarized in table 2. In this connection, some comments will be made on a subject which essentially is philosophical but which continues to plague many medical discussions; namely, the problem of comparing the efficacy of different therapeutic measures. Such comparisons are implicitly based on the following conceptual scheme: We postulate disease "A," from which many patients suffer. Therapies "B," "C," and "D" are given to groups of patients suffering with disease "A," and the results are compared. It is usually

Table 2
Analysis of the concepts of "disease," "treatment," and "therapeutic result."

Doctor-patient relationship	Meaning of "treatment"	"Therapeutic result"	Notions of disease and health	In medicine (illustrative examples)	In psychiatry (illustrative examples)
1. Activity-passivity	Whatever the physician does; the actual operations (procedures) which he employs	Alteration in the structure and/or function of the patient's body (or behavior, as determined by the physician's judgment); the patient's judgment does not enter into the evaluation of results; e.g., T & A is "successful" irrespective of how patient feels afterward	The presence or absence of some unwanted structure or function The actual state of affairs The same state without the disability	1. Treatment of the unconscious patient; for example, the patient in diabetic coma; cerebral hemorrhage; shock due to acute injury; etc. 2. Major surgical operation under general anesthesia	1. Hypnosis 2. Convulsive treatments (electroshock, insulin, etc.) 3. Surgical treatments (lobotomy, etc.)

2. Guidance-cooperation	Whatever the physician does; similar to the above	Similar to the above, albeit patient's judgment is no longer completely irrelevant; success of therapy is still the physician's private decision; if patient agrees, he is a good patient, but if he disagrees he is bad or "uncooperative"	The presence or absence of "signs" and "symptoms"; the physician's particular concept of "disease" "health" (e.g., (usually, infection) no disease; e.g., no infection)	Most of general medicine and the postoperative care of surgical patients (e.g., prescription of drugs, "advice" to smoke less, etc.)	1. "Suggestion," counseling, therapy based on "advice," etc. 2. Some modifications of psychoanalytic therapy 3. So-called psychotherapy "combined" with physical therapies (e.g., electric shock)
3. Mutual participation	An abstraction of one aspect of the relationship, embodying the activities of both participants; "treatment" cannot be said to take place unless both participants orient themselves to the task ahead	Much more poorly defined than in the previous models: evaluation of the result will depend on both the physician's and the patient's judgments and is further complicated by the fact that these may change in the very process of treatment	The notions of disease and health lose most of their relevance in this context; the notions of more or less successful (for certain purposes) modes of behavior, adaptation, or integration take the place of the earlier, more categorical concepts	The treatment of patients with certain chronic diseases or structural defects; for example, the management of diabetes mellitus or of myasthenia gravis; "rehabilitation" of patients with orthopedic defects, such as learning the use of prostheses, etc.	1. Psychoanalysis 2. Some modifications of psychoanalytic therapy

overlooked that, for the results to be meaningful, significant conceptual similarities must exist between the operations which are compared. The three categories of the doctor-patient relationship are concretely useful in delineating areas within which meaningful comparisons can be made. Comparisons between therapies belonging to different categories are philosophically (and logically) meaningless and lead to fruitless controversy.

To illustrate this thesis let us consider some examples. A typical comparison, with which we can begin, is that of the various agents used in the treatment of lobar pneumonia: type-specific antisera, sulfonamides, and penicillin. Each superseded the other, as the increased efficacy of the newer preparations was demonstrated. This sort of comparison is meaningful because there is agreement as to what is being treated and as to what constitutes a "successful" result. There should be no need to belabor this point. What is important is that this conceptual model of therapeutic comparisons is constantly used in situations in which it does not apply; that is, in situations in which there is clear-cut disagreement as to what constitutes "cure." In this connection, the problem of peptic ulcer will exemplify a group of illnesses in which several therapeutic approaches are possible.

This question is often posed: Is surgical, medical, or psychiatric treatment the "best" for peptic ulcer?[3] Unless we specify conditions, goals, and the "price" we are willing to pay (in the largest sense of the word), the question is meaningless. In the case of peptic ulcer, it is immediately apparent that each therapeutic approach implies a different conception of "disease" and correspondingly divergent notions of "cure." At the risk of slight overstatement, it can be said that according to the surgical viewpoint the disease is the "lesion," treatment aims at its eradication (by surgical means), and cure consists of its persistent absence (nonrecurrence). If a patient undergoes a vagotomy and all evidence of the lesion disappears, he is considered cured even if he develops another (apparently unrelated) illness six months later. It should be emphasized that no criticism of this frame of reference is intended. The foregoing (surgical) approach is entirely appropriate, and accusations of "narrowness" are no more (nor less) justified than they would be against any other specialized branch of knowledge.

To continue our analysis of therapeutic comparisons, let us consider the same patient (with peptic ulcer) in the hands of an internist. This specialist might have a somewhat different idea of what is wrong with him than did the surgeon. He might regard peptic ulcer as an essentially chronic disease (perhaps due to heredity and other "predispositions"), with which the patient probably will have to live as comfortably as possible for years. This point is emphasized to demonstrate that the surgeon and the internist do not treat the "same disease." How then can the two methods of treatment and their results be compared? The most that can be hoped for is to be able to determine to what extent each method is appropriate and successful within its own frame of reference.

If we take our hypothetical patient to a psychoanalyst, the situation is even more radically different. This specialist will state that he is not treating the "ulcer" and might even go so far as to say that he is not treating the patient for his ulcer. The psychoanalyst (or psychiatrist) has his own ideas about what constitutes "disease," "treatment," and "cure" (Zilboorg 1941; Bowman and Rose 1954).

Conclusions

Comments have been made on some factors which provide satisfactions to both patient and physician in various therapeutic relationships. In conclusion, we call attention to two important considerations regarding the complementary situations described.

First, it might be thought that one of the three basic models of the doctor-patient relationship is in some fundamental (perhaps ethical) way "better" than another. In particular, it might be considered that it is better to identify with the patient than to treat him like a helplessly sick person. We have tried to avoid such an inference. In our opinion, each of the three types of therapeutic relationship is entirely appropriate under certain circumstances and each is inappropriate under others.

Secondly, we will comment on the therapeutic relationship as a situation (more or less fixed in time) and as a process (leading to change in one or both participants). Most of our previous comments have dealt with the relationship as a situation. It is, however, also a process in that the patient may change not only in terms of his symptoms but also in the way he wishes to relate to his doctor. A typical example is the patient with diabetes mellitus who, when first seen, is in coma. At this time, the relationship must be based on the activity-passivity model. Later, he has to be educated (guided) at the level of cooperation. Finally, ideally, he is treated as a full-fledged partner in the management of his own health (mutual participation). Confronted by a problem of this type, the physician is called upon to change through a corresponding spectrum of attitudes. If he cannot make these changes, he may interfere with the patient's progress and may promote an arrest at some intermediate stage in the evolution toward relative self-management. The other possibility in this situation is that both physician and patient will become dissatisfied with each other. This outcome, however unfortunate, is probably the commonest one. Most of us can probably verify it firsthand in the roles of both physician and patient (Pinner and Miller 1952).

At such juncture, the physician usually feels that the patient is "uncooperative" and "difficult," whereas the patient regards the physician as "unsympathetic" and lacking in understanding of his personally unique needs. Both are correct. Bot are confronted by the wish to induce changes in the other. As we well know, this is no easy task. The dilemma is usually resolved when the patient seeks another physician, one who is more attuned to his (new) needs. Conversely, the physician will "seek" a new patient, usually one who will benefit from the physician's (old) needs and corresponding attitudes. And so life goes on.

The pattern described accounts for the familiar fact that patients often choose physicians not solely, or even primarily, on the basis of technical skill. Considerable weight is given to the type of human relationship which they foster. Some patients prefer to be "unconscious" (figuratively speaking), irrespective of what ails them. Others go to the other extreme. The majority probably falls somewhere between these two polar opposites. Physicians, motivated by similar personal "conflicts" form a complementary series. Thus, there is an interlocking integration of the sick and his healer.

Summary

The introduction of the construct of "human relationship" represents an addition to the repertoire of fundamental medical concepts.

Three basic models of the doctor-patient relationship have been described, with examples. The models are (1) Activity-passivity. The comatose patient is completely helpless. The physician must take over and do something to him. (2) Guidance-cooperation. The patient with an acute infectious process seeks help and is ready and willing to cooperate. He turns to the physician for guidance. (3) Mutual participation. The patient with a chronic disease is aided to help himself.

The physician's own inner needs (and satisfactions) form a complementary series with those of the patient.

The general problem usually referred to with the question "what is good medicine?" has been briefly considered. Different types of doctor-patient relationships imply different concepts of "disease," "treatment," and "cure." This is of importance in comparing diverse therapeutic methods. Meaningful comparisons can be made only if interventions are based on the same frame of reference.

It has been emphasized that different types of doctor-patient relationships are necessary and appropriate for various circumstances. Problems in human contact between physician and patient often arise if in the course of treatment changes require an alteration in the pattern of the doctor-patient relationship. This may lead to a dissolution of the relationship.

Notes

1. In our approach to this subject we have been influenced by psychologic (psychoanalytic), sociologic, and philosophic considerations. See in this connection Dewey and Bentley 1949; Russell 1938; Szasz 1955; Szasz 195X.

2. We omit any discussion of the physician's technical skill, training, equipment, etc. These factors, of course, are of importance, and we do not minimize them. The problem of what is "good medicine" can be considered from a number of viewpoints (e.g., technical skill, economic considerations, social roles, human relationships, etc.). Our scope in this essay is limited to but one—sometimes quite unimportant— aspect of the contact between physician and patient.

3. Such a question is roughly comparable to asking, "Is an automobile or an airplane better—without specifying for what. See Rapoport 1954.

References

Bowman, K. M., and M. Rose. 1954. Do Our Medical Colleagues Know What to Expect from Psychotherapy? *Am. J. Psychiat.* 111: 401.

Dewey, J., and A. F. Bentley. 1949. *Knowing and the Known.* Beacon.

Dubos, R. J. 1955. Second Thoughts on the Germ Theory. *Sci. Am.* 192: 31.

Jones, E. 1951. The God Complex. In E. Jones, *Essays in Applied Psychoanalysis,* vol. 2. Hogarth.

Marmor, J. 1953. The Feeling of Superiority: An Occupational Hazard in the Practice of Psychotherapy. *Am. J. Psychiat.* 110: 370.

Pinner, M., and B. F. Miller, eds. 1952 *When Doctors Are Patients.* Norton.

Rapoport, A. 1954. *Operational Philosophy.* Harper.

Ruesch, J., and G. Bateson. 1951. *Communication: The Social Matrix of Psychiatry.* Norton.

Russell, B. 1938. *Power: A New Social Analysis.* Norton.

Szasz, T. S. 1955. Entropy, Organization, and the Problem of the Economy of Human Relationships. *Int. J. Psychoanal.* 36: 289.

Szasz, T. S. 1957. On the Theory of Psychoanalytic Treatment. *Int. J. Psychoanal.* 38.

4

Client Control and Medical
Practice[1]
Eliot Freidson

That the medical practitioner is typically a colleague in a structure of
institutions and organizations, the patient being an essentially minor
contingency, is the picture presented in the general discussions of
Carr-Saunders and Wilson,[2] Parsons,[3] Merton,[4] and Goode,[5] as well
as in studies of medical practice by Hall,[6] Solomon,[7] Hyde,[8] Peterson,[9] and Coleman, Menzel, and Katz.[10] The nature of medical
practice is seen as determined largely by the practitioner's relation to
his colleagues and their institutions and by the profession's relation to
the state.

But practice cannot exist without clients, and clients often have
ideas about what they want that differ markedly from those supposedly held by the professionals they consult. As anthropologists
have so copiously illustrated,[11] the client's choice is guided by norms
that differ from culture to culture and even within a single complex
culture.[12] And, after the client has exercised his choice to see a
practitioner, normative or cultural differences between patient and
physician qualify the relationship considerably.[13] These characteristics, in the client, obviously are a systematic source of pressure on the
practitioner. To understand medical practice, therefore, one must
learn the circumstances in which the pressure is initiated and sustained, and this requires regarding the client and the practitioner in a
single analytical system in which one explores the sources of strength
of each.

To bring the two together, analysis must proceed on a model of
society that is more common to anthropological than to sociological
studies. Practice seems usefully analyzed not only as a set of practitioners interacting with each other[14] but as a concrete local situation
in which two systems touch to form a larger whole in which there are

characteristic norms, positions, and movements. To isolate the whole, the model is not that of a society within which there are practitioners and clients,[15] or of a consultation room in which there are a practitioner and a client,[16] but of a system in which representatives of the medical profession practice in consultation rooms located in local communities of prospective clients. In recognizing practitioners as members of a profession, reference may be made to their organization and culture. In recognizing clients are members of a specific local community, reference may be made to their own organization and culture. In joining the two within a community, instances studied by anthropologists in which professional practitioners find it difficult to get clients can find as much of a place in the analysis as instances in which professional practice is so thoroughly accepted by clients as to be almost (but never quite) routine.

It is the purpose of this paper to use such a model to organize analysis of aspects of client experience that may significantly affect medical practice and to outline a descriptive typology of such practice, the analysis being put in a sufficiently general fashion to allow application to other types of professional practice.

Characteristically, the professional practitioner claims that his skills are so esoteric that the client is in no position to evaluate them. From this stems his privilege to be somewhat removed from the marketplace and to accept the evaluation of his colleagues rather than of his clients.[17] And this claim is one mark of his separation as a member of a professional "community."[18]

But, while his own "community" may be without physical locus, he must *practice* in a spatially located community among more or less organized potential clients. Thus, while he is a member of a professional "community," accepting its norms and formally dependent on its institutions, the practitioner is always a kind of stranger in the community of his practice, for his reference group is his colleagues, not his clients.

However, while the physician may share special knowledge, identity, and loyalty with his colleagues rather than with laymen, he is dependent upon laymen for his livelihood. Where he does not have the power to force them to use his services, he depends upon the free choice of prospective patients.[19] But, since these prospective clients are in no position to evaluate his services as would his colleagues, and insofar as they do exercise choice, it follows that they must evaluate him by nonprofessional criteria and that they will interact with him on the basis of nonprofessional norms. Hence practice generically consists in interaction between two different, sometimes conflicting, sets of norms.

Consequently, we have two systems, the professional and the lay. In any concrete situation the two touch: the local physician may be seen as the "hinge" between a local lay system and an "outside" professional system. Structurally, the practitioner's support theoretically lies outside the community in which he practices, in the hands of his colleagues, while his prospective clientele are organized by the community itself. Culturally, the professional's referent is by definition "the great tradition" of his supralocal profession, while his prospective clientele's referent is the "little tradition" of the local community or neighborhood.[20] The lay tradition of the local community may, in one place or another, absorb varying amounts of the professional tradition, but by the nature of the case, as Saunders and Hewes have so persuasively argued,[21] lay medical culture seems unlikely ever to become identical with professional medical culture.

How are the physician and his prospective clientele brought together? How is consultation initiated and sustained? Obviously, the prospective client must perceive some need for help and that it is a physician who can help him. And, if solo practice is the rule, he must determine who is a "good" practitioner. These perceptions seem to emerge from a process of interpersonal influence similar to that studied in other areas of life, a process organized by the culture and structure of the community or neighborhood through which "outside" knowledge and evaluation is strained.

In one locality,[22] conceiving the need for "outside" help for a physical disorder seems to be initiated by purely personal, tentative self-diagnoses that stress the temporary character of the symptoms and to end by the prescribing of delay to see what happens. If the symptoms persist, simple home remedies such as rest, aspirin, antacids, laxatives, and change of diet will be tried. At the point of trying some remedy, however, the potential patient attracts the attention of his household, if he has not asked for attention already. Diagnosis then is shared, and new remedies may be suggested, or a visit to a physician. If a practitioner is not seen, but the symptoms continue (and in most cases the symptoms do not continue), the diagnostic resources of friends, neighbors, relatives, and fellow workers may be explored. This is rarely very deliberate; it takes place in daily intercourse, initiated first by inquiries about health and only afterward about the weather.

This casual exploring of diagnoses, when it is drawn out and not stopped early by the cessation of symptoms or by resort to a physician, typically takes the form of referrals through a hierarchy of authority. Discussion of symptoms and their remedies is referral as much as prescription—referral to some other layman who himself had and cured the same symptoms, to someone who was once a nurse and therefore knows about such things, to a druggist who once fixed someone up with a wonderful brown tonic, and, of course, to a marvelous doctor who treated the very same thing successfully.

Indeed, the whole process of seeking help involves a network of potential consultants, from the intimate and informal confines of the nuclear family through successively more select, distant, and authoritative laymen, until the "professional" is reached.[23] This network of consultants, which is part of the structure of the local lay community and which imposes form on the seeking of help, might be called the "lay referral structure." Taken together with the cultural understandings involved in the process, we may speak of it as the "lay referral system."

There are as many lay referral systems as there are communities, but it is possible to classify all systems by two critical variables—the degree of congruence between the culture of the clientele and that of the profession and the relative number of lay consultants who are interposed between the first perception of symptoms and the decision to see a professional. Considerations of culture have relevance to the diagnoses and prescriptions that are meaningful to the client and to the kinds of consultants considered authoritative. Consideration of the extensiveness of the lay referral structure has relevance to the channeling and reinforcement of lay culture and to the flowing-in of "outside" communications.

These variables may be combined so as to yield four types of lay referral system, of which only two need be discussed here—first, a system in which the prospective clients participate primarily in an indigenous lay culture and in which there is a highly extended lay referral structure and, second, a system in which the prospective clients participate in a culture of maximum congruence with that of the profession in which there is a severely truncated referral structure or none at all.

The indigenous, extended system is an extreme instance in which the clientele of a community may be expected to show a high degree of resistance to using medical services. Insofar as the idea of diagnostic authority is based on an assumed hereditary or divine "gift" or on intrinsically personal knowledge of one's "own" health, necessary for effective treatment, professional authority is unlikely to be recognized at all. And, insofar as the cultural definitions of illness contradict those of professional culture, the referral process will not often lead to the professional practitioner. In turn, with an extended lay referral structure, lay definitions are supported by a variety of lay consultants, when the sick man looks about for help. Obviously, here the folk practitioner will be used by most, the professional practitioner being called for minor illnesses only, or, in illness considered critical, called only by the socially isolated deviate, and by the sick man desperately snatching at straws.

The opposite extreme of the indigenous extended system is found when the lay culture and the professional culture are much alike and when the lay referral system is truncated or there is none at all. Here, the prospective client is pretty much on his own, guided more or less by cultural understandings and his own experience, with few lay consultants to support or discourage his search for help. Since his knowledge and understandings are much like the physician's, he may take a great deal of time trying to treat himself, but nonetheless will go directly from self-treatment to a physician.

Of these extreme cases, the former is exemplified by the behavior of primitive people and the latter by the behavior of physicians or nurses when taken ill. (Paradoxically, they are notoriously "uncooperative" patients, given to diagnosing and treating themselves.) Between these two extremes, in the United States at least, members of the lower class participate in lay referral systems resembling the indigenous case, and members of the professional class tend toward the other pole, with the remaining classes taking their places in the middle ranges of the continuum.[24]

As Goode has noted, "Client choices are a form of social control. They determine the survival of a profession or a specialty, as well as the career success of particular professionals."[25] The concept of lay referral system, thus, provides a basis not only for organizing knowledge about the patient's behavior but also for understanding conditions under which he, a layman, to some extent controls professional practice. Indeed, the lay referral system illuminates the ways in which the client's choice is qualified and channeled and how the physician's sex, race, and ethnic background affect his success—though it is often said that professions rest upon achieved status.[26] We can see now why a practitioner may never get any clients, and why, on the other hand, he may get clients but then lose them; for the lay referral system not only channels the client's choice but also sustains it or, later on, leads him to change his mind. Interviews with urban patients reveal that the first visit to a practitioner is often tentative, a tryout. Whether the physician's prescription will be followed or not, and whether the patient will come back, seems to rest at least partly on his retrospective assessment of the professional consultation. The client may form an opinion by himself, or, as is often the case, he may compare notes with others—indeed, he passes through the referral structure not only on his way to the physician but also on his way back, discussing the doctor's behavior, diagnosis, and prescription with his fellows, with the possible consequence that he may never go back.

One might assume that all but the most thick-skinned practitioner soon become aware of lay evaluations, whether through repeated requests of their patients for vitamins or wonder drugs or through repeated disappearances or protests following the employment of scientifically acceptable prescriptions such as calomel or bleeding. Whether their motive be to heal the patient or to survive professionally, they will feel pressure to accept or manipulate lay expectations, whether by administering harmless placebos[27] or by giving up unpopular drugs.[28]

In a relatively organized community, channels of influence and authority that exist independently of the profession may guide the patient toward or away from the physician and may more or less control not only the latter's success but, to some extent, also his professional technique and manner;[29] in short, the lay referral system is a major contingency of medical practice. Practice in an indigenous extended system must adjust itself to the system in order to exist: when involving patients who are themselves professionals, it may make fewer adjustments.

The above discussion of the lay referral system should be taken to show that, in being *relatively* free, the medical profession should not be mistaken for being *absolutely* free from control by patients. Indeed, we may classify various kinds of professional practice on the basis of relative freedom from client control. But, to do so, we must examine sources of professional freedom that lie not in a complaisant clientele but in the nature of professional organization itself.

Enough has been written about the privileged position that the organized power of the state grants the practitioner. (Indeed, this support by power located outside the community is often crucial to practice in "underdeveloped" countries where the prospective patients do not have a high opinion of modern physicians.) At the same time, political support sets severe limitations on competition,[30] both by prosecuting irregular "folk" or "quack" practice and by allowing restriction of the number of professional practitioners, two measures which greatly contribute to the stability and independence of the professional role.

Beyond these measures, however, we must note an additional important source of strength: Insofar as there are two "traditions" and two structures in a community, the lay referral system is one, and what we might call the "professional referral system" is the other. The professional referral system is a structure or network of relationships with colleagues that often extends beyond the local community and tends to converge upon professionally controlled organizations such as hospital and medical schools. Professional prestige and power radiate out from the latter and diminish with distance from them. The authoritative source of professional culture—that is, medical knowledge—also lies in these organizations, partly created by them and partly flowing to them from the outside.

The farther this professional referral system is penetrated, the more free it is of any particular local community of patients. A layman seeking help finds that, the farther within it he goes, the fewer choices can he make and the less can he control what is done to him. Indeed, it is not unknown for the "client" to be a petitioner, asking to be chosen: the organizations and practitioners who stand well within the professional referral system may or may not "take the case," according to their judgment of its interest.

This fundamental symmetry, in which the client chooses his professional services when they are in the lay referral system and in which the physician chooses the patient to whom to give his services when he is in the professional referral system, demonstrates additional circumstances of the seeking of help. When he first feels ill, the patient thinks he is competent to judge whether he is actually ill and what general class of illness it is. On this basis he treats himself. Failure of his initial prescriptions leads him into the lay referral structure, and the failure of other lay prescriptions leads him to the physician. Upon this preliminary career of failures the practical authority of the physician rests, though it must be remembered that the client may still think he knows what is wrong with him.

This movement through the lay referral system is predicated upon the client's conception of what he needs. The practitioner standing at the apex of the lay referral system is the last consultant chosen on the basis of those lay conceptions.[31] When that chosen practitioner cannot himself handle the problem, it becomes *his* function, not that of the patient or his lay consultants, to refer to another practitioner. At this point the professional referral system is entered. Choice, and therefore positive control, is now taken out of the hands of the client and comes to rest in the hands of the practitioner, and the use of professional services is no longer predicated on the client's lay understandings—indeed, the client may be given services for which he did not ask, whose rationale is beyond him. Obviously, the patient by now is relatively helpless, divorced from his lay supports.

From the point of view of the physician, position in the process of referrals is also of importance. If he is the first practitioner seen in the lay referral structure, and if he sends no cases further on, he is subjected only to the lay evaluation of his patients as they pass back through the hands of their lay consultants after they leave him. If he refers a case to another practitioner, however, his professional behavior becomes subject to the evaluation of the consultant. In turn, when the patient leaves the consultant, he often passes back to the referring practitioner, so in this sense the professional consultant is subjected to the evaluation of the referring physician. Thus the physician who subsists on patients referred by colleagues is almost always subject to evaluation and control by his colleagues, while the practitioner who attracts patients himself and need not refer them to others is subject primarily to evaluation and control at the hands of his patients.

These observations suggest two extreme types of practice, differing in the relation of practice to the lay and to the professional referral systems. At one extreme is a practice that can operate independently of colleagues, its existence predicated on attracting its own lay clientele.[32] In order to do so, this "independent practice" must offer services for which those in a lay referral system themselves feel the need. In reality, of course, it will be conditioned both by the existence of competitors and by the particular lay system in which it finds itself, but on the whole, one should expect it to be incapable of succeeding unless conducted in close accord with lay expectations. To survive without colleagues, it must be located within a lay referral system and, as such, is *least* able to resist control by clients, and *most* able to resist control by colleagues.

At the other extreme is postulated a "dependent practice" that does not in and by itself attract its own clientele but, instead, serves the needs of other practices, individual or organizational. The lay clientele with whom the practice must sometimes deal does not choose the service involved. A professional colleague or organization decides that a client needs the services of a professional in a dependent practice and transmits the client to him. The colleague or organization alone, in many cases, is told the results of the consultation.

Obviously, by definition, dependent practice could not exist in a lay referral system. To survive without self-selected clients, it must be in a professional referral system where clients are so helpless that they may be merely transmitted. As such, dependent practice is *most* able to resist control by clients and *least* able to resist control by colleagues.

The logical extreme of independent practice does not seem fully applicable to any professional practice, if only because a professional practitioner is trained outside the lay community before he enters it to practice and because his license to practice ultimately depends upon his colleagues "outside" and may be revoked. The "quack" seems to fit this logical extreme, for not only does he not require outside certification but, as Hughes defined him, he is one "who continues through time to please his customers but not his colleagues." [33] He, like the folk practitioner, is a consultant relatively high in the structure of lay referrals, with no connection with an outside professional referral system.

Close to this extreme in the United States is the independent neighborhood or village practice (usually general in nature) that Hall calls "individualistic," [34] with, at best, loose cooperative ties to colleagues and to loosely organized points in the professional referral system. All else being equal in this situation of minimal observability by colleagues and maximum dependence on the lay referral system, we should expect to find the least sensitivity to formal professional standards.[35] and the greatest sensitivity to the local lay standards.[36] This differential sensitivity should show up best where the lay referral system is indigenous and extended.

Moving toward the position of dependent practice is what Hall called the "colleague practice," in close connection with a well-organized "inner fraternity" of colleagues and rigidly organized service institutions.[37] This practice tends to revolve around specialties, which in itself makes for location outside particular neighborhoods or villages, and therefore reduces the possibility of organized control by the clients.

Finally, the closest to the extreme of dependent practice is a type that overlaps somewhat with the "colleague practice" but that seems sufficiently significant to consider separately. It might be called "organizational practice." Found in hospitals, clinics, and other professional bureaucracies,[38] it involves maximal restriction on the client's choice of individuals or services. Clients are referred by other practitioners to the organization, or, if they are seeking help on their own, they exercise choice only in selecting the organization itself, functionaries of which then screen them and refer them to a practitioner. Here, practice is dependent upon organizational auspices and equipment. The client's efforts at control are most likely to take the form of evasion. The events of the referral process being systematically recorded and scrutinized, and ordered by hierarchical supervision, the practitioner is highly vulnerable to his colleagues' evaluations. We should expect him to be most sensitive to professional standards and controls and least sensitive to the expectations of his patient.

This paper has stressed two notions—that variation in the culture and organization of patients and in the location of medical practice in the community is decisive in the introducing and sustaining of practice and in the technical and interpersonal modes of procedure in established practice. These closely interrelated notions were derived by conceiving of practice in relation to organized lay communities as well as to organized professional systems and by following the prospective patient through the two referral systems. The outcome emphasized was the relative extent to which control lay in the client's or in the practitioner's hands.

Like any analysis in which one must hold much of reality in abeyance, this has produced a certain amount of exaggeration. Where practice is already established, as opposed to where it is struggling to establish itself, much of what goes on is routine and conflict between the patient and the physician is rarely open but is masked by evasion and depends upon the practitioner's justified assumption that incompatible clientele will stay away or can be discouraged easily. Within this routine, such breaks and irritations as do exist are, of course, strategic areas to study, but the very routine, with the stable set of selected patients it implies, when compared from place to place, practice to practice, should reveal the compromises necessary to establish and maintain practice in the face of varying lay systems and varying positions in the lay and professional systems. Thus, the abstractly conceived professional role as described by such writers as Parsons may be qualified—indeed, sometimes, compromised—by the cultural and structural conditions in which it must be played.

Notes and References

1. Revision of a paper read at the 1959 meetings of the American Sociological Society, Chicago.

2. A. M. Carr-Saunders and P. A. Wilson, *The Professions* (Oxford: Clarendon Press, 1933).

3. Talcott Parsons, "The Professions and Social Structure," in his *Essays in Sociological Theory Pure and Applied* (Glencoe, Ill.: Free Press, 1949), pp. 185–99.

4. Robert K. Merton, "Some Preliminaries to a Sociology of Medical Education," in Robert K. Merton, George G. Reader, and Patricia L. Kendall (eds.), *The Student-Physician* (Cambridge, Mass.: Harvard University Press, 1957), pp. 73–79.

5. William J. Goode, "Community within a Community: The Professions," *American Sociological Review* 22 (April, 1957), 194–200.

6. Oswald Hall, "The Informal Organization of the Medical Profession," *Canadian Journal of Economics and Political Science* 12 (February, 1946), 30–41; "The Stages of the Medical Career," *American Journal of Sociology* 53 (March, 1948), 327–36; and "Types of Medical Careers," *ibid* 55 (November, 1949), 243–53.

7. David N. Solomon, "Career Contingencies of Chicago Physicians" (unpublished Ph.D. dissertation, University of Chicago, 1952).

8. David R. Hyde and Payson Wolff, with Anne Gross and Elliott L. Hoffman, "The American Medical Association: Power, Purpose and Politics in Organized Medicine," *Yale Law Journal* 63 (May, 1954), 938–1022.

9. Osler L. Peterson *et al.*, "An Analytical Study of North Carolina General Practice, 1953–1954." *Journal of Medical Education* 31, Part II (December, 1956), 1–165.

10. Herbert Menzel and Elihu Katz, "Social Relations and Innovation in the Medical Profession: The Epidemiology of a New Drug," *Public Opinion Quarterly* 19 (Winter, 1955–56), 337–52; James Coleman, Elihu Katz, and Herbert Menzel, "The Diffusion of an Innovation among Physicians," *Sociometry* 20 (December, 1957), 253–70; Herbert Menzel, James Coleman, and Elihu Katz, "Dimensions of Being 'Modern' in Medical Practice," *Journal of Chronic Diseases* 19 (January, 1959), 20–40.

11. E.g., Benjamin D. Paul (ed.), *Health Culture and Community* (New York: Russell Sage Foundation, 1955), and the studies cited in George M. Foster, *Problems in Intercultural Health Programs* ("Social Science Research Council Pamphlets," No. 12 [New York, 1958]).

12. E.g., Earl L. Koos, *The Health of Regionville* (New York: Columbia University Press, 1954), and the excellent summary and bibliography in Ozzie G. Simmons, *Social Status and Public Health* ("Social Science Research Council Pamphlets," No. 13 [New York, 1958]).

13. E.g., Lyle W. Saunders, *Cultural Differences and Medical Care* (New York: Russell Sage Foundation, 1954).

14. Hall's stress on the "inner fraternity" implies this even though he has some important things to say about clients (see Hall "Informal Organization," *op. cit.*, pp. 30–31). He is primarily concerned with how a physician obtains a clientele already organized into practices.

15. Goode (*op. cit.*) exploits this perspective.

16. Cf. Talcott Parsons, *The Social System* (Glencoe, Ill.: Free Press, 1954), pp. 428–73.

17. See Everett C. Hughes, "Licence and Mandate," in Everett C. Hughes, *Men and Their Work* (Glencoe, Ill.: Free Press, 1958), pp. 78–87.

18. Goode, *op. cit., passim.* Goode uses the term "community" in the sense of shared interests and identity. Thus all American physicians belong to the medical "com-

munity," just as all American Catholics belong to the Catholic "community." I use the term to mean locality.

19. It is not predicated here that clients choose particular practitioners—that is, that practice is characteristically solo, fee-for-service in nature. Choice of physician is made to some degree by clients in the United States but hardly in other countries (cf., on Israel, J. Ben-David, "The Professional Role of the Physician in Bureaucratized Medicine: A Study in Role Conflict," *Human Relations* 11 [1958], 255–74). The choice the client must make everywhere is not which doctor to see but whether to see one at all.

20. The terms and image are those of Robert Redfield. See his *Peasant Society and Culture* (Chicago: University of Chicago Press, 1956), pp. 43–45, and his "A Community within Communities," *The Little Community* (Chicago: University of Chicago Press, 1955), pp. 113–51. In industrial society the "little tradition" seems less stable than in peasant society and more dependent upon the "great tradition" for its content.

21. L. Saunders and G. H. Hewes, "Folk Medicine and Medical Practice," *Journal of Medical Education* 28 (September, 1953), 43–46.

22. The following sketch stems from intensive interviews with 71 patients of a metropolitan medical group, in which they were asked to give detailed chronological accounts of the way in which they were led to seek medical care. It is not intended to describe the average experience but is a synthetic construct designed to portray the full length to which the process may go before professional practice is reached. The data suggest that the longer the process that intervenes between first perception of difficulty and contact with a practitioner, the greater the likelihood that the symptoms are ambiguous and not unbearable: a broken leg has different consequences from a "cold" of excessive duration.

23. For data on the referral process and the network of consultants see E. E. Evans-Pritchard, *Witchcraft, Oracles and Magic Among the Azande* (Oxford: Clarendon Press, 1937); M. R. Yarrow, C. G. Schwartz, H. S. Murphy, and L. C. Deasy, "The Psychological Meaning of Mental Illness in the Family," *Journal of Social Issues* 11 (1955), 12–24; John A. Clausen and M. R. Yarrow, "Paths to the Mental Hospital," *Journal of Social Issues* 11 (1955), 25–32; Erving Goffman, "The Moral Career of the Mental Patient," *Psychiatry* 22 (May, 1959), 123–42.

24. See the review of studies in Simmons, *op. cit.*

25. *Op. cit.*, p. 198.

26. E.g., Talcott Parsons, "The Professions," *op. cit.*, pp. 189 and 193; note the qualification on p. 197.

27. The placebo might be used as an index of control by the client of the terms of practice. On rationalizing sleight-of-hand as the placebo see Evans-Pritchard, *op. cit.*, pp. 235–36.

28. "This helplessness of regular physicians, coupled with popular distaste for bleeding and vile medicines, goes far to explain the success enjoyed by large groups of irregular practitioners.... A not uncommon shingle advertisement in those early years was: Dr. John Doe; No Calomel" (Thomas Neville Bonner, *Medicine in Chicago, 1850–1950* [Madison, Wis.: American History Research Center, 1957], p. 12). When doctors began to do less dosing in the late eighteenth and early nineteenth centuries, the public went out and bought its own medicine (Richard Harrison Shryock, *The Development of Modern Medicine* [New York: Alfred A. Knopf, 1947], pp. 248 ff.).

29. Cf. the devices used in China and in Europe to avoid offending the patient's sense of modesty—Howard Dittrick, "Chinese Medical Dolls," *Bulletin of the History of Medicine* 26 (September–October, 1952), 422–29; Julius Friedenwald and Samuel Morrison, "The History of the Enema with Some Notes on Related Procedures," *Bulletin of the History of Medicine* 8 (January, 1940), 68–114, and *ibid.*, February, 1940, pp. 239–76. On modern practice, articles in *Medical Economics* provide evidence.

30. To cite a dramatic instance of earlier competition: Two tenth-century physicians who were competing for the favor of a king ended by poisoning each other at the king's dinner table. The one who knew the antidotes obtained the king's patronage (L. C. MacKinney, "Tenth Century Medicine as Seen in the *Historia* of Richter of Rheims," *Bulletin of the History of Medicine* 2 [August, 1934], 367–68). The veracity of this is questioned in P. O. Kristeller, "The School of Salerno," *Bulletin of the History of Medicine* 17 (February, 1945), 143–44, but as the historian Louis Gottschalk once said, "Se non è vero è ben trovato." For modern times Hall's observations on the "individualistic career" are relevant.

31. The actual specialty of the practitioner's standing in the lay referral system varies; certainly, the general practitioner is almost always within it. Often pediatricians, gynecologists, internists, and ophthalmologists are to be found within it, particularly in communities of the professional classes; pathologists, anesthesiologists, and radiologists are unlikely ever to be within it.

32. See my paper "Specialties without Roots: The Utilization of New Services," *Human Organization* 18 (Fall, 1959).

33. Hughes, *op. cit.*, p. 98.

34. See Hall, "Types of Medical Career," *op. cit.*, pp. 249–52, and Solomon, *op. cit.*, chaps. vi and vii on physicians connected with Group II hospitals.

35. This, rather than medical education, might be an important determinant of the findings in Peterson *et al.*; *op cit.*

36. As examples of the effect of clients' prejudices on success and location see Josephine J. Williams, "Patients and Prejudice: Attitudes toward Women Physicians," *American Journal of Sociology* 51 (January, 1946), 283–87; and Stanley Lieberson, "Ethnic Groups and the Practice of Medicine," *American Sociological Review* 23 (October, 1958), 542–49. For the effect of the type of legal practice on participation in community affairs see Walter I. Wardwell and Arthur L. Wood, "The Extra-Professional Role of the Lawyer," *American Journal of Sociology* 61 (January, 1956), 304–7; Arthur Lewis Wood, "Informal Relations in the Practice of Criminal Law," *American Journal of Sociology* 62 (July, 1956), 48–55.

37. See Hall, "Types of Medical Careers," *op. cit.*, pp. 246–49; see also Solomon, *op. cit.*, chaps vi and vii, on physicians connected with Group I hospitals. In "colleague practice" it seems that the colleagues' racial or ethnic prejudice determines success, not the clients'.

38. This term is defined in Dennis C. McElrath, "Prepaid Group Medical Practice: A Comparative Analysis of Organizations and Perspectives" (unpublished Ph.D. dissertation, Yale University, 1958); its problems are analyzed in Mary E. W. Goss, "Physicians in Bureaucracy: A Case Study of Professional Pressures on Organizational Roles" (unpublished Ph.D. dissertation, Columbia University, 1959). See also Ben-David, *op. cit.* Unfortunately for our present purposes, none of these studies paid much attention to the role of the client.

5

Negotiating Reality: Notes on Power in the Assessment of Responsibility
Thomas J. Scheff

The use of interrogation to reconstruct parts of an individual's past history is a common occurrence in human affairs. Reporters, jealous lovers, and policemen on the beat are often faced with the task of determining events in another person's life, and the extent to which he was responsible for those events. The most dramatic use of interrogation to determine responsibility is in criminal trials. As in everyday life, criminal trials are concerned with both act and intent. Courts, in most cases, first determine whether the defendant performed a legally forbidden act. If it is found that he did so, the court then must decide whether he was "responsible" for the act. Reconstructive work of this type goes on less dramatically in a wide variety of other settings, as well. The social worker determining a client's eligibility for unemployment compensation, for example, seeks not only to establish that the client actually is unemployed, but that he has actively sought employment, i.e., that he himself is not responsible for being out of work.

This paper will contrast two perspectives on the process of reconstructing past events for the purpose of fixing responsibility. The first perspective stems from the common-sense notion that interrogation, when it is sufficiently skillful, is essentially neutral. Responsibility for past actions can be fixed absolutely, independent of the method of reconstruction. This perspective is held by the typical member of society, engaged in his day-to-day tasks. It is also held, in varying degrees, by most professional interrogators. The basic working doctrine is one of *absolute* responsibility. This point of view actually entails the comparison of two different kinds of items: first, the fixing of actions and intentions, and second, comparing these

Reprinted, with permission, from *Social Problems* 16 (1968): 3 ff.

actions and intentions to some predetermined criteria of responsibility. The basic premise of the doctrine of absolute responsibility is that both actions and intentions, on the one hand, and the criteria of responsibility, on the other, are absolute, in that they can be assessed independent of social context.[1]

An alternative approach follows from the sociology of knowledge. From this point of view, the reality within which members of society conduct their lives is largely of their own construction.[2] Since much of reality is a construction, there may be multiple realities, existing side by side, in harmony or in competition. It follows, if one maintains this stance, that the assessment of responsibility involves the construction of reality by members; construction of actions and intentions, on the one hand, and of criteria of responsibility, on the other. The former process, the continuous reconstruction of the normative order, has long been the focus of sociological concern.[3] The discussion in this paper will be limited, for the most part, to the former process, the way in which actions and intentions are constructed in the act of assessing responsibility.

My purpose is to argue that responsibility is at least partly a product of social structure. The alternative to the doctrine of absolute responsibility is that of relative responsibility: the assessment of responsibility always includes a process of negotiation. In this process, responsibility is in part constructed by the negotiating parties. To illustrate this thesis, excerpts from two dialogues of negotiation will be discussed: a real psychotherapeutic interview, and an interview between a defense attorney and his client taken from a work of fiction. Before presenting these excerpts it will be useful to review some prior discussions of negotiation, the first in courts of law, the second in medical diagnosis.[4]

The negotiation of pleas in criminal courts, sometimes referred to as "bargain justice," has been frequently noted by observers of legal processes.[5] The defense attorney, or (in many cases, apparently) the defendant himself, strikes a bargain with the prosecutor—a plea of guilty will be made, provided that the prosecutor will reduce the charge. For example, a defendant arrested on suspicion of armed robbery may arrange to plead guilty to the charge of unarmed robbery. The prosecutor obtains ease of conviction from the bargain; the defendant, leniency.

Although no explicit estimates are given, it appears from observers' reports that the great majority of criminal convictions are negotiated. Newman states:

A major characteristic of criminal justice administration, particularly in jurisdictions characterized by legislatively fixed sentences, is charge reduction to elicit pleas of guilty. Not only does the efficient functioning of criminal justice rest upon a high proportion of guilty pleas, but plea bargaining is closely linked with attempts to individualize justice, to obtain certain desirable conviction consequences, and to avoid undesirable ones such as "undeserved" mandatory sentences.[6]

It would appear that the bargaining process is accepted as routine. In the three jurisdictions Newman studied, there were certain meeting places where the defendant, his client, and a representative of the prosecutor's office routinely met to negotiate the plea. It seems clear that in virtually all but the most unusual cases, the interested parties expected to, and actually did, negotiate the plea.

From these comments on the routine acceptance of plea bargaining in the courts, one might expect that this process would be relatively open and unambiguous. Apparently, however, there is some tension between the fact of bargaining and moral expectations concerning justice. Newman refers to this tension by citing two contradictory statements: an actual judicial opinion ("Justice and liberty are not the subjects of bargaining and barter") and an off-the-cuff statement by another judge ("All law is compromise"). A clear example of this tension is provided by an excerpt from a trial and Newman's comments on it:

The following questions were asked of a defendant after he had pleaded guilty to unarmed robbery when the original charge was armed robbery. This reduction is common, and the judge was fully aware that the plea was negotiated:

Judge: You want to plead guilty to robbery unarmed?

Defendant: Yes, Sir.

Judge: Your plea of guilty is free and voluntary?

Defendant: Yes, Sir.

Judge: No one has promised you anything?

Defendant: No.

Judge: No one has induced you to plead guilty?

Defendant: No.

Judge: You're pleading guilty because you are guilty?

Defendant: Yes.

Judge: I'll accept your plea of guilty to robbery unarmed and refer it to the probation department for a report and for sentencing Dec. 28.[7]

The delicacy of the relationship between appearance and reality is apparently confusing, even for the sociologist-observer. Newman's comment on this exchange has an Alice-in-Wonderland quality:

This is a routine procedure designed to satisfy the statutory requirement and is not intended to disguise the process of charge reduction.[8]

If we put the tensions between the different realities aside for the moment, we can say that there is an explicit process of negotiation between the defendant and the prosecution which is a part of the legal determination of guilt or innocence, or, in the terms used above, the assessment of responsibility.

In medical diagnosis a similar process of negotiation occurs, but is much less self-conscious than plea bargaining. The English psychoanalyst Michael Balint refers to this process as one of "offers and responses":

Some of the people who, for some reason or other, find it difficult to cope with problems of their lives resort to becoming ill. If the doctor has the opportunity of seeing them in the first phases of their being ill, i.e. before they settle down to a definite "organized" illness, he may observe that the patients, so to speak, offer or propose various illnesses, and that they have to go on offering new illnesses until between doctor and patient an agreement can be reached resulting in the acceptance by both of them of one of the illnesses as justified.[9]

Balint gives numerous examples indicating that patients propose reasons for their coming to the doctor which are rejected, one by one, by the physician, who makes counterproposals until an "illness" acceptable to both parties is found. If "definition of the situation" is substituted for "illness," Balint's observations become relevant to a wide variety of transactions, including the kind of interrogation discussed above. The fixing of responsibility is a process in which the client offers definitions of the situation, to which the interrogator responds. After a series of offers and responses, a definition of the situation acceptable to both the client and the interrogator is reached.

Balint has observed that the negotiation process leads physicians to influence the outcome of medical examinations, independent of the patient's condition. He refers to this process as the "apostolic function" of the doctor, arguing that the physician induces patients to have the kind of illness that the physician thinks is proper:

Apostolic mission or function means in the first place that every doctor has a vague, but almost unshakably firm, idea of how a patient ought to behave when ill. Although this idea is anything but explicit and concrete, it is immensely powerful, and influences, as we have found, practically every detail of the doctor's work with his patients. It was almost as if every doctor had revealed knowledge of what was right and what was wrong for patients to expect and to endure, and further, as if he had a sacred duty to convert to his faith all the ignorant and unbelieving among his patients.[10]

Implicit in this statement is the notion that interrogator and client have unequal power in determining the resultant definition of the situation. The interrogator's definition of the situation plays an important part in the joint definition of the situation which is finally negotiated. Moreover, his definition is more important than the client's in determining the final outcome of the negotiation, principally because he is well trained, secure, and self-confident in his role in the transaction, whereas the client is untutored, anxious, and uncertain about his role. Stated simply, the subject, because of these conditions, is likely to be susceptible to the influence of the interrogator.

Note that plea bargaining and the process of "offers and responses" in diagnosis differ in the degree of self-consciousness of the participants. In plea bargaining, the process is at least partly visible to the participants themselves. There appears to be some ambiguity about the extent to which the negotiation is morally acceptable to some of the commentators, but the parties to the negotiations appear to be aware that bargaining is going on, and accept the process as such. The bargaining process in diagnosis, however, is much more subterranean. Certainly neither physicians nor patients recognize the offers and responses process as bargaining. There is no commonly accepted vocabulary for describing diagnostic bargaining, such as there is in the legal analogy, e.g. "copping out" or "copping a plea." It may be that in legal processes there is some appreciation of the different kinds of reality, i.e. the difference between the public (official, legal) reality and private reality, whereas in medicine this difference is not recognized.

The discussion so far has suggested that much of reality is arrived at by negotiation. This thesis was illustrated by materials on legal processes presented by Newman and materials on medical processes presented by Balint. These processes are similar in that they appear to represent clear instances of the negotiation of reality. The instances are different in that the legal bargaining processes appear to be more open and accepted than the diagnostic process. In order to outline some of the dimensions of the negotiation process and to establish some of the limitations of the analyses by Newman and Balint, two excerpts of cases of bargaining will be discussed: the first taken from an actual psychiatric "intake" interview, the second from a fictional account of a defense lawyer's first interview with his client.

The Process of Negotiation

The psychiatric interview to be discussed is from the first interview in *The Initial Interview in Psychiatric Practice*.[11] The patient is a 34-year-old nurse who feels, as she says, "irritable, tense, depressed." She appears to be saying from the very beginning of the interview that the external situation in which she lives is the cause of her troubles. She focuses particularly on her husband's behavior. She says he is an alcoholic, is verbally abusive, and won't let her work. She feels that she is cooped up in the house all day with her two small children, but that when he is home at night (on the nights when he *is* at home) he will have nothing to do with her and the children. She intimates, in several ways, that he does not serve as a sexual companion. She has thought of divorce, but has rejected it for various reasons (for example, she is afraid she couldn't take proper care of the children, finance the babysitters, etc.). She feels trapped.[12]

In the concluding paragraph of their description of this interview, Gill, Newman, and Redlich give this summary:

The patient, pushed by we know not what or why at the time (the children—somebody to talk to) comes for help apparently for what she thinks of as help with her external situation (her husband's behavior as she sees it). The therapist does not respond to this but seeks her role and how it is that she plays such a role. Listening to the recording it sounds as if the therapist is at first bored and disinterested and the patient defensive. He gets down to work and keeps asking, "What is it all about?" Then he becomes more interested and sympathetic and at the same time very active (participating) and demanding. *It sounds as if she keeps saying " This is the trouble."* He says, "*No! Tell me the trouble.*" She says, "*This is it!*" He says, "*No, tell me,*" until the patient finally says, "*Well I'll tell you.*" Then the therapist says, "*Good! I'll help you.*"[13]

From this summary it is apparent that there is a close fit between Balint's idea of the negotiation of diagnosis through offers and responses and what took place in this psychiatric interview. It is difficult, however, to document the details. Most of the psychiatrist's responses, rejecting the patient's offers, do not appear in the written transcript, but they are fairly obvious as one listens to the recording. Two particular features of the psychiatrist's responses especially stand out: (1) the flatness of intonation in his responses to the patient's complaints about her external circumstances; and (2) the rapidity with which he introduces new topics, through questioning, when she is talking about her husband.

Some features of the psychiatrist's coaching are verbal, however:

T: Has anything happened recently that makes it . . . you feel that . . . ah . . . you're sort of coming to the end of your rope? I mean I wondered what led you . . .

P: (Interrupting.) It's nothing special. It's just everything in general.

T: What led you to come to a . . .

P: (Interrupting.) It's just that I . . .

T: . . . a psychiatrist just now?

P: Because I felt that the older girl was getting tense as a result of . . . of my being stewed up all the time.

T: Mmmhnn.

P: Not having much patience with her.

T: Mmmhnn. (Short Pause.) Mmm. And how had you imagined that a psychiatrist could help with this? (Short pause.)

P: Mmm . . . maybe I could sort of get straightened out . . . straighten things out in my own mind. I'm confused. Sometimes I can't remember things that I've done, whether I've done 'em or not or whether they happened.

T: What is it that you want to straighten out? (Pause)

P: I think I seem mixed up.

T: Yeah? You see that, it seems to me, is something that we really should talk about because . . . ah . . . from a certain point of view somebody might say, "Well now, it's all very simple. She's unhappy and disturbed because her husband is behaving this way, and unless something can be done about that how could she expect to feel any other way." But, instead of that, you come to the psychiatrist, and you say that you think there's something about you that needs straightening out. I don't quite get it. Can you explain that to me? (Short pause.)

P: I sometimes wonder if I'm emotionally grown up.

T: By which you mean what?

P: When you're married you should have one mate. You shouldn't go around and look at other men.

T: You've been looking at other men?

P: I look at them, but that's all.

T: Mmmhnn. What you mean ... you mean a grown-up person should accept the marital situation whatever it happens to be?

P: That was the way I was brought up. Yes. (Sighs.)

T: You think that would be a sign of emotional maturity?

P: No.

T: No. So?

P: Well, if you rebel against the laws of society you have to take the consequences.

T: Yes?

P: And it's just that I ... I'm not willing to take the consequences. I ... I don't think it's worth it.

T: Mmhnn. So in the meantime then while you're in this very difficult situation, you find yourself reacting in a way that you don't like and that you think is ... ah ... damaging to your children and yourself? Now what can be done about that?

P: (Sniffs; sighs.) I dunno. That's why I came to see you.

T: Yes. I was just wondering what you had in mind. Did you think a psychiatrist could ... ah ... help you face this kind of a situation calmly and easily and maturely? Is that it?

P: More or less. I need somebody to talk to who isn't emotionally involved with the family. I have a few friends, but I don't like to bore them. I don't think they should know ... ah ... all the intimate details of what goes on.

T: Yeah?

P: It becomes food for gossip.

T: Mmmhnn.

P: Besides they're in ... they're emotionally involved because they're my friends. They tell me not to stand for it, but they don't understand that if I put my foot down it'll only get stepped on.

T: Yeah.

P: That he can make it miserable for me in other ways. ...

T: Mmm.

P: ... which he does.

T: Mmmhnn. In other words, you find yourself in a situation and don't know how to cope with it really.

P: I don't.

T: You'd like to be able to talk that through and come to understand it better and learn how to cope with it or deal with it in some way. Is that right?

P: I'd like to know how to deal with it more effectively.

T: Yeah. Does that mean you feel convinced that the way you're dealing with it now ...

P: There's something wrong of course.

T: ... something wrong with that. Mmmhnn.

P: There's something wrong with it.[14]

Note that the therapist reminds her *four times* in this short sequence that she has come to see a *psychiatrist*. Since the context of these reminders is one in which the patient is attributing her difficulties to an external situation, particularly her husband, it seems plausible to hear these reminders as subtle requests for analysis of her own contributions to her difficulties. This interpretation is supported by the therapist's subsequent remarks. When the patient once again describes external problems, the therapist tries the following tack:

T: I notice that you've used a number of psychiatric terms here and there. Were you specially interested in that in your training, or what?

P: Well, my great love is psychology.

T: Psychology?

P: Mmmhnn.

T: How much have you studied?

P: Oh (Sighs.) what you have in your nurse's training, and I've had general psych, child and adolescent psych, and the abnormal psych.

T: Mmmhnn. Well, tell me ... ah ... what would you say if you had to explain yourself what is the problem?

P: You don't diagnose yourself very well, at least I don't.

T: Well you can make a stab at it. (Pause.)[15]

This therapeutic thrust is rewarded: the patient gives a long account of her early life which indicates a belief that she was not "adjusted" in the past. The interview continues:

T: And what conclusions do you draw from all this about why you're not adjusting now the way you think you should?

P: Well, I wasn't adjusted then. I feel that I've come a long way, but I don't think I'm still ... I still don't feel that I'm adjusted.

T: And you don't regard your husband as being the difficulty? You think it lies within yourself?

P: Oh he's a difficulty all right, but I figure that even ... ah ... had ... if it had been other things that ... that this probably—this state—would've come on me.

T: Oh you do think so?

P: (Sighs.) I don't think he's the sole factor. No.

T: And what are the factors within ...

P: I mean ...

T: ... yourself?

P: Oh it's probably remorse for the past, things I did.

T: Like what? (Pause.) It's sumping hard to tell, hunh? (Short pause.)[16]

After some parrying, the patient tells the therapist what he wants to hear. She feels guilty because she was pregnant by another man when her present husband proposed. She cries. The therapist tells the patient she needs and will get psychiatric help, and the interview ends, the patient still crying. The negotiational aspects of the process are clear: After the patient has spent most of the interview blaming her current difficulties on external circumstances, she tells the therapist a deep secret about which she feels intensely guilty. The patient, and not the husband, is at fault. The therapist's tone and manner change abruptly. From being bored, distant, and rejecting, he becomes warm and solicitous. Through a process of offers and responses, the therapist and patient have, by implication, negotiated a shared definition of the situation—the patient, not the husband, is responsible.

A Contrasting Case

The negotiation process can, of course, proceed on the opposite premise, namely that the client is not responsible. An ideal example would be an interrogation of a client by a skilled defense lawyer. Unfortunately, we have been unable to locate a verbatim transcript of a defense lawyer's initial interview with his client. There is available, however, a fictional portrayal of such an interview, written by a man with extensive experience as defense lawyer, prosecutor, and judge. The excerpt to follow is taken from the novel *Anatomy of a Murder*.[17]

The defense lawyer, in his initial contact with his client, briefly questions him regarding his actions on the night of the killing. The client states that he discovered that the deceased, Barney Quill, had raped his wife; he then goes on to state that he then left his wife, found Quill, and shot him.

"... How long did you remain with your wife before you went to the hotel bar?"
"I don't remember."
"I think it is important, and I suggest you try."
After a pause. "Maybe an hour."
"Maybe more?"
"Maybe."
"Maybe less?"
"Maybe."
I paused and lit a cigar. I took my time. I had reached a point where a few wrong answers to a few right questions would leave me with a client—if I took his case—whose cause was legally defenseless. Either I stopped now and begged off and let some other lawyer worry over it or I asked him the few fatal questions and let him hang himself. Or else, like any smart lawyer, I went into the Lecture. I studied my man, who sat as inscrutable as an Arab, delicately fingering his Ming holder, daintily sipping his dark mustache. He apparently did not realize how close I had him to admitting that he was guilty of first degree murder, that is, that he "feloniously, wilfully and of his malice afore-thought did kill and murder one Barney Quill." The man was a sitting duck.[18]

The lawyer here realizes that his line of questioning has come close to fixing the responsibility for the killing on his client. He therefore shifts his ground by beginning "the lecture":

The Lecture is an ancient device that lawyers use to coach their clients so that the client won't quite know he has been coached and his lawyer can still preserve the face-saving illusion that he hasn't done any coaching. For coaching clients, like robbing them, is not only frowned upon, it is downright unethical and bad, very bad. Hence the Lecture, an artful device as old as the law itself, and one used constantly by some of the nicest and most ethical lawyers in the land. "Who, me? I didn't tell him what to say," the lawyer can later comfort himself. "I merely explained the law, see." It is a good practice to scowl and shrug here and add virtuously; "That's my duty, isn't it?"
... "We will now explore the absorbing subject of legal justification or excuse," I said.
... "Well, take self-defense," I began. "That's the classic example of justifiable homicide. On the basis of what I've so far heard and read about your case I do not think we need pause too long over that. Do you?"
"Perhaps not," Lieutenant Manion conceded. "We'll pass it for now."
"Let's," I said dryly. "Then there's the defense of habitation, defense of

property, and the defense of relatives or friends. Now there are more ramifications to these defenses than a dog has fleas, but we won't explore them
now. I've already told you at length why I don't think you can invoke the
possible defense of your wife. When you shot Quill her need for defense had
passed. It's as simple as that."

"Go on," Lieutenant Manion said, frowning.

"Then there's the defense of a homicide committed to prevent a felony—
say you're being robbed—; to prevent the escape of the felon—suppose he's
getting away with your wallet—; or to arrest a felon—you've caught up
with him and he's either trying to get away or has actually escaped." ...

... "Go on, then; what are some of the other legal justifications or excuses?"

"Then there's the tricky and dubious defense of intoxication. Personally
I've never seen it succeed. But since you were not drunk when you shot Quill
we shall mercifully not dwell on that. Or were you?"

"I was cold sober. Please go on."

"Then finally there's the defense of insanity." I paused and spoke abruptly, airily: "Well, that just about winds it up." I arose as though making ready
to leave.

"Tell me more."

"There is no more." I slowly paced up and down the room.

"I mean about this insanity."

"Oh, insanity," I said, elaborately surprised. It was like luring a trained
seal with a herring. "Well, insanity, where proven, is a complete defense to
murder. It does not legally justify the killing, like self-defense, say, but rather
excuses it." The lecturer was hitting his stride. He was also on the home
stretch. "Our law requires that a punishable killing—in fact, any crime—
must be committed by a sapient human being, one capable, as the law
insists, of distinguishing between right and wrong. If a man is insane, legally
insane, the act of homicide may still be murder but the law excuses the
perpetrator."

Lieutenant Manion was sitting erect now, very still and erect. "I see—and
this—this perpetrator, what happens to him if he should—should be
excused?"

"Under Michigan law—like that of many other states—if he is acquitted
of murder on the grounds of insanity it is provided that he must be sent to a
hospital for the criminally insane until he is pronounced sane." ...

... Then he looked at me. "Maybe," he said, "maybe I was insane."

... Thoughtfully: "Hm. ... Why do you say that?"

"Well, I can't really say," he went on slowly. "I—I guess I blacked out. I
can't remember a thing after I saw him standing behind the bar that night
until I got back to my trailer."

"You mean—you mean you don't remember shooting him?" I shook my
head in wonderment.

"Yes, that's what I mean."

"You don't even remember driving home?"

"No."

"You don't remember threatening Barney's bartender when he followed
you outside after the shooting—as the newspaper says you did?" I paused
and held my breath. "You don't remember telling him, 'Do you want some,
too, Buster?' ?"

The smoldering dark eyes flickered ever so little. "No, not a thing."

"My, my," I said blinking my eyes, contemplating the wonder of it all. "Maybe you've got something there."

The Lecture was over; I had told my man the law; and now he had told me things that might possibly invoke the defense of insanity. . . .[19]

The negotiation is complete. The ostensibly shared definition of the situation established by the negotiation process is that the defendant was probably not responsible for his actions.

Let us now compare the two interviews. The major similarity between them is their negotiated character: they both take the form of a series of offers and responses that continue until an offer (a definition of the situation) is reached that is acceptable to both parties. The major difference between the transactions is that one, the psychotherapeutic interview, arrives at an assessment that the client is responsible; the other, the defense attorney's interview, reaches an assessment that the client was not at fault, i.e., not responsible. How can we account for this difference in outcome?

Discussion

Obviously, given any two real cases of negotiation which have different outcomes, one might construct a reasonable argument that the difference is due to the differences between the cases—the finding of responsibility in one case and lack of responsibility in the other, the only outcomes which are reasonably consonant with the facts of the respective cases. Without rejecting this argument, for the sake of discussion only, and without claiming any kind of proof or demonstration, I wish to present an alternative argument: that the difference in outcome is largely due to the differences in technique used by the interrogators. This argument will allow us to suggest some crucial dimensions of negotiation processes.

The first dimension, consciousness of the bargaining aspects of the transaction, has already been mentioned. In the psychotherapeutic interview, the negotiational nature of the transaction seems not to be articulated by either party. In the legal interview, however, certainly the lawyer, and perhaps to some extent the client as well, is aware of and accepts the situation as one of striking a bargain, rather than as a relentless pursuit of the absolute facts of the matter.

The dimension of shared awareness that the definition of the situation is negotiable seems particularly crucial for assessments of responsibility. In both interviews, there is an agenda hidden from the client. In the psychotherapeutic interview, it is probably the psychiatric criteria for acceptance into treatment, the criterion of "insight." The psychotherapist has probably been trained to view patients with "insight into their illness" as favorable candidates for psychotherapy, i.e., patients who accept, or can be led to accept, the problems as internal, as part of their personality, rather than seeing them as caused by external conditions.

In the legal interview, the agenda that is unknown to the client is the legal structure of defenses or justifications for killing. In both the legal and psychiatric cases, the hidden agenda is not a simple one. Both involve fitting abstract and ambiguous criteria (insight, on the one hand; legal justification, on the other) to a richly specific, concrete case. In the legal interview, the lawyer almost immediately broaches this hidden agenda; he states clearly and concisely the major legal justifications for killing. In the psychiatric interview, the hidden agenda is never revealed. The patient's offers during most of the interview are rejected or ignored. In the last part of the interview, her last offer is accepted and she is told that she will be given treatment. In no case are the reasons for these actions articulated by either party.

The degree of shared awareness is related to a second dimension which concerns the format of the conversation. The legal interview began as an interrogation, but was quickly shifted away from that format when the defense lawyer realized the direction in which the questioning was leading the client, i.e., toward a legally unambiguous admission of guilt. On the very brink of such an admission, the defense lawyer stopped asking questions and started, instead, to make statements. He listed the principle legal justifications for killing, and, in response to the *client's* questions, gave an explanation of each of the justifications. This shift in format put the client, rather than the lawyer, in control of the crucial aspects of the negotiation. It is the client, not the lawyer, who is allowed to pose the questions, assess the answers for their relevance to his case, and, most crucially, to determine himself the most advantageous tack to take. Control of the definition of the situation, the evocation of the events and intentions relevant to the assessment of the client's responsibility for the killing, was given to the client by the lawyer. The resulting client-controlled format of negotiation gives the client a double advantage. It not only allows the client the benefit of formulating his account of actions and intentions in their most favorable light, it also allows him to select, out of a diverse and ambiguous set of normative criteria concerning killing, that criterion which is most favorable to his own case.

Contrast the format of negotiation used by the psychotherapist.

The form is consistently that of interrogation. The psychotherapist poses the questions; the patient answers. The psychotherapist then has the answers at his disposal. He may approve or disapprove, accept or reject, or merely ignore them. Throughout the entire interview, the psychotherapist is in complete control of the situation. Within this framework, the tactic that the psychotherapist uses is to reject the patient's "offers" that her husband is at fault—first by ignoring them; later, and ever more insistently, by leading her to define the situation as one in which she is at fault. In effect, what the therapist does is to reject her offers, and to make his own counteroffers.

These remarks concerning the relationship between technique of interrogation and outcome suggest an approach to assessment of responsibility somewhat different than that usually followed. The common-sense approach to interrogation is to ask how accurate and fair is the outcome. Both Newman's and Balint's analyses of negotiation raise this question. Both presuppose that there is an objective state of affairs that is independent of the technique of assessment. This is quite clear in Newman's discussion, as he continually refers to defendants who are "really" or "actually" guilty or innocent.[20] The situation is less clear in Balint's discussion, although occasionally he implies that certain patients are really physically healthy but psychologically distressed.

The type of analysis suggested by this paper seeks to avoid such presuppositions. It can be argued that, *independent* of the facts of the case, the technique of assessment plays a part in determining the outcome. In particular, one can avoid making assumptions about actual responsibility by utilizing a technique of textual criticism of a transaction. The key dimension in such work would be the relative power and authority of the participants in the situation.[21]

As an introduction to the way in which power differences between interactants shape the outcome of negotiations, let us take as an example an attorney in a trial dealing with "friendly" and "unfriendly" witnesses. A friendly witness is a person whose testimony will support the definition of the situation the attorney seeks to convey to the jury. With such a witness the attorney does not employ power, but treats him as an equal. His questions to such a witness are open and allow the witness considerable freedom. The attorney might frame a question such as "Could you tell us about your actions on the night of———?"

The opposing attorney, however, interested in establishing his own version of the witness' behavior on the same night, would probably approach the task quite differently. He might say: "You felt angry and offended on the night of ———, didn't you?" The witness frequently will try to evade so direct a question with an answer like: "Actually, I had started to...." The attorney quickly interrupts, addressing the judge: "Will the court order the witness to respond to the question, yes or no?" That is to say, the question posed by the opposing attorney is abrupt and direct. When the witness attempts to answer indirectly and at length, the attorney quickly invokes the power of the court to coerce the witness to answer as he wishes, directly. The witness and the attorney are not equals in power; the attorney uses the coercive power of the court to force the witness to answer in the manner desired.

The attorney confronted by an "unfriendly" witness wishes to control the format of the interaction, so that he can retain control of the definition of the situation that is conveyed to the jury. It is much easier for him to neutralize an opposing definition of the situation if he retains control of the interrogation format in this manner. By allowing the unfriendly witness to respond only by yes or no to his own verbally conveyed account, he can suppress the ambient details of the opposing view that might sway the jury, and thus maintain an advantage for his definition over that of the witness.

In the psychiatric interview discussed above, the psychiatrist obviously does not invoke a third party to enforce his control of the interview. But he does use a device to impress the patient that she is not to be his equal in the interview that is reminiscent of the attorney with an unfriendly witness. The device is to pose abrupt and direct questions to the patient's open-ended accounts, implying that the patient should answer briefly and directly; through that implication, the psychiatrist controls the whole transaction. Throughout most of the interview the patient seeks to give detailed accounts of her behavior and her husband's, but the psychiatrist almost invariably counters with a direct and, to the patient, seemingly unrelated question.

The first instance of this procedure occurs when the psychiatrist asks the patient, "What do you do?" She replies "I'm a nurse, but my husband won't let me work." Rather than responding to the last part of her answer, which would be expected in conversation between equals, the psychiatrist asks another question, changing the subject: "How old are you?" This pattern continues throughout most of the interview. The psychiatrist appears to be trying to teach the patient to follow his lead. After some thirty or forty exchanges of this kind, the patient apparently learns her lesson; she cedes control of the transaction competely to the therapist, answering briefly and directly to direct questions and elaborating only on cue from the therapist. The therapist thus implements his control of the interview not by direct coercion, but by subtle manipulation.

All of the discussion above, concerning shared awareness and the format of the negotiation, suggests several propositions concerning control over the definition of the situation. The professional interrogator, whether lawyer or psychotherapist, can maintain control if the client cedes control to him because of his authority as an expert, because of his manipulative skill in the transaction, or merely because the interrogator controls access to something the client wants, e.g. treatment or a legal excuse. The propositions are:

1a. Shared awareness of the participants that the situation is one of negotiation. (The greater the shared awareness, the more control the client gets over the resultant definition of the situation.)

1b. Explicitness of the agenda. (The more explicit the agenda of the transaction, the more control the client gets over the resulting definition of the situation.)

2a. Organization of the format of the transaction, offers and responses. (The party to a negotiation who responds, rather than the party who makes the offers, has more power in controlling the resultant shared definition of the situation.)

2b. Counteroffers. (The responding party who makes counteroffers has more power than the responding party who limits his response to merely accepting or rejecting the offers of the other party.)

2c. Directness of questions and answers. (The more direct the questions of the interrogator, and the more direct the answers he demands and receives, the more control he has over the resultant definition of the situation.)

These concepts and hypotheses are only suggestive until such times as operational definitions can be developed. Although such terms as offers and responses seem to have an immediate applicability to most conversation, it is likely that a thorough and systematic analysis of any given conversation would show the need for clearly stated criteria of class inclusion and exclusion. Perhaps a good place for such research would be in the transactions for assessing responsibility discussed above. Since some 90 percent of all criminal convictions in the United States are based on guilty pleas, the extent to which techniques of interrogation subtly influence outcomes would have immediate policy implication. There is considerable evidence that interrogation techniques influence the outcome of psychotherapeutic interviews also.[22] Research in both of these areas would probably have implications for both the theory and practice of assessing responsibility.

Conclusion: Negotiation in Social Science Research

More broadly, the application of the sociology of knowledge to the negotiation of reality has ramifications which may apply to all of social science. The interviewer in a survey, or the experimenter in a social psychological experiment, is also involved in a transaction with a client—the respondent or subject. Recent studies by Rosenthal and others strongly suggest that the findings in such studies are negotiated and are influenced by the format of the study.[23] Rosenthal's review of bias in research suggests that such bias is produced by a pervasive and subtle process of interaction between the investigator and his source of data. Those errors which arise because of the investigator's influence over the subject (the kind of influence discussed in this paper as arising out of power disparities in the process of negotiation) Rosenthal calls "expectancy effects." In order for these errors to occur, there must be direct contact between the investigator and the subject.

A second kind of bias Rosenthal refers to as "observer effects." These are errors of perception or reporting which do not require that the subject be influenced by investigation. Rosenthal's review leads one to surmise that even with techniques that are completely nonobtrusive, observer error could be quite large.[24]

The occurrence of these two kinds of bias poses an interesting dilemma for the lawyer, the psychiatrist, and the social scientist. The investigator of human phenomena is usually interested in more than a sequence of events; he wants to know why the events occurred. Usually this quest for an explanation leads him to deal with the motivation of the persons involved. The lawyer, clinician, social psychologist, or survey researcher try to elicit motives directly, by questioning the participants. But in the process of questioning, as suggested above, he becomes involved in a process of negotiation, perhaps subtly influencing the informants through expectancy effects. A historian, on the other hand, might try to use documents and records to determine motives. He would certainly avoid expectancy effects in this way, but, since he would not elicit motives directly, he might find it necessary to collect and interpret various kinds of evidence which are only indirectly related, at best, to determine motives of the participants. Thus, through his choice in the selection and interpretation of the indirect evidence, he may be as susceptible to error as the interrogator, survey researcher, or experimentalist—his error being due to observer effects, however, rather than expectancy effects.

The application of the ideas outlined here to social and psychological research needs to be developed. The five propositions suggested above might be used, for example, to estimate the validity of surveys using varying degrees of open-endedness in their interview format. If some technique could be developed which would yield an independent assessment of validity, it might be possible to demonstrate, as Aaron Cicourel has suggested, that the more reliable the technique, the less valid the results.

The influence of the assessment itself on the phenomena to be assessed appears to be an ubiquitous process in human affairs, whether in ordinary daily life, in the determination of responsibility in legal or clinical interrogation, or in most types of social science research. The sociology-of-knowledge perspective, which suggests that people go through their lives constructing reality, offers a framework within which the negotiation of reality can be seriously and constructively studied. This paper has suggested some of the avenues of the problem that might require further study. The prevalence of the problem in most areas of human concern recommends it to our attention as a substantial field of study, rather than as an issue that can be ignored or, alternatively, be taken as the proof that rigorous knowledge of social affairs is impossible.

Acknowledgments

The author wishes to acknowledge the help of the following persons who criticized earlier drafts: Aaron Cicourel, Donald Cressey, Joan Emerson, Erving Goffman, Michael Katz, Lewis Kurke, Robert Levy, Sohan Lal Sharma, and Paul Weubben. The paper was written during a fellowship provided by the Social Science Research Institute, University of Hawaii.

Notes

1. The doctrine of absolute responsibility is clearly illustrated in psychiatric and legal discussions of the issue of "criminal responsibility," i.e., the use of mental illness as an excuse from criminal conviction. An example of the assumption of absolute criteria of responsibility is found in the following quotation: "The finding that someone is criminally responsible means to the psychiatrist that the criminal must change his behavior before he can resume his position in society. *This injunction is dictated not by morality, but, so to speak, by reality.*" See Edward J. Sachar, "Behavioral Science and Criminal Law," *Scientific American* 209 (1963), pp. 39–45. (Emphasis added.)

2. Cf. Peter L. Berger and Thomas Luckmann. *The Social Construction of Reality: A Treatise in the Sociology of Knowledge* (New York: Doubleday, 1966).

3. The classic treatment of this issue is found in E. Durkheim, *The Elementary Forms of the Religious Life*.

4. A sociological application of the concept of negotiation, in a different context, is found in Anselm Strauss et al., "The Hospital and its Negotiated Order," in Eliot Freidson, editor, *The Hospital in Modern Society* (New York: Free Press, 1963).

5. Newman reports a study in this area, together with a review of earlier work, in "The Negotiated Plea," in Donald J. Newman, *Conviction: The Determination of Guilt or Innocence Without Trial* (Boston: Little, Brown, 1966).

6. Ibid., p. 76.

7. Ibid., p. 83.

8. Idem.

9. Michael Balint, *The Doctor, His Patient, and The Illness* (New York: International Universities Press, 1957), p. 18. A description of the negotiations between patients in a tuberculosis sanitarium and their physicians is found in Julius A. Roth, *Timetables: Structuring the Passage of Time in Hospital Treatment and Other Careers* (Indianapolis: Bobbs-Merrill, 1963), pp. 48–59. Obviously, some cases are more susceptible to negotiation than others. Balint implies that the great majority of cases in medical practice are negotiated.

10. Balint, op. cit., p. 216.

11. Merton Gill, Richard Newman, and Fredrick C. Redlich, *The Initial Interview in Psychiatric Practice* (New York: International Universities Press, 1954).

12. Since this interview is complex and subtle, the reader is invited to listen to it himself and compare his conclusions with those discussed here. The recorded interview is available on the first L.P. record that accompanies Gill, Newman, and Redlich, op. cit.

13. Ibid., p. 133. (Italics added.)

14. Ibid., pp. 176–182.

15. Ibid., pp. 186–187.

16. Ibid., pp. 192–194.

17. Robert Traver, *Anatomy of a Murder* (New York: Dell, 1959).

18. Ibid., p. 43.

19. Ibid., pp. 46–47, 57–60.

20. In his foreword the editor of the series, Frank J. Remington, comments on one slip that occurs frequently, the "acquittal of the guilty," noting that this phrase is contradictory from the legal point of view. He goes on to say that Newman is well aware of this but uses the phrase as a convenience. Needless to say, both Remington's comments and mine can both be correct: The phrase is used as a convenience, but it also reveals the author's presuppositions.

21. Berger and Luckmann (op. cit., p. 100) also emphasize the role of power, but at the societal level. "The success of particular conceptual machineries is related to the power possessed by those who operate them. The confrontation of alternative symbolic universes implies a problem of power—which of the conflicting definitions of

reality will be 'made to stick' in the society." Haley's discussions of control in psychotherapy are also relevant. See Jay Haley, "Control in Psychoanalytic Psychotherapy." *Progress in Psychotherapy* 4 (1959), pp. 48–65.

22. Thomas J. Scheff, *Being Mentally Ill* (Chicago: Aldine, 1966).

23. Robert Rosenthal, *Experimenter Effects in Behavioral Research* (New York: Appleton-Century-Crofts, 1966). Friedman, reporting a series of studies of expectancy effects, seeks to put the results within a broad sociological framework; see Neil Friedman, *The Social Nature of Psychological Research: The Psychological Experiment as Social Interaction* (New York: Basic Books, 1967).

24. Critics of "reactive techniques" often disregard the problem of observer effects. See, for example, Eugene J. Webb, Donald T. Campbell, Richard D. Schwartz, and Lee Sechrest, *Unobtrusive Measures: Nonreactive Research in Social Science* (Chicago: Rand-McNally, 1966).

6

Behavior in Private Places: Sustaining Definitions of Reality in Gynecological Examinations
Joan P. Emerson

In *The Social Construction of Reality*, Berger and Luckmann discuss how people construct social order and yet construe the reality of everyday life to exist independently of themselves.[1] Berger and Luckmann's work succeeds in synthesizing some existing answers with new insights. Many sociologists have pointed to the importance of social consensus in what people believe; if everyone else seems to believe in something, a person tends to accept the common belief without question. Other sociologists have discussed the concept of legitimacy, an acknowledgment that what exists has the right to exist, and delineated various lines of argument which can be taken to justify a state of affairs. Berger and Luckmann emphasize three additional processes that provide persons with evidence that things have an objective existence apart from themselves. Perhaps most important is the experience that reality seems to be out there before we arrive on the scene. This notion is fostered by the nature of language, which contains an all-inclusive scheme of categories, is shared by a community, and must be learned laboriously by each new member. Further, definitions of reality are continuously validated by apparently trivial features of the social scene, such as details of the setting, persons' appearance and demeanor, and "inconsequential" talk. Finally, each part of a systematic world view serves as evidence for all the other parts, so that reality is solidified by a process of intervalidation of supposedly independent events.

Because Berger and Luckmann's contribution is theoretical, their units of analysis are abstract processes. But they take these processes to be grounded in social encounters. Thus, Berger and Luckmann's theory provides a framework for making sense of social interaction. In this paper observations of a concrete situation will be interpreted to

Reprinted, with the permission of the author, from *Recent Sociology* no. 2 (1970): 74–97.

show how reality is embodied in routines and reaffirmed in social interaction.

Situations differ in how much effort it takes to sustain the current definition of the situation. Some situations are relatively stable; others are precarious.[2] Stability depends on the likelihood of three types of disconforming events. Intrusions on the scene may threaten definitions of reality, as when people smell smoke in a theater or when a third person joins a couple and calls one member by a name the second member does not recognize. Participants may deliberately decline to validate the current reality, like Quakers who refused to take off their hats to the king. Sometimes participants are unable to produce the gestures which would validate the current reality. Perhaps a person is ignorant of the relevant vocabulary of gestures. Or a person, understanding how he should behave, may have limited social skills so that he cannot carry off the performance he would like to. For those who insist on "sincerity," a performance becomes especially taxing if they lack conviction about the trueness of the reality they are attempting to project.

A reality can hardly seem self-evident if a person is simultaneously aware of a counterreality. Berger and Luckmann write as though definitions of reality were internally congruent. However, the ordinary reality may contain not only a dominant definition, but in addition counterthemes opposing or qualifying the dominant definition. Thus, several contradictory definitions must be sustained at the same time. Because each element tends to challenge the other elements, such composite definitions of reality are inherently precarious even if the probability of disconfirming events is low.

A situation where the definition of reality is relatively precarious has advantages for the analysis proposed here, for processes of sustaining reality should be more obvious where that reality is problematic. The situation chosen, the gynecological examination,[3] is precarious for both reasons discussed above. First, it is an excellent example of multiple contradictory definitions of reality, as described in the next section. Second, while intrusive and deliberate threats are not important, there is a substantial threat from participants' incapacity to perform.

Dramaturgical abilities are taxed in gynecological examinations because the less convincing reality internalized by secondary socialization is unusually discrepant with rival perspectives taken for granted in primary socialization.[4] Gynecological examinations share similar problems of reality-maintenance with any medical procedure, but the issues are more prominent because the site of the medical task is a woman's genitals. Because touching usually connotes personal intimacy, persons may have to work at accepting the physician's privileged access to the patient's genitals.[5] Participants are not entirely convinced that modesty is out of place. Since a woman's genitals are commonly accessible only in a sexual context, sexual connotations come readily to mind. Although most people realize that sexual responses are inappropriate, they may be unable to dismiss the sexual reaction privately and it may interfere with the conviction with which they undertake their impersonal performance. The structure of a gynecological examination highlights the very features which the participants are supposed to disattend. So the more attentive the participants are to the social situation, the more the unmentionable is forced on their attention.

The next section will characterize the complex composition of the definition of reality routinely sustained in gynecological examinations. Then some of the routine arrangements and interactional maneuvers which embody and express this definition will be described. A later section will discuss threats to the definition which arise in the course of the encounter. Measures that serve to neutralize the threats and reaffirm the definition will be analyzed. The concluding section will turn to the theoretical issues of precariousness, multiple contradictory definitions of reality, and implicit communication.

The Medical Definition and Its Counterthemes

Sometimes people are in each other's presence in what they take to be a "gynecological examination." What happens in a gynecological examination is part of the common stock of knowledge. Most people know that a gynecological examination is when a doctor examines a woman's genitals in a medical setting. Women who have undergone this experience know that the examination takes place in a special examining room where the patient lies with her buttocks down to the edge of the table and her feet in stirrups, that usually a nurse is present as a chaperone, that the actual examining lasts only a few minutes, and so forth. Besides knowing what equipment to provide for the doctor, the nurse has in mind a typology of responses patients have to this situation, and a typology of doctors' styles of performance. The doctor has technical knowledge about the examining procedures, what observations may be taken to indicate, ways of getting patients to relax, and so on.

Immersed in the medical world where the scene constitutes a routine, the staff assume the responsibility for a credible performance.

The staff take part in gynecological examinations many times a day, while the patient is a fleeting visitor. More deeply convinced of the reality themselves, the staff are willing to convince skeptical patients. The physician guides the patient through the precarious scene in a contained manner: taking the initiative, controlling the encounter, keeping the patient in line, defining the situation by his reaction, and giving cues that "this is done" and "other people go through this all the time."

People must continue to believe not only that "this is a gynecological examination," but also that "this is a gynecological examination going right." The major definition to be sustained for this purpose is "this is a medical situation" (not a party, sexual assault, psychological experiment, or anything else). If it is a medical situation, then it follows that "no one is embarrassed"[6] and "no one is thinking in sexual terms."[7] Anyone who indicates the contrary must be swayed by some nonmedical definition.

The medical definition calls for a matter-of-fact stance. One of the most striking observations about a gynecological examination is the marked implication underlying the staff's demeanor toward the patient: "Of course, you take this as matter-of-factly as we do." The staff implicitly contend: "In the medical world the pelvic area is like any other part of the body; its private and sexual connotations are left behind when you enter the hospital." The staff want it understood that their gazes take in only medically pertinent facts, so they are not concerned with an aesthetic inspection of a patient's body. Their nonchalant pose attempts to put a gynecological examination in the same light as an internal examination of the ear.

Another implication of the medical definition is that the patient is a technical object to the staff. It is as if the staff work on an assembly line for repairing bodies; similar body parts continually roll by and the staff have a particular job to do on them. The staff are concerned with the typical features of the body part and its pathology rather than with the unique features used to define a person's identity. The staff disattend the connection between a part of the body and some intangible self that is supposed to inhabit that body.

The scene is credible precisely because the staff act as if they have every right to do what they are doing. Any hint of doubt from the staff would compromise the medical definition. Since the patient's nonchalance merely serves to validate the staff's right, it may be dispensed with without the same threat. Furthermore, the staff claim to be merely agents of the medical system, which is intent on providing good health care to patients. This medical system imposes procedures and standards which the staff are merely following in this particular instance. That is, what the staff do derives from external coercion— "We have to do it this way"—rather than from personal choices which they would be free to revise in order to accommodate the patient.

The medical definition grants the staff the right to carry out their task. If not for the medical definition, the staff's routine activities could be defined as unconscionable assaults on the dignity of individuals. The topics of talk—particularly inquiries about bodily functioning, sexual experience, and death of relatives—might be taken as offenses against propriety. As for exposure and manipulation of the patient's body, it would be a shocking and degrading invasion of privacy were the patient not defined as a technical object. The infliction of pain would be mere cruelty. The medical definition justifies the request that a presumably competent adult give up most of her autonomy to persons often subordinate in age, sex, and social class. The patient needs the medical definition to minimize the threat to her dignity; the staff need it in order to inveigle the patient into cooperating.

Yet definitions that appear to contradict the medical definition are routinely expressed in the course of gynecological examinations. Some gestures acknowledge the pelvic area as special; other gestures acknowledge the patient as a person. These counterdefinitions are as essential to the encounter as the medical definition. We have already discussed how an actor's lack of conviction may interfere with his performance. Implicit acknowledgments of the special meaning of the pelvic area help those players hampered by lack of conviction to perform adequately. If a player's sense of "how things really are" is implicitly acknowledged, he often finds it easier to adhere outwardly to a contrary definition.

A physician may gain a patient's cooperation by acknowledging her as a person. The physician wants the patient to acknowledge the medical definition, cooperate with the procedures of the examination, and acknowledge his professional competence. The physician is in a position to bargain with the patient in order to obtain this cooperation. He can offer her attention and acknowledgment as a person. At times he does so.

Although defining a person as a technical object is necessary in order for medical activities to proceed, it constitutes an indignity in itself. This indignity can be canceled or at least qualified by simultaneously acknowledging the patient as a person.

The medical world contains special activities and special perspectives. Yet the inhabitants of the medical world travel back and forth to the general community, where modesty, death, and other medically relevant matters are regarded quite differently. It is not so easy to dismiss general community meanings for the time one finds oneself in a medical setting. The counterthemes that the pelvic area is special and that patients are persons provide an opportunity to show deference to general community meanings at the same time that one is disregarding them.

Sustaining the reality of a gynecological examination does not mean sustaining the medical definition, then. What is to be sustained is a shifting balance between medical definition and counterthemes.[8] Too much emphasis on the medical definition alone would undermine the reality, as would a flamboyant manifestation of the counterthemes apart from the medical definition. The next three sections will suggest how this balance is achieved.

Sustaining the Reality

The appropiate balance between medical definition and counterthemes has to be created anew at every moment. However, some routinized procedures and demeanor are available to participants in gynecological examinations. Persons recognize that if certain limits are exceeded, the situation will be irremediably shattered. Some arrangements have been found useful because they simultaneously express medical definition and countertheme. Routine ways of meeting the task requirements and also dealing with "normal trouble" are available. This section will describe how themes and counterthemes are embodied in routinized procedures and demeanor.

The pervasiveness of the medical definition is expressed by indicators that the scene is enacted under medical auspices.[9] The action is located in "medical space" (hospital or doctor's office). Features of the setting such as divisions of space, decor, and equipment are constant reminders that it is indeed "medical space." Even background details such as the loudspeaker calling "Dr. Morris, Dr. Armand Morris" serve as evidence for medical reality. (Suppose the loudspeaker were to announce instead: "Five minutes until post time.") The staff wear medical uniforms, don medical gloves, use medical instruments. The exclusion of laypersons, particularly visitors of the patient who may be accustomed to the patient's nudity at home, helps to preclude confusion between the contact of medicine and the contact of intimacy.[10]

Some routine practices simultaneously acknowledge the medical definition and qualify it by making special provision for the pelvic area. For instance, rituals of respect express dignity for the patient. The patient's body is draped so as to expose only that part which is to receive the technical attention of the doctor. The presence of a nurse acting as "chaperone" cancels any residual suggestiveness of male and female alone in a room.[11]

Medical talk stands for and continually expresses allegiance to the medical definition. Yet certain features of medical talk acknowledge a nonmedical delicacy. Despite the fact that persons present on a gynecological ward must attend to many topics connected with the pelvic area and various bodily functions, these topics are generally not discussed. Strict conventions dictate what unmentionables are to be acknowledged under what circumstances. However, persons are exceptionally free to refer to the genitals and related matters on the obstetrics-gynecology service. If technical matters in regard to the pelvic area come up, they are to be discussed nonchalantly.

The special language found in staff-patient contacts contributes to depersonalization and desexualization of the encounter. Scientific-sounding medical terms facilitate such communication. Substituting dictionary terms for everyday words adds formality. The definite article replaces the pronoun adjective in reference to body parts, so that, for example, the doctor refers to "the vagina" and never "your vagina." Instructions to the patient in the course of the examination are couched in language that bypasses sexual imagery; the vulgar connotation of "spread your legs" is generally metamorphosed into the innocuous "let your knees fall apart."

While among themselves the staff generally use explicit technical terms, explicit terminology is often avoided in staff-patient contacts.[12] The reference to the pelvic area may be merely understood, as when a patient says "I feel so uncomfortable there right now" or "They didn't go near to this area, so why did they have to shave it?" In speaking with patients the staff frequently uses euphemisms. A doctor asks: "When did you first notice difficulty down below?" and a nurse inquires: "Did you wash between your legs?" Persons characteristically refer to pelvic examinations euphemistically in staff-patient encounters. "The doctors want to take a peek at you," a nurse tells a patient. Or "Dr. Ryan wants to see you in the examining room."

In one pelvic examination there was a striking contrast between the language of staff and patient. The patient was graphic; she used action words connoting physical contact to refer to the examination procedure: feeling, poking, touching, and punching. Yet she never located this action in regard to her body, always omitting to state where the physical contact occurred. The staff used impersonal medical language and euphemisms: "I'm going to examine you"; "I'm just cleaning out some blood clots"; "He's just trying to fix you up a bit."

Sometimes the staff introduce explicit terminology to clarify a patient's remark. A patient tells the doctor "It's bleeding now" and the doctor answers: "You? From the vagina?" Such a response indicates the appropriate vocabulary, the degree of freedom permitted in technically oriented conversation, and the proper detachment. Yet the common avoidance of explicit terminology in staff-patient contacts suggests that, despite all the precautions to assure that the medical definition prevails, many patients remain somewhat embarrassed by the whole subject. To avoid provoking this embarrassment, euphemisms and understood references are used when possible.

Highly specific requirements for everybody's behavior during a gynecological examination curtail the leeway for the introduction of discordant notes. Routine technical procedures organize the event from beginning to end, indicating what action each person should take at each moment. Verbal exchanges are also constrained by the technical task, in that the doctor uses routine phrases of direction and reassurance to the patient. There is little margin for ad-libbing during a gynecological examination.

The specifications for demeanor are elaborate. Foremost is that both staff and patient should be nonchalant about what is happening. According to the staff, the exemplary patient should be "in play," showing she is attentive to the situation by her bodily tautness, facial expression, direction of glance, tone of voice, tempo of speech and bodily movements, and timing and appropriateness of responses. The patient's voice should be controlled, mildly pleasant, self-confident, and impersonal. Her facial expression should be attentive and neutral, leaning toward the mildly pleasant and friendly side, as if she were talking to the doctor in his office, fully dressed and seated in a chair. The patient is to have an attentive glance upward, at the ceiling or at other persons in the room, eyes open, not dreamy or "away," but ready at a second's notice to revert to the doctor's face for a specific verbal exchange. Except for such a verbal exchange, however, the patient is supposed to avoid looking into the doctor's eyes during the actual examination because direct eye contact between the two at this time is provocative. Her role calls for passivity and self-effacement. The patient should show willingness to relinquish control to the doctor. She should refrain from speaking at length and from making inquiries that would require the doctor to reply at length. So as not to point up her undignified position, she should not project her personality profusely. The self must be eclipsed in order to sustain the definition that the doctor is working on a technical object and not a person.

The physician's demeanor is highly stylized. He intersperses his examination with remarks to the patient in a soothing tone of voice: "Now relax as much as you can"; "I'll be as gentle as I can"; "Is that tender right there?" Most of the phrases with which he encourages the patient to relax are routine, even though his delivery may suggest a unique relationship. He demonstrates that he is the detached professional, and the patient demonstrates that it never enters her mind that he could be anything except detached. Since intimacy can be introduced into instrumental physical contact by a "loving" demeanor (lingering, caressing motions and contact beyond what the task requires), a doctor must take special pains to ensure that his demeanor remains a brisk, no-nonsense show of efficiency.[13]

Once I witnessed a gynecological examination of a 40-year-old woman who played the charming and scatterbrained Southern belle. The attending physician stood near the patient's head and carried on a flippant conversation with her while a resident and a medical student performed the actual examination. The patient completely ignored the examination, except for brief answers to the examining doctor's inquiries. Under these somewhat trying circumstances she attempted to carry off a gay, attractive pose, and the attending physician cooperated with her by making a series of bantering remarks.

Most physicians are not so lucky as to have a colleague conversing in cocktail-hour style with the patient while they are probing her vagina. Ordinarily the physician must play both parts at once, treating the patient as an object with his hands while simultaneously acknowledging her as a person with his voice. In this incident, where two physicians simultaneously deal with the patient in two distinct ways, the dual approach to the patient usually maintained by the examining physician becomes more obvious.[14]

The doctor needs to communicate with the patient as a person for technical reasons. Should he want to know when the patient feels pain in the course of examination, or information about other medical matters, he must address her as a person. Also, the doctor may want to instruct the patient on how to facilitate the examination. The most reiterated instruction refers to relaxation. Most patients are not sufficiently relaxed when the doctor is ready to begin. He then reverts to a primitive level of communication and treats the patient almost like a young child. He speaks in a soft, soothing voice, probably calling the patient by her first name, and it is not so much the words as his manner that is significant. This caressing voice is routinely used by hospital staff members to patients in critical situations, as when the patient is overtly frightened or disoriented. By using it here, the doctor heightens his interpersonal relation with the patient, trying to reassure her as a person in order to get her to relax.

Moreover, even during a gynecological examination, failing to acknowledge another as a person is an insult. It is insulting to be entirely instrumental about instrumental contacts. Some acknowledgment of the intimate connotations of touching must occur. Therefore, a measure of "loving" demeanor is subtly injected. A doctor cannot employ the full gamut of loving insinuations that a lover might infuse into instrumental touching, so he indirectly implies a hint of intimacy which is intended to counter the insult and make the procedure acceptable to the woman. The doctor conveys this loving demeanor not by lingering or superfluous contact, but by radiating concern in his general manner, offering extra assistance, and occasionally sacrificing the task requirements to "gentleness."

In short, the doctor must convey an optimal combination of impersonality and hints of intimacy and simultaneously avoid the insult of sexual familiarity and the insult of unacknowledged identity. The doctor must manage this even though the behaviors emanating from these definitions are contradictory. If the doctor can achieve this feat, it will contribute to keeping the patient in line. In the next section, we will see how the patient may threaten this precarious balance.

Precariousness in Gynecological Examinations

Threats to the reality of a gynecological examination may occur if the balance of opposing definitions is not maintained as described above. Reality in gynecological examinations is challenged mainly by patients. Occasionally a medical student, who might be considerably more of a novice than an experienced patient, seemed uncomfortable in the scene.[15] Experienced staff members were rarely observed to undermine the reality.

Certain threatening events that could occur in any staff-patient encounter bring an added dimension of precariousness to a gynecological examination because the medical aegis screens so much more audacity at that time. In general, staff expect patients to remain poised and in play like a friendly office receptionist; any show of emotion except in a controlled fashion is objectionable. Patients should not focus on identities of themselves or the staff outside those relevant to the medical exchange. Intractable patients may complain about the pain, discomfort, and indignities of submitting to medical treatment and care. Patients may go so far as to show reluctance to comply with the staff. Even if they are complying, they may indirectly challenge the expert status of the staff, as by "asking too many questions."

Failure to maintain a poised performance is a possible threat in any social situation. Subtle failures of tone are common, as when a performer seems to lack assurance. Performers may fumble for their lines, hesitate, begin a line again, or correct themselves. A show of embarrassment, such as blushing, has special relevance in gynecological examinations. On rare occasions when a person shows signs of sexual response, he or she really has something to blush about. A more subtle threat is an indication that the actor is putting an effort into the task of maintaining nonchalant demeanor; if it requires such an effort, perhaps it is not a "natural" response.

Such effort may be indicated, for example, in regard to the direction of glance. Most situations have a common visual focus of attention, but in a gynecological examination the logical focus (the patient's internal organs) is not accessible and none of the alternatives, such as staring at the patient's face, locking glances with others, or looking out the window, are feasible. The unavailability of an acceptable place to rest the eyes is more evident when the presence of several medical students creates a "crowd" atmosphere in the small cubicle. The lack of a visual focus of attention and the necessity to shift the eyes from object to object requires the participants to remain vaguely aware of their directions of glance. Normally the resting place of the eyes is a background matter automatically managed without conscious attention. Attentiveness to this background detail is a constant reminder of how awkward the situation is.

Certain lapses in a patient's demeanor are so common as hardly to be threatening. When a patient expresses pain, it can be overlooked if the patient is giving other signs of trying to behave well, because it can be taken that the patient is temporarily overwhelmed by a physiological state. The demonstrated presence of pain recalls the illness framework and counters sexual connotations. Crying can be accredited to pain and dismissed in a similar way. Withdrawing attention from the scene, so that one is not ready with an immediate comeback when called upon, is also relatively innocuous because it is close to the required "passive but in play" demeanor.

Some threats derive from the patient's ignorance of how to strike an acceptable balance between medical and nonmedical definitions, despite her willingness to do so. In two areas in particular, patients stumble over the subtleties of what is expected: physical decorum (proprieties of sights, sounds, and smells of the body) and modesty. While the staff are largely concerned with behavioral decorum and not with lapses in physical decorum, patients are more concerned about the latter, whether due to their medical condition or to the procedure. Patients sometimes even let behavioral decorum lapse in order to express their concern about unappealing conditions of their bodies, particularly discharges and odors. This concern is a vestige of a nonmedical definition of the situation, for an attractive body is relevant only in a personal situation and not in a medical one.

Some patients fail to know when to display their private parts unashamedly to others and when to conceal them like anyone else. A patient may make an "inappropriate" show of modesty, thus not granting the staff the right to view what medical personnel have the right to view and others do not. But if a patient acts as though she literally accepts the medical definition, this also constitutes a threat. If a patient insists on acting as if exposing her breasts, buttocks, and pelvic area is no different from exposing her arm or leg, she is "immodest." The medical definition is supposed to be in force only as necessary to facilitate specific medical tasks. If a patient becomes nonchalant enough to allow herself to remain uncovered for much longer than is technically necessary, she becomes a threat. This also holds for verbal remarks about personal matters. Patients who misinterpret the license by exceeding its limits unwittingly challenge the definition of reality.[16]

Neutralizing Threatening Events

Most gynecological examinations proceed smoothly, and the definition of reality is sustained without conscious attention.[17] Sometimes subtle threats to the definition arise, and occasionally staff and patient struggle covertly over the definition throughout the encounter.[18] The staff take more preventive measures where they anticipate the most trouble: young, unmarried girls; persons known to be temporarily upset; and persons with reputations as uncooperative. In such cases the doctor may explain the technical details of the procedure more carefully and offer direct reassurance. Perhaps he will take extra time to establish personal rapport, as by medically related inquiries ("How are you feeling?" "Do you have as much pain today?"), personal inquiries ("Where do you live?"), addressing the patient by her first name, expressing direct sympathy, praising the patient for her behavior in this difficult situation, speaking in a caressing voice, and affectionate gestures. Doctors also attempt to reinforce rapport as a response to threatening events.

The foremost technique in neutralizing threatening events is to sustain a nonchalant demeanor even if the patient is blushing with embarrassment, blanching from fear, or moaning in pain. The patient's inappropriate gestures may be ignored as the staff convey "We're waiting until you are ready to play along." Working to bring the scene off, the staff may claim that this is routine, or happens to patients in general; invoke the "for your own good" clause; counter-claim that something is less important than the patient indicates; assert that the unpleasant medical procedure is almost over; and contend that the staff do not like to cause pain or trouble to patients (as by saying "I'm sorry" when they appear to be causing pain). The staff may verbally contradict a patient, give an evasive answer to a question, or try to distract the patient. By giving a technical explanation or rephrasing in the appropriate hospital language something the patient has referred to in a nonmedical way, the staff member reinstates the medical definition.

Redefinition is another tactic available to the staff. Signs of embarrassment and sexual arousal in patients may be redefined as "fear of pain." Sometimes sexual arousal will be labeled "ticklishness." After one examination the doctor thanked the patient, presumably for her cooperation, thus typifying the patient's behavior as cooperative and so omitting a series of uncooperative acts he had previously acknowledged.

Humor may be used to discount the line the patient is taking. At the same time, humor provides a safety valve for all parties whereby the sexual connotations and general concern about gynecological examinations may be expressed by indirection. Without taking the responsibility that a serious form of the message would entail, the participants may communicate with each other about the events at hand. They may discount the derogatory implications of what would be an invasion of privacy in another setting by dismissing the procedure with a laugh. A person who can joke on a topic demonstrates to others a laudatory degree of detachment.

For example, in one encounter a patient vehemently protests: "Oh, Dr. Raleigh, what are you doing?" Dr. Raleigh, exaggerating his southern accent, answers: "Nothin'." His levity conveys: "However much you may dislike this, we have to go on with it for your own good. Since you know that perfectly well, your protest could not be calling for a serious answer." Dr. Raleigh also plays the seducer claiming innocence, thus obliquely referring to the sexual connotations of where his hand is at the moment. In another incident, Dr. Ryan is attempting to remove some gauze which has been placed in the vagina to stop bleeding. He flippantly announces that the remaining piece of gauze has disappeared inside the patient. After a thorough search, Dr. Ryan holds up a piece of gauze on the instrument triumphantly: "Well, here it is. Do you want to take it home and put it in your scrapbook?" By this remark, Dr. Ryan ridicules the degree of involvement in one's own medical condition that would induce a patient to save this kind of memento. Later in the same examination Dr. Ryan announces he will do a rectal examination and the (elderly) patient protests: "Oh, honey, don't bother." Dr. Ryan assures her jokingly: "It's no bother, really." The indirect message of all three jokes is that one should take gynecological procedures casually. Yet simultaneously an undercurrent of each joke acknowledges a perspective contrary to the medical definition.

While in most encounters the nurse remains quietly in the background, she comes forward to deal actively with the patient if the definition of reality is threatened. In fact, one of the main functions of her presence is to provide a team member for the doctor in those occasional instances where the patient threatens to get out of line. Team members can create a more convincing reality than one person alone. Doctor and nurse may collude against an uncooperative patient, as by giving each other significant looks. If things reach the point of staff collusion, however, it may mean that only by excluding the patient can the definition of reality be reaffirmed. A more drastic form of solidifying the definition by excluding a recalcitrant participant is to cast the patient in the role of an "emotionally disturbed person." Whatever an "emotionally disturbed person" may think or do does not count against the reality the rest of us acknowledge.

Perhaps the major safeguard of reality is that challenge is channeled outside the examination. Comments about the unpleasantness of the procedure and unaesthetic features of the patient's body occur mainly between women—two patients, or a nurse and a patient. Such comments are most frequent while the patient gets ready for the examination and waits for the doctor or after the doctor leaves. The patient may establish a momentary "fellow-woman aura" as she quietly voices her distaste for the procedure to the nurse. "What we women have to go through," the patient may say. Or, "I wish all gynecologists were women." Why? "They understand because they've been through it themselves." The patient's confiding manner implies: "I have no right to say this, or even feel it, and yet I do." This phenomenon suggests that patients actually have strong negative reactions to gynecological examinations which belie their acquiescence in the actual situation. Yet patients' doubts are expressed in an innocuous way that does not undermine the definition of reality when it is most needed.

To construct the scene convincingly, participants constantly monitor their own behavior and that of others. The tremendous work of producing the scene is contained in subtle maneuvers in regard to details that may appear inconsequential to the layman. Since awareness may interfere with a convincing performance, the participants may have an investment in being as un-self-conscious as possible. But the sociologist is free to recognize the significance of "inconsequential details" in constructing reality.

Conclusion

In a gynecological examination the reality sustained is not the medical definition alone, but a dissonance of themes and counterthemes. What is done to acknowledge one theme undermines the others. No theme can be taken for granted, because its opposite is always in mind. That is why the reality of a gynecological examination can never be routinized but always remains precarious.

The gynecological examination should not be dismissed as an anomaly. The phenomenon is revealed more clearly in this case because it is an extreme example, but the gynecological examination merely exaggerates the internally contradictory nature of definitions of reality found in most situations. Many situations where the dominant definition is occupational or technical have a secondary theme of sociality which must be implicitly acknowledged (as in buttering up the secretary, small talk with sales clerks, or the undertaker's show of concern for the bereaved family). In "business entertaining" and conventions of professional associations a composite definition of work and pleasure is sustained. Under many circumstances, a composite definition of action as both deviant and unproblematic prevails. For example, while Donald Ball stresses the claim of respectability in his description of an abortion clinic, his material illustrates the interplay of the dominant theme of respectability and a countertheme wherein the illicitness of the situation is acknowledged.[19] Internally inconsistent definitions of who persons are and what their relationships with one another are also are sustained in many settings.

Sustaining a sense of the solidness of a reality composed of multiple contradictory definitions takes unremitting effort. The required balance among the various definitions fluctuates from moment to moment. The appropriate balance depends on what the participants are trying to do at that moment. As soon as one matter is dealt with, something else comes into focus, calling for a diferent balance. Sometimes, even before one issue is completed, another may impose itself as taking priority. Further, each balance contains the seeds of its own demise, in that a temporary emphasis on one theme may disturb the long-run balance unless subsequent emphasis on the countertheme negates it. Because the most effective balance depends on many unpredictable factors, it is difficult to routinize the balance into formulas that prescribe a specific balance for given conditions. Routinization is also impractical because the particular forms by which the themes are expressed are opportunistic. That is, persons seize opportunities for expression according to what would be a suitable move at each unique moment of an encounter. Therefore, a person constantly must attend to how to express the balance of themes via the currently available means.

Multiple contradictory realities are expressed on various levels of explicitness and implicitness. Sustaining a sense of solidness of reality depends on the right balance of explicit and implicit expressions of each theme through a series of points in time. The most effective gestures express a multitude of themes on different levels. The advantages of multiple themes in the same gesture are simultaneous qualification of one theme by another, hedging (the gesture lacks one definite meaning), and economy of gestures.

Rational choices of explicit and implicit levels would take the following into account: The explicit level carries the most weight, unless countered by deliberate effort. Things made explicit are harder to dismiss or discount than what is left implicit. In fact, if the solidification of explication is judged to be nonreversible, use of the explicit level may not be worth the risk. On the other hand, when participants sense that the implicit level is greatly in use, their whole edifice of belief may be shaken. "I sense that a lot is going on underneath" makes a person wonder about the reality he is accepting. There must be a lot he does not know, some of which might be evidence which would undermine what he currently accepts.

The invalidation of one theme by the concurrent expression of its countertheme must be avoided by various maneuvers.. The guiding principle is that participants must prevent a definition that a contradiction exists between theme and countertheme from emerging. Certain measures routinely contribute to this purpose. Persons must try to hedge on both theme and countertheme by expressing them tentatively rather than definitely and simultaneously alluding to and discounting each theme. Theme and countertheme should not be presented simultaneously or contiguously on the explicit level unless it is possible to discount their contradictory features. Finally, each actor must work to keep the implicit level out of awareness for the other participants.

The technique of constructing reality depends on good judgment about when to make things explicit and when to leave them implicit, how to use the implicit level to reinforce and qualify the explicit level, distributing themes among explicit and implicit levels at any one moment, and seizing opportunities to embody messages. To pursue further these tentative suggestions on how important explicit and implicit levels are for sustaining reality, implicit levels of communication must be explored more systematically.

Acknowledgments

Arlene K. Daniels has applied her talent for editing and organizing to several drafts of this paper. Robert M. Emerson, Roger Pritchard, and Thomas J. Scheff have also commented on the material. The investigation was supported in part by a predoctoral fellowship from the National Institute of Mental Health (Fellowship Number MPM-18,239) and by Behavioral Sciences Training Grant MH-8104 from the National Institute of Mental Health, as well as General Research Support Grant I-SOI-FR-05441 from the National Institutes of Health, U.S. Department of Health, Education and Welfare, to the School of Public Health, University of California, Berkeley.

Notes

1. Peter Berger and Thomas Luckmann, *The Social Construction of Reality* (Garden City, N.Y.: Doubleday, 1966).

2. The precarious nature of social interaction is discussed throughout the work of Erving Goffman.

3. The data in this article are based on observations of approximately 75 gynecological examinations conducted by male physicians on an obstetrics-gynecology ward and some observations from a medical ward for comparison. For a full account of this study, see Joan P. Emerson, Social Functions of Humor in a Hospital Setting, doctoral dissertation, University of California at Berkeley, 1963. For a sociological discussion of a similar setting, see William P. Rosengren and Spencer DeVault, The sociology of time and space in an obstetrical hospital, in *The Hospital in Modern Society*, Eliot Freidson, ed. (New York: Free Press of Glencoe, 1963).

4. It takes severe biographical shocks to disintegrate the massive reality internalized in early childhood; much less to destroy the realities internalized later. Beyond this, it is relatively easy to set aside the reality of the secondary internalizations." Berger and Luckmann, op. cit., p. 142.

5. As stated by Lief and Fox: "The amounts and occasions of bodily contact are carefully regulated in all societies, and very much so in ours. Thus, the kind of access to the body of the patient that a physician in our society has is a uniquely privileged one. Even in the course of a so-called routine physical examination, the physician is permitted to handle the patient's body in ways otherwise permitted only to special intimates, and in the case of procedures such as rectal and vaginal examinations in ways normally not even permitted to a sexual partner." Harold I. Lief and Renee C. Fox, Training for "detached concern" in medical students, in Harold I. Lief et al. (eds.), *The Psychological Basis of Medical Practice* (New York: Harper & Row, 1963), p. 32. As Edward Hall remarks, North Americans have an inarticulated convention that discourages touching except in moments of intimacy. Edward T. Hall, *The Silent Language* (Garden City, N.Y.: Doubleday, 1959), p. 149.

6. For comments on embarrassment in the doctor-patient relation, see Michael Balint, *The Doctor, His Patient, and the Illness* (New York: International Universities Press, 1957), p. 57.

7. Physicians are aware of the possibility that their routine technical behavior may be interpreted as sexual by the patient. The following quotation states a view held by some physicians: "It is not unusual for a suspicious hysterical woman with fantasies of being seduced to misinterpret an ordinary movement in the physical examination as an amorous advance." E. Weiss and O. S. English, *Psychosomatic Medicine* (Philadelphia: Saunders, 1949), quoted in Marc Hollender, *The Psychology of Medical Practice* (Philadelphia: Saunders, 1958), p. 22. An extreme case suggests that pelvic examinations are not without their hazards for physicians, particularly during training: "A third-year student who had prided himself on his excellent adjustment to the stresses of medical school developed acute anxiety when about to perform, for the first time, a pelvic examination on a gynecological patient. Prominent in his fantasies were memories of a punishing father who would unquestionably forbid any such explicitly sexual behavior." Samuel Bojar, Psychiatric problems of medical students, in *Emotional Problems of the Student*, Graham B. Blaine, Jr., et al., eds. (Garden City, N.Y.: Doubleday, 1961), p. 248.

8. Many other claims and assumptions are being negotiated or sustained in addition to this basic definition of the situation. Efforts in regard to some of these other claims and assumptions have important consequences for the fate of the basic definition. That is, in the actual situation any one gesture usually has relevance for a number of realities, so that the fates of the various realities are intertwined with each other. For example, each participant is putting forth a version of himself which he wants validated. A doctor's claims about competence may reinforce the medical definition, and so may a patient's interest in appearing poised. But a patient's ambition to "understand what is really happening" may lead to undermining of the medical definition. Understanding that sustaining the basic definition of the situation is intertwined with numerous other projects, however, we will proceed to focus on that reality alone.

9. Compare Donald Ball's account of how the medical definition is conveyed in an abortion clinic, where it serves to counter the definition of the situation as deviant.

Donald W. Ball, An abortion clinic ethnography, *Social Problems* 14 (winter 1967): 293–301.

10. Glaser and Strauss discuss the hospital prohibition against examinations and exposure of the body in the presence of intimates of the patient. Barney Glaser and Anselm Strauss, *Awareness of Dying* (Chicago: Aldine, 1965), p. 162.

11. Sudnow reports that at the county hospital he studied, male physicians routinely did pelvic examinations without nurses present, except in the emergency ward. David Sudnow, *Passing On: The Social Organization of Dying* (Englewood Cliffs, N.J.: Prentice-Hall, 1967), p. 78.

12. The following quotation suggests that euphemisms and understood references may be used because the staff often has the choice of using "lewd words" or not being understood. "Our popular vocabulary for describing sexual behavior has been compounded of about equal parts of euphemism and obscenity, and popular attitude and sentiment have followed the same duality. Among both his male and female subjects, the interviewers found many who knew only the lewd words for features of their own anatomy and physiology." Nelson N. Foote, Sex as play, in Jerome Himelhock and Sylvia F. Fava, *Sexual Behavior in American Society* (New York: Norton, 1955), p. 239.

13. The doctor's demeanor typically varies with his experience. In his early contacts with patients, the young medical student may use an extreme degree of impersonality generated by his own discomfort in his role. By the time he has become accustomed to doctor-patient encounters, the fourth-year student and intern may use a newcomer's gentleness, treating the scene almost as an intimate situation by relying on elements of the "loving" demeanor previously learned in nonprofessional situations. By the time he is a resident and focusing primarily on the technical details of the medical task, the physician may be substituting a competent impersonality, although he never reverts to the extreme impersonality of the very beginning. The senior doctor, having mastered not only the technical details but an attitude of detached concern as well, reintroduces a mild gentleness without the involved intimacy of the intern.

14. The management of closeness and detachment in professional-client relations is discussed in Charles Kadushin, Social distance between client and professional, *American Journal of Sociology* 67 (March 1962): 517–531. Wilensky and Lebeaux discuss how intimacy with strangers in the social worker–client relation is handled by accenting the technical aspects of the situation, limiting the relationship to the task at hand, and observing the norms of emotional neutrality, impartiality, and altruistic service. Harold L. Wilensky and Charles N. Lebeaux, *Industrial Society and Social Welfare* (New York: Russell Sage Foundation, 1958), pp. 299–303.

15. For a discussion of the socialization of medical students toward a generally detached attitude, see Lief and Fox, op. cit., pp. 12–35. See also Morris J. Daniels, Affect and its control in the medical intern, *American Journal of Sociology* 66 (November 1960): 259–267.

16. The following incident illustrates how a patient may exceed the limits: Mrs. Lane, a young married woman, was considered by the physicians a "seductive patient," although her technique was subtle and her behavior never improper. After examining Mrs. Lane, an intern privately called my attention to a point in the examination when he was pressing on the patient's ovaries and she remarked to the nurse: "I have this pain in intercourse until my insides are about to come out." The intern told me

that Mrs. Lane said that to the nurse, but she wanted him to hear. He didn't want to know that, he said; it wasn't necessary for her to say that. The intern evidently felt that Mrs. Lane's remark had exceeded the bounds of decorum. A specific medical necessity makes the imparting of private information acceptable, the doctor's reaction suggests, and not merely the definition of the situation as medical.

17. There is reason to think that those patients who would have most difficulty in maintaining their poise generally avoid the situation altogether. Evidence that some uncool women avoid pelvic examinations is found in respondents remarks quoted by Rainwater: "I have thought of going to a clinic for a diaphragm, but I'm real backward about doing that. I don't even go to the doctor to be examined when I'm pregnant. I never go until about a month before I have the baby." "I tell you frankly, I'd like a diaphragm but I'm just too embarrassed to go get one." Lee Rainwater, *And the Poor Get Children* (Chicago: Quadrangle, 1960), pp. 10, 31.

18. An example of such a struggle is analyzed in Joan P. Emerson, Nothing unusual is happening, in Tamotsu Shibutani, editor, *Human Nature and Collective Behavior: Papers in Honor of Herbert Blower* (Englewood Cliffs, N.J.: Prentice-Hall, 1970).

19. Donald Ball, op. cit.

7

The Captive Professional: Bureaucratic Limitations in the Practice of Military Psychiatry
Arlene K. Daniels

When a member of one of the "free" professions becomes an employee of a bureaucratic organization, the organization often supersedes the ultimate control and authority normally invested in his professional colleagues, and the professional thus becomes a "captive." The captivity of employment may then create conflicts for the professional caught between the value systems of his profession and those of the organization to which he submits. This paper delineates some of the conflicts inherent in differing value systems and describes how the conflicts engendered by captivity may be resolved.[1] The example provided for this description is that of the military psychiatrist.[2]

The professional model of activity has always been that of the free agent contracting to perform a service for his client. (Carr-Saunders and Wilson 1933; Scott 1966, p. 268) Thus the client can choose his own professional, and the first loyalty of the professional is to his client. However, this model gives little attention to the vast numbers of professionals who have always been employed by organizations and the changes which such employment brings about in the client-professional relationship. The argument which inhibits the change in this focus of attention has been that the independence, initiative, and professional judgment of the practitioner are strongly instilled through specialized training. Therefore the professional character of the service rendered by the practitioner remains essentially unchanged regardless of the context and circumstances in which it occurs. In this view, the assumption can be made that the military officer, the county clinic physician, the schoolteacher, and the court-appointed public defender will adhere to the ideas of public service instilled in their training despite pressures from either personal or organizational

Reprinted, with permission, from *Journal of Health and Social Behavior* 10 (1969): 255–265. Copyright 1969 by American Sociological Association.

interests. As a result of this assumption, practitioners in these and similar categories have been treated as though they were "free professionals," self-employed and independently formulating their theories and practices for the benefit of their clients. (Scott 1966, p. 270) Unfortunately, such a view ignores the ways in which conflicting values exert pressures upon the practitioner, particularly where third parties intervene in some manner for the serviced client. Professions with a basic mandate to provide a personal service to the individual—for example, the medical profession—may find this mandate directly or indirectly challenged by organizational priorities which require either the practitioner or his client to place other considerations first[3] (Freidson 1963, p. 316).

This situation has led to a literature produced by the professions in which one often finds expressed the assumption that professionals enforce their definition of appropriate professional activity over the view of an organization employing them. However, studies by sociologists of professionals in organizations raise doubts about this assumption. Kornhauser (1962) shows, for example, that scientists in industry are pressured to subordinate their basic research interests to applied commercial problems of concern to their employers. Where the rewards are high enough, professionals may adapt their own professional ideas of competence, rewards, and status to the value system of the organization they serve. Coldner and Ritti (1967, pp. 489–502) show how readily professionals abandon their own work for administrative duties so as to rise within the status hierarchy of their employing organization. Merton (1957, pp. 207–224) has suggested that intellectuals who enter governmental service face similar predicaments. When they accept the value system and the task as given by bureaucracy chiefs, they perform as technical advisors. Some intellectuals who are more professionally innovative many try to influence the existing bureaucratic system of priorities and values to conform to their professional definitions. But the effectiveness of these attempts is open to question; defeated or disillusioned intellectuals often leave government service. These studies suggest that it cannot be assumed that organizational goals will give way to professional goals. Professionals who wish to succeed may well respond to the specific immediate pressures of their employing organization before the more abstract and distant expectations of their profession. Further, conflict resolution may be so successful that professionals may no longer perceive even the potential existence of that conflict. Burchard (1954, pp. 528–535) shows, for instance, that conflicts in basic differences between professional and organizational values are so readily resolved in favor of the organization that no conflict is seen. When he asked military chaplains how they managed conflicts between their loyalty to the biblical commandment against killing and their loyalty to the military organization, most did not see any conflict.

The changes or modifications in professional practice which result from adaptations to organizational requirements are not superficial; rather, such changes often affect the core functions of the profession. In the case of psychiatry, as Szasz (1963, p. 1967) has argued, once the profession moves into a bureaucratic setting it becomes unrecognizable. The focus of the practitioner's concern can no longer be on helping the patient, because his professional rights and duties have been redefined by the organization.

The organization and practice of psychiatry is particularly vulnerable to organizational requirements. But in this respect psychiatry is similar to any profession offering a value-oriented service. Normally, when everyone agrees about the value (e.g., health) no problem arises. The problem of the value orientation arises when the professional practitioner is employed to mediate between conflicting sets of values. The value of health, for example, may be in conflict with the need for available manpower (Field 1960). In such situations the practitioner is subject to pressures by the groups represented, and is likely to make decisions which favor the client who has the most power. Thus professionals hired by organizations tend to support the dominant bureaucratic perspective rather than dissident elements within it. Paradoxically, this tendency appears even when the avowed function of professionals in the organization is to mitigate the bureaucratic perspective by offering advocacy or representation to those dissident elements.

In the case of psychiatry, vulnerability to the bureaucratic definition stems, at least in part, from the way in which psychiatric practice depends upon commonsense notions of illness (Garfinkel 1956, pp. 181–195). The very process of identifying patients for psychiatric treatment requires that commonsense judgments and diagnoses be made by laypersons. Eccentric behavior must be "diagnosed" as "symptoms" by friends, family, work associates, or neighbors before a person enters one of the psychiatric referral routes. Neighbors may suggest that one needs "help" (Mechanic 1967). In juvenile proceedings, probation officers sometimes explain a case to be presented to a psychiatrist so that the psychiatrist can "see" that the case is or is not one that would benefit from psychiatric intervention (Emerson 1968).

Vulnerabilities to bureaucratic definitions are compounded by the

ambiguities in psychiatric theory. These ambiguities allow justification for opposing positions taken about the proper relationship
between psychiatrist and patient. The ambiguities can be used to
provide ammunition to an already existing power structure where the
patient is subordinate to the psychiatrist. Patients may complain
about abrogation of their civil liberties, while doctors speak of resistance to treatment. Negroes may see themselves as persecuted in
situations where white hospital staff speak of paranoid delusions.

Ordinarily, in the private practice of psychiatry, this relation
between psychiatric practice and the commonly held values in the
society does not become an issue. The patient and the psychiatrist, for
example, usually share the same value system, and so they agree not
only that a certain type of behavior is wrong (or bad) but also that it is
pathological (or symptomatic). They can then agree on a course of
treatment because they agree that the patient's own behavior has led
to his unhappiness. Thus, the patient can present himself to the
psychiatrist for help. The existence of agreement in this case is
important because of its consequences. If differences should arise,
either party is free to terminate the relationship. However, when
psychiatry is practiced within an institutional setting, neither the
agreement nor this pattern for the resolution of differences can be
taken for granted.

In the institutional setting, it is not up to the patient to decide to
accept or reject the psychiatrist's evaluations. Nor is it left to the
patient to decide whether to utilize these evaluations in making
decisions about his own life. Though the patient may reject them, the
psychiatrist may be sought out and listened to by other members of
the organization who will accept his evaluation and attempt to
implement it. The contrast between private office practice and
organization-based psychiatry is particularly acute in the military
setting. Who may and who must see the psychiatrist, what kind of
treatment may be given, and when it must be given are all matters
defined by the military organization rather than areas of negotiation
open to the parties directly involved.[4]

The Place of Psychiatry in the Military Organization

Psychiatrists were introduced into the armed forces in order to aid or
manage the control of deviant behavior in new ways (Morgan 1961).
They are required because military service has never been popular
with the rank-and-file. A certain amount of coercion has always been
necessary in order to extract obedience; recalcitrance to orders from

those above one in the hierarchy is not tolerated, and insubordination is severely punished (deserters are sometimes shot). In the modern American military organization, such punishment of insubordinate behavior is somewhat restricted. Here, as in the civilian world, police and judicial functions of catching and punishing deviants are supplemented by the psychiatrist and his mental-hygiene-clinic team. They are expected to be the representatives of "modern humane" influences. They bring a permissiveness from the middle-class civilian value system into the harsh and disciplinary framework of a military bureaucracy. In such a context, permissiveness may be introduced when psychiatric diagnoses are accepted as a mitigating or excusing explanation for some unacceptable behavior.

However, as both the psychiatrists and their clients are in the military, it is the military, not the psychiatric profession, that defines the distinction between appropriate or inappropriate permissiveness and leniency. And it is the military organization, not the client, that decides how much of a psychiatric evaluation to accept. It is under these conditions that a transformation and a subordination of professional interpretations of behavior to organizational ones occur. The range of independent decisions and negotiations open to any professional, even though it exists, is constrained and delimited by the structure of organizational goals and values.[5]

To show the process by which psychiatric goals have been transformed by organizational goals, let us examine some of the core or prescribed duties required of the psychiatrist by the military, and then the range of situations the military psychiatrist faces and the adaptations to them that he is able to make.

The Basic Requirements of the Situation: Processing Referrals

Ideally, a patient in private practice comes voluntarily for an interview. But in military actions, the patient is not a patient; rather he is a "referral" in a system of channels. In this situation he comes not so much for an interview (which may be a prelude to psychotherapy) as for an interview (or examination) which will lead to a recommendation and disposition. He is usually sent by his commanding officer or by a medical corps officer, a chaplain, or a staff member from the Judge Advocate Corps (a lawyer). Thus, in the system it is by military officers that one is defined as in need of medical care. Should an individual desire to see the doctor on his own, he must go through "proper channels"; i.e., he is expected to request permission from his officers, so that by the time he reaches the psychiatrist the patient has become a referral from command.

It is so taken for granted that patients do not go directly to the psychiatrist that those who do present themselves are specially named: self-referrals. But even the self-referrals who make a direct request for an interview are seen first by the psychiatrist's agent (an enlisted-man technician), who screens them and decides on the reasonableness of the request before passing it on. Consequently, in one way or another, all patients go through a processing screening, which turns them into referrals. If a patient does not "need" to see the psychiatrist (i.e., does not require a psychiatric signature for some processing), he may be shunted out of the channel. In this case he is either counselled by the technician or referred to other services which the technician thinks appropriate.

The psychiatrist reviews the collection of facts prepared for him on those who survive the preliminary screening. He sees these persons very briefly and makes his recommendations (Maillet 1966, p. 168). Thus, the psychiatrist sees those who are defined by the organization as in need of his services. In military terms, the psychiatrist is needed so that he may evaluate all persons "requiring" a mental-health examination. He is not needed to perform psychotherapy on suitable patients. Only after the psychiatrist has dealt with the referrals can he consider what number and kind of patients he will select to see in therapy. There are a variety of situations in which military personnel are automatically referred to the psychiatrist for his recommendation. Three of the most common are discussed below.

The Psychiatric Evaluation for Administrative Separation
One of the main responsibilities of the military psychiatrist is examination of all candidates for administrative separation from the military. These candidates are men who are leaving the service for reasons other than those permitting a regular, honorable discharge yet are not seen as deserving the bad-conduct or dishonorable discharge.[6] Since separation leading to anything other than an honorable discharge casts some doubt on the ability or motivation for military service of the discharged, the psychiatrist must evaluate the relation of mental status to responsible action. This action is taken so that persons judged not entirely responsible due to some mental defect shall be exempt from the more harsh and punitive measures. In all cases where a man is under consideration for administrative separation, the signature of the psychiatrist must be on file before the man is retained or processed out of the service. This signature accompanies

the evaluation and a recommendation based upon the psychiatrist's opinion of the attention due the mental health of the referral in giving him a new assignment. For those considered unsuitable for retention, a psychiatric opinion affects the type of separation to be awarded. Such men (once separated) are released at the discretion of military authorities under either an honorable, a general, or an undesirable discharge. (The separation is, in bureaucratic terms, the first stage in release from service. It does not govern, though it strongly influences, the type of discharge awarded.)

Psychiatric Evaluation of the Accused Awaiting Trial
Psychiatrists in the military provide much the same kind of advice to the legal branch (the Judge Advocate Corps) of the service that forensic psychiatrists offer in civilian courts. Most commonly—as with the administrative separations—the task is a routine one. The general view is that all general courts martial require a psychiatric pretrial evaluation. But such evaluations are optional for any other, lesser court martial. The evaluation is similar to that in administrative separations; it involves screening persons accused of crimes in order to determine if any mental disease or defect is present. If none is found during pretrial evaluations, proceedings against the accused may continue according to military regulations.

Psychiatric Responsibility in Medical Separations
In the role of medical officer in the military, the psychiatrist serves on medical evaluation boards to decide whether or not a candidate should receive special status or disability retirement. These decisions are based on the extent of the disability and the psychiatric opinion as to the origin of the disability (prior to service or during duty). The psychiatrist thus facilitates or hinders a restrictive duty—military separation—and the granting of pension and disability benefits attendant upon such a separation. Here, as in the two other situations presented, the psychiatric opinion has fateful consequences for the patient.

Limitations on Psychiatric Practice Introduced by Basic Requirements of the Military Setting

The psychiatrist decides what consideration should be given to the mental status of each referral in cases of separation from or retention in the service and in cases of disciplinary or criminal trials. But he is not free to make the decision (or diagnosis) strictly in terms of his own professional judgment. Military regulations provide standards, which the psychiatrist must follow. These rules provide the meaning of the facts on which the psychiatrist is supposed to base his decision. For example, the kinds of behavior defined as relevant to psychiatry, and their diagnostic interpretations, are described in the Separations Manual (Personnel Separations Army Regulations: No. 636–212, 1966). These become the basic "facts of the case" as reported by or about the referral to the psychiatrist. Even though the psychiatrist may not have to recommend the type of separation by name, he is made aware of the effect of his report (or the report of others corroborated or denied by his examination) on the specific disposition of a case.[7] Thus, the psychiatrist learns to foresee that terms like "mental illness or incapacity" will be translated by other officers as "inability to soldier"; i.e., the Separations Officer in the Adjutant General's office will complete the separation forms under AR 635–212b.

Another way in which the organization constrains professional decisions is that the psychiatrist performs a specific role; he becomes an agent in the process of controlling and eliminating deviants. For example, a company commander must have the evaluation of the psychiatrist on record before he can initiate a separation request for one of his men. If the psychiatrist recommends a "further trial of duty," the commander will have difficulty persuading higher channels to honor his request to separate a man. The psychiatrist lends weight to the commander's request for a separation if his evaluation suggests that some kind of mental incapacity is present. The psychiatrist's expertise can be used to justify a separation where otherwise the question of the commander's leadership and judgment in the management of a difficult soldier might have been raised. Such considerations in the situation may be reflected directly in the diagnosis of the case. Thus, all parties involved come to understand that the requirement for a psychiatrist's evaluation may affect not only the future career of a difficult soldier but also, on occasion, the career of his commanding officer. However, in all likelihood, the most serious or fateful consequences are those which will befall the patient-referral.

The requirements and specifications which surround the psychiatric evaluation are not only more likely to be fateful to the direct referral, they are also likely to affect him disadvantageously. This consequence of psychiatric evaluation is seen most clearly in the psychiatrist's assistance in military court actions. The military organization requires service from psychiatrists to protect its judicial-criminal division from possible later charges of inhumane treatment. Theoretically, the psychiatrist either sifts mentally ill persons out of the judicial process or testifies on their behalf. However, there are very few cases where the restrictive military definitions of mental illness actually permit him to intervene for the referral. As a consequence, he is far more likely to be a witness for the prosecution, stating that no sign of mental disease or defect has been found. The following field-note excerpts are illustrative. As one officer in the Judge Advocate Corps put it,

The whole key is the seriousness of the offense. The more serious, the less credit prosecution is going to give a psychiatrist unless he says the guy is sane anyway.... Now ... this (is) the weakness of the system. Too great a pressure on (the) psychiatrist.

In general, this view of the existing pressures in the military system makes lawyers cautious about seeking psychiatric help for the defense of an accused. In commenting on this position, another member of the Judge Advocate Corps stated:

(The military psychiatrist) is not retained to be sympathetic.... He really isn't your doctor.... I don't think they're agents of the government so much as ... they just don't have as much time to spend on the individual.

The tendencies of the military system to marshal the support of the psychiatrist to a less sympathetic view of mental illness can also be seen in the management of criminals or accused persons caught in the disciplinary network of the system. As one psychiatrist put it,

At the stockade all the guys ask for an appointment, but we refuse to see them, because they know the psychiatrist is a way out.

In general, then, the likelihood that psychiatric evaluation will work to the advantage of the referral is slim.

Whatever the variety of administrative-legal processing responsibilities, the military psychiatrist remains primarily an evaluator and a maker of recommendations about a referral rather than a therapist offering him service. As a consequence, he makes more significant decisions about the lives of patients than his confreres do in most situations they meet in private practice. Moreover, the nature of the evaluations and their uses for bureaucratic requirements change the nature of the psychiatric function altogether. Gradually, then, the psychiatrist is transformed from a counseling agent into a controlling agent. Even when the psychiatrist does not specifically recommend a particular disposition of a referral, he cannot avoid the problem of judgment. In the military bureaucracy, when the psychiatrist makes a diagnosis or evaluation his professional decision (according to regulations) influences the specific award of one or another disposition of the case. Thus, even if he tries to avoid participation in issues, he in effect makes a decision. An Army psychiatrist who was chief of his service at a large post in 1968 illustrates this point in his discussion of the management of conscientious objectors:

There is a regulation which says that if a person wants to apply for conscientious objector [status] he has to go through a rigmarole and one of the rigmaroles he has to go through is to get a psychiatric evaluation. Now my own policy has been—which nobody has decided to question particularly— is that we will do a psychiatric evaluation. [But] we will not "pass" on the decision as to whether he is a conscientious objector or not. We will pass on whether we find any psychiatric illness. . . . So the majority of the people we see, the only thing that goes out is [date of evaluation and diagnosis of no psychiatric illness]. We do not say if he is or is not a CO because that is not our business. I couldn't tell a CO from anybody else. . . . I have never . . . recommended that a guy be discharged because he is a CO. I have recommended that he be put in a noncombat unit. Normally I just say NPD (no psychiatric disease).

The problem here is that the psychiatrist ignores the fact that, as a result of his diagnosis, the referral will be subjected to the harsher disciplinary measures available under military law. There is no way for the psychiatrist to avoid participation in the ultimate disposition of a case. Whether or not he objects to this consequence of his action, his compliance smoothes the path by which the military control system operates.

The following example demonstrates some of the problems of an Army psychiatry officer (at a basic training post in 1966) when he evaluates a conscientious objector:

A guy . . . went through a couple of trials here; said he was a conscientious objector, though registered and [then enlisted in the Army].
I evaluated him [as] NPD although well motivated to be a pacifist. His religious background was Church of Christ. Pacifism was part of this; although he hadn't practiced his religion, it was there in the background. I thought it was sincere. He wouldn't touch a gun, although willing to do other things. And they sentenced him to two or three years at Leavenworth and a DD [dishonorable discharge]. . . . I was called a couple of days before his trial, and trial counsel said: I want to warn you that defense counsel is thinking of calling you. I explained to him how detailed I had made my certificate. But he said defense counsel wants to challenge and you may have to prove the man is *not* mentally ill. . . . The only thing that made me worry

about [the possibility of his mental illness was that he accepted military counsel. I would have screamed for [Clarence Darrow]. . . .

In such a case, the psychiatrist may feel genuinely concerned over the fate of some referral. Nonetheless, he may not be able to find an opportunity within the system to argue for mercy in either the judgment or the sentencing.

Contingent Limitations on the Psychiatrist's Judgments
There are a number of shifting or variable contingencies which influence the interpretation of the "true and proper" meaning of the regulations under which the psychiatrist works. The final evaluation that he makes is influenced by the climate of opinion, the situational requirements, and the specific wishes of commanders or their key personnel.

The Effect of Climate of Opinion on Psychiatric Decisions in the Military
At the most general level, the climate of opinion often limits freedom to initiate and complete administrative actions. Ordinarily, in peacetime, officials in the military organization can cull out marginal and "difficult" servicemen. But during manpower shortages caused by acute or continued crises, only the strictest and most cautious interpretation of such categories as "unsuitable" or "inapt" may be permitted[8] (Ginsberg et al. 1953). On the other hand, a rash of suicides or an epidemic of meningitis may cause a reverse reaction and leniency in evaluations will be demanded. Even during a manpower shortage, public opinion and pressures from high officials may combine to push psychiatrists toward evaluations which permit easy or quick administrative separations.

In discussing a suicide "epidemic" at his post, one chief of a psychiatric unit made the following remarks:

There was an excessive number of suicides over a short period. . . . We had six in three months. The post Commanding General was very concerned about suicides. So we found that . . . we were getting a number of referrals of guys saying that I'm going to kill myself unless you get me out of the Army. . . . The General . . . thought this was important. . . . He said in his Command Conference [that] we've got to get rid of those guys and get them out of the Army. . . . I thought that we should at least be able to discuss . . . what is legitimate depression . . . what does a potential suicide look like?. . . . However I couldn't convince my next level commander . . . (that we should be selective in evaluating threats of suicide).

The Delimitations on Psychiatric Decisions Provided by Situational Events
In addition to the contingencies created by climate of opinion, the
processing of administrative separations is limited by such situational
factors as logistics and organizational specialization. An example of
the limitations caused by logistics is the general military policy not to
transfer active-duty personnel—with their belongings and depen-
dents—over long distances without a very good reason. Arrival and
departure at an overseas post is supposed to coincide with the assigned,
full tour of duty (generally a period of 1–3 years). This expectation
may be waived for very "good" reasons (e.g. hardship, legal-criminal,
medical). But the kinds of reasons governing the administrative
separation are not seen as within this category. A recommendation
for an otherwise routine administrative separation if initiated from a
garrison post in the continental U.S. may be impractical from combat
or occupation areas in Asia or Europe. A man who is "unfit" or
"inapt" will not meet the expectations governing the general or
honorable discharge once he is overseas, even though his case might
meet these expectations if he were still in the U.S.

The second limitation—organizational specialization—arises because military regulations allow various types of actions to be initiated
only at given posts. This means that in separations a man should be
examined by a psychiatrist at or near his own post; examination by a
group of more specialized psychiatrists at the large military hospital
centers is not considered necessary. The likelihood that an administrative separation will be allowed under the auspices of a distant
hospital is problematical at best, for medical boards will see the
referral as inappropriate and return the man to the "proper level for
action." A resident explains:

> The way we handle [inappropriate transfer for administrative action here]
> is to send a guy back [to the field] for what we call trial of duty—meaning
> that your decision is back in your lap.... They can send him right back to
> us.... I know of some of the other ... residents [who] did have fellows who
> bounced back and forth.... We got tired and finally gave them the type of
> discharge we thought they deserved or else we have them assigned some
> place and a fresh doctor or a fresh unit took them over.

Problems Created by Idiosyncratic Commanders
In addition to the foregoing limitations on the psychiatrist's discretion, one must consider that commanders of hospitals, posts, or
departments sometimes have powers similar to those of feudal barons
in their fiefs. Current "official" policy about regulations may be
overturned or "reinterpreted" by local commanders or their key

administrators. Here are two examples of such contingencies:

We generally recommend [the less punitive separation]. But having to live under post policy, we just recommend "discharge under appropriate recommendation" because [otherwise] this double-binds the intermediate CO [commanding officer]. He may agree and want to give the man a general discharge. But the attitudes or policy of higher command is if you make it too easy, everyone will try to get out. So you got to punish. Kind of turns my stomach. But that is the way life is here.

The Chief of Staff is ... probably one of the most powerful people on a military post as far as decision-making and policy changing and so on.... He has some effect. And in this [administrative separation] business he did.... For a while they asked us not to make any recommendations whatsoever ... not to name a regulation. And ... what was happening was some little girl who was working in the office in AG [the Adjutant General division] ... we called her "Lieutenant Colonel" Thomas ... she was a civil service employee. And she was typing these [separation forms] for the general's signature, supposedly getting all the information (for) the more punitive separation. And making a final recommendation which the general was to sign. Now she liked to [give] everyone [the punitive separation].... And that's the way it worked.... And the AG even disagreed with her.

And, in accord with general principles of command, psychiatrists under the direction of a chief psychiatrist have to abide by the chief's interpretations, irrespective of their own individual views:

Under Major E. (when he was chief in my second year) you didn't make any ... commitments. [You] let the unit recommend.... But in general, people did not get out [through psychiatric recommendation for an administrative discharge] even if [their line officers] wanted them out. If you also agreed that they ought to get out, you allowed their [commanding officer's] recommendation to stand ... [which type of separation] was not a medical decision. It had nothing to do with psychiatry but [rather] how angry he made [his officers] or how bad [he was] for the Army, and that was the information other people had, not the psychiatrist.

Such delimitations, then, will often affect the psychiatrist's activity in irregular ways, even when he wishes to perform his duties conscientiously.

Conclusions

The foregoing discussion illustrates the crucial dilemma of both the organization and the professional in military psychiatry. Officially, the psychiatrist is supposed to diagnose exclusively within the military psychiatry classification system. Given the special requirements of the organization and the vague and ambiguous nature of the psychiatric nosology, this expectation loses clarity. By observing the letter of the regulation, the psychiatrist may find himself an unhappy witness for the prosecution and the upholder of stringent military discipline. These are the costs of captivity for the military psychiatrist.

For those who define the core responsibility of the professional psychiatrist to be the maintenance of a private relation of trust with a patient, an attitude of resignation or acceptance of captivity might be questionable. A common view expressed by private practitioners is that "you can't do psychiatry in the Army." But the growth of military psychiatry indicates that the bureaucratic limitations are not considered unduly restrictive and that such practice is legitimate. Perhaps the difference in opinion derives from the definition of core responsibilities in psychiatry. For the military organization, these responsibilities are seen as diagnosing or curing illnesses (or deviances) within a system. The direct, primal relation to an individual client is not requisite. But the traditional mandate in psychiatry—as developed in private practice—does place the direct client or patient first. For those who see the advisory and helper role to the patient as predominant, the overtones of control and manipulation introduced by institutional practice are repugnant. As the professional functions (as in the practice of military psychiatry), the question arises whether advice and control activities can both be legitimated under the original advisory mandate—the medical-psychiatric mandate to help or heal the direct client.

In generalizing from this case to the larger problem of professionals captive in bureaucracies, one could argue that a considerable readjustment in client priorities and professional validation seems to be required. For a successful bureaucratic adaptation, professionals need to develop a primary commitment to the larger aims or general rationale of the organization they serve. In this way the greater concern may be transferred from serving the direct client to serving the larger agency. If this transfer of loyalties is accomplished successfully, the professional need have no qualms about whether or not he is engaging in unprofessional behavior. And he may not feel that he is a captive of the organization as he goes about his work. In Gouldner's terms (1957), one might say the professionals who insist on treating the direct client first are the unreconstructed cosmopolitans. They persist in viewing other professional psychiatrists in other locations as their primary audience. The successful or well-adjusted captives become locals; they carry on the necessary work of the bureaucracy.

And their primary audience may come to include many colleagues in the bureaucratic hierarchy who are not psychiatrists at all. And so cosmopolitans and locals, in performing their professional responsibilities differently, may have to look to different audiences for validation. In this way they can be supported as they come to have different definitions about what those professional responsibilities should entail.

Acknowledgments

This paper is a by-product of various grants: A Study of Social Factors Affecting Acceptable and Unacceptable Responses to Army Life in the Trainee Population, U.S. Army Research and Development Command, Contract DA–DM–49–193–66–G181; NIMH post-doctoral fellowship to study the relationship between military psychiatry and military legal procedures, 1F3-8885-01. The paper was completed under the auspices of NIH grant HD02776-02 to study problems of social change and control in professions, for which the author is principal investigator. I am extremely grateful to Rachel Kahn-Hut and Edwin Lemert for their help in organizing and editing this paper. I would also like to thank Neil Friedman and Warren Hagstrom for their suggestions. Finally, thanks are due my chief friends and advisors in military psychiatry, Colonels Roy E. Clausen, Ralph W. Morgan, and Vincent Sweeney, for their encouragement and assistance at virtually every stage of data collection.

Notes

1. The data for this paper were gathered from interviews, military documents, and a limited amount of nonparticipant observation. The interviews were collected in 1964–68. They include interviews with all 15 supervisors and 48 residents in psychiatry at two large military training hospitals. Regular and reserve officers at a variety of other posts (approximately 35) were also interviewed. Where not otherwise indicated by brackets, all illustrations from interview material are verbatim transcripts.

2. Throughout this paper, references to military psychiatry are primarily to Army military psychiatry. The great majority of interviews and observations were located in Army contexts. However, interviews, research into published materials, and the observations suggest that the conditions of practice in other branches of military psychiatry are substantially similar, even though minor variations exist. Army military psychiatry was chosen as the focus for study because the Army is the largest branch of the armed forces. Its services, including those pertaining to military psychiatry, are the most elaborate and extensive of the three major branches of the armed forces.

3. Freidson has suggested that the confrontation of professional autonomy and bureaucratic authority provides an important way to study the resolutions of conflicting value systems: "The physician with his high social status, his strong subjective sense of importance and the immediate fateful consequences and the privacy of his daily work seems better able to resist bureaucratic authority than any of the other professionals. Consequently, careful study of bureaucratic practice should shed much light on the parieties of influence and authority which can exist in a bureaucratic organization and can demonstrate some of the limits of professional freedom in a bureaucratic setting."

4. Sometimes, of course, military psychiatrists do offer therapy in a context much like private practice. And sometimes, also, private practitioners participate in organizational psychiatry settings which resemble the military in some respects. Nonetheless, these settings are differentiated here to suggest the value of the "ideal types" they represent. A more detailed discussion of the rationale for a distinction between military and other types of psychiatry is presented in A. K. Daniels. Military psychiatry: The emergence of a sub specialty," in Eliot Freidson and Judith Lorber, eds., *Medical Men and Their Work* (Chicago: Aldine, 1971).

5. Space does not permit a discussion of all the methods available to the practitioner to moderate the demands of the system and even to defy it.

6. The examination by the psychiatrist is a requirement under military regulations. In the Army they are called AR 635–212. These regulations are subdivided into 212 a and 212 b. They supersede 635–208 and 635–209, which were in effect from April 8, 1959, to July 15, 1966. The older regulations were in effect during most of the period during which data were collected for this study. But the general understandings remain the same.

7. Negotiating a diagnosis so that a particular disposition may ultimately occur is a delicate matter.

8. Ginsberg and others have documented the relation of changes in military policy concerning the rigidity or flexibility of interpretations permitted for any discharge to manpower requirements.

References

Burchard, W. W. 1954. Role conflicts of military chaplains. *American Sociological Review* 19: 528–535.

Carr-Saunders, A. M., and P. A. Wilson. 1933. *The Professions*. Clarendon.

Emerson, R. M. 1968. The Juvenile Court: Labeling and Institutional Careers. Ph.D. dissertation, Brandeis University.

Field, M. 1960. Approaches to mental illness in Soviet society. *Social Problems* 7 (spring): 277–297.

Freidson, E. 1963. The organization of medical practice. In *Handbook of Medical Sociology*, ed. H. Freeman et al. (Prentice-Hall).

Garfinkel, H. 1956. Some sociological concepts and methods for psychiatrists. *Psychiatric Research Reports* 6: 181–195.

Ginsberg. E., et al. 1953. *Psychiatry and Military Manpower Policy*. King's Crown Press.

Goldner, F. H., and R. R. Ritti. 1967. Professionalization as career immobility. *American Journal of Sociology* 72 (March): 489–502.

Gouldner, A. W. 1957. Cosmopolitans and locals: Toward an analysis of latent social roles. *Administrative Science Quarterly* 2 (December).

Headquarters, Department of the Army. 1966. Discharge: Unfitness and Unsuitability. Personnel Separations. Army Regulations, no. 635–212. Washington, D. C.

Kornhauser, W. 1962. *Scientists in Industry: Conflicts and Accomodation.* University of California Press.

Maillet, E. L. 1966. A Study of the Readiness of Troop Commanders to Use the Service of the Army Mental Hygiene Consultation Service. D.S.W. dissertation, Catholic University of America.

Mechanic, D. 1967. Some factors in identifying and defining mental illness. In *Mental Illness and Social Processes*, ed. T. Scheff (Harper & Row).

Merton, R. K. 1957. Role of the intellectual in public bureaucracy. In *Social Theory and Social Structure* (Free Press).

Morgan, R. W. 1961. Clinical Social Work in the U.S. Army, 1947–1959. Dissertation, Catholic University.

Scott, W. R. 1966. Professionals in bureaucracies—Areas of Conflict. In *Professionalization*, ed. H. Vollmer and D. L. Mills (Prentice-Hall).

Szasz, T. S. 1963. Classification in psychiatry. In *Law, Liberty, and psychiatry* (Macmillan).

Szasz, T. S. 1967. The psychiatrist as a double-agent. *Trans-action* 4 (October): 16–25.

III

The Nature of the Communication

In comparison with other dyadic encounters, such as those between husband and wife, taxi driver and fare, guard and prisoner, or lawyer and client, probably more is known about the communication between doctor and patient, even though the encounter has traditionally been conducted privately and is, or has been, circumscribed by secrecy, so that it is known only to the participants and through their gossip, anecdotes, and writings about it (though nowadays all sorts of medical and administrative personnel read the patient's medical record, and there is much routine transmittal of records to insurers, law courts, lawyers, and welfare agencies).

The writings on this subject are of two kinds: from inside and from outside the relation. First, doctors have always had the proclivity to write about the patient, and often, in passing, about the relation. (Indeed, talking about the relationship is an easy way to talk about oneself indirectly, and doctors, by old tradition, are reluctant to disclose themselves directly.) Second, whether for criticism or improvement, the relation has been directly examined and systematically studied by independent and participant observers outside the relation (using tape and video recordings and sitting in encounters) more than have many other professional encounters, such as those in law and education.

Most reports continue to come from the doctor, as the patient reconstructs the experience of illness when interrogated by the doctor taking the medical history. Derived from the patient's story and verbal responses, the narrative is then organized in the conventional topics of a complete medical history, a largely standardized format since the 1920s. Thus, today's office record and the more complete hospital medical record are, in effect, the most common everyday account of the relation and of the topics doctors and patients cover (if not discuss) at their encounters—namely, patients' complaints, current sicknesses, and medical histories, along with the histories of their families and their social backgrounds. Audio recordings of the consultations, first made in the 1940s (and videotapes, made since the 1960s) confirm that the doctor discusses such items as the experience of bodily complaints and the use of medications that make up the present illness (not all of which is written down), while asking about family and social history, gossiping some, listening to personal feelings and concerns, and often closing with medical explanation, advice, and medical directions (including suggestions about behavior or how to live better, such as "Stop smoking").

Retrospective survey studies of what went on from the patient's perspective confirm that these topics are covered (or not covered, as the case may be) at the medical visit (M. Wadsworth and D. Robinson, *Studies in Everyday Medical Life* [Martin Robertson, 1976]). While these several items are the content that doctors and patients often report about the medical visit, the emerging observational studies and tape recordings of consultations may reveal still other dimensions (D. Tuckett, *The Patient Project* [London: Health Education Council, 1982]). Recordings reveal dissonances between the participants, in what Elliot Mishler (*Discourse of Medicine* [Ablex, 1983]) refers to as the voices of medicine (the medical inquiries) and the voices of lay world (the patient's experiences), where the doctor often fails to hear the lay world—or, if hearing it, does not respond. In the case of behavioral science observers, they will note communication regularities between doctor and patient, e.g., interruptions by the doctor or by the patient, and patterns of nonverbal behavior. In the case of clinical teachers, they will rate the doctor's interview performance for the proper norms of such processes as listening, looking, questioning, and explaining. Despite these many direct observations, however, we know little about variations in doctors' responses to patients' requests, complaints, expectations, attributions, psychological distress, and personal concerns, or how doctors and patients conduct their encounters over time as the relation ages.

One exceptional example of early studies that recorded doctor-patient communication is that of Vida Francis, Barbara M. Korsch, and Marie J. Morris, "Gaps in Doctor-Patient Communication" (included in this volume). Its emphasis is on an important feature of the encounter, the doctor's explanation about illness and treatment and its impact on patient satisfaction at a single session of a walk-in clinic setting.

Arthur Kleinman, a psychiatrist and anthropologist, has also looked at the explanatory work of the doctor from an anthropological and cross-cultural perspective. In the paper reprinted here, he early observed that what the doctor (or the medical system itself) does for patients is to label, explain, or construct the nature of their illness, even though patients carry and bring their own fixed (but not immutable) explanatory models as well as what the anthropologist Allan Young refers to in "The Anthropologies of Illness and Sickness" (*Ann. Rev. Anthropol.* 11 [1983]: 257) as "prototype" and "chain events," transient explanations or attributions that accompany acute symptoms and that are less fixed than medical beliefs. Such explanations, in effect, provide patients with a meaning for their own illness experience. Because explanations give meaning to illness, they provide the patients with control. Knowing an explanation of the illness, its attribution, can reduce the patient's helplessness aroused by the uncertainty of what the illness is; these causal notions, in turn, indicate the activities (self-treatment or medical consultation) that may be pursued to control the illness, also decreasing the helplessness.

Indeed, the nature of much of the doctor's communicative acts with patients is the explanation of illness (P. L. Entralgo, *The Therapy of the Word in Classical Antiquity* [Yale University Press, 1976]). In explaining the cause of an illness, the doctor may be confronted with the meanings the patients derives from his popular and folk medical beliefs. With case examples, Kleinman's paper illustrates the significance of these cognitive acts, which are part of nearly all encounters. Moreover, he details, as was also done by J. D. Stoeckle and A. J. Barsky ("Attributions: Use of Social Science in the 'Doctoring' of Primary Care," in *The Relevance of Social Science in Medicine*, ed. A. Kleinman and L. Eisenberg [Reidel, 1980]), how the doctor can use the patient's explanation in the clinical tasks of care. Unfortunately, because communication is not a technical act, it is often viewed as "trivial." In effect, doctors are seemingly "doing nothing" when giving names and labels (diagnoses) to patients' "minor complaints," even though their explanations may appear somewhat more important when given to patients who have advanced organic diseases where the prognosis and long-term treatment are uncertain. Kleinman's paper and others are useful correctives to the traditional dim view of the significance of doctor-patient communication (see A. Kleinman, P. Kunstadter, R. E. Alexander, and J. Gale, eds., *Culture and Healing in Asian Societies* [Schenkman, 1978])—a notion also being challenged as internists, in particular, seek to get paid for such cognitive work.

Besides their attributions and interpretations, patients have requests that are negotiated in the relationship more often implicitly than directly. Aaron Lazare and his colleagues ("Patient Requests in a Walk-in Clinic," *Comprehensive Psychiatry* 16 [1975]: 467) have reported on these in a psychiatric walk-in service, and others have examined them in family practice (M. Good and B. D. Good, "Patient Requests in Primary Care Clinics," in *Clinical Applied Anthropology*, ed. N. J. Chrisman and T. W. Maretzki [Reidel]; M. J. Good, B. D. Good, and A. M. Massi, "Patient Requests in Primary Care Health Settings: Development and Validation of Research Instrument," *J. Behav. Medicine* 6 [1983]: 151; R. Like, Patient Requests in Family Practice: An Exploratory Study, thesis, Case Western Reserve University) and in internal medicine practice (C. Koopman, S. Eisenthal, and J. D. Stoeckle, The Patient's Perspective: Complaints and Requests in a General Medicine Practice and Walk-In Unit, mimeo, Primary Care Program, Massachusetts General Hospital). In medical and psychiatric settings requests are little different. Besides asking for diagnoses, physical exams, drugs, and tests, medical patients (like those seeking help in "psychiatric" settings) request succor, ventilation of their feelings, confession, explanations, and simple or complex administrative help.

8

Gaps in Doctor-Patient Communication: Patients' Response to Medical Advice
Vida Francis, Barbara M. Korsch, and Marie J. Morris

Medical care is increasingly fragmented and complex, and the warmth of a long-term association with a single physician has become a luxury for a few rather than the customary setting for the delivery of health care. In the light of this development it seems imperative to consider various aspects of doctor-patient interaction objectively and scientifically, instead of leaning completely on teaching by precept and intuition as the basis for clinical practices. This study represents an effort at subjecting the verbal communication between doctor and patient to scientific inquiry to learn what features of the interaction can be shown to influence the patient's responses to what his physician told him.

To this end, a large-scale investigation of the verbal interaction between physician and patient in a pediatric clinic was carried out at Childrens Hospital of Los Angeles.[1] This investigation furnished data on patient satisfaction with medical visits and also documented the extent to which patients followed medical advice.

Review of Literature

The degree to which factors such as patients' personal attributes, the severity or kind of illness for which the doctor is consulted, the type of regimen prescribed, and the doctor-patient relation influence response to medical advice has been studied by a number of investigators.

Patient Attributes
Cultural factors and patient beliefs have been shown to influence the outcome of medical visits to varying degrees.[2-4] It has also been

Reprinted, with permission, from *New England Journal of Medicine* 280 (1969): 535–540.

found that personality and social influences determine response to medical advice.[5,6] Findings related to socioeconomic factors are conflicting: Elling et al.[7] reported that low education leads to poor understanding and cooperation in patients with rheumatic heart disease. In a study of cardiac patients by Davis and Eichhorn[8] a greater proportion of patients with high education reported failures in compliance over a given period; however, Johnson[9] found that cardiac patients with higher education were more compliant in carrying out recommendations regarding smoking. Gordis and Markowitz[10] could not demonstrate meaningful relations between demographic data and patients' cooperation in penicillin prophylaxis. Davis[11] observed no demonstrable effects of patient background on compliance.

Severity or Kind of Illness

Regarding the illness, the findings are again conflicting. Berkowitz et al.[12] reported that patients with difficult illnesses were less compliant, whereas Donabedian and Rosenfeld[13] associated severe illness with increased compliance. Davis and Eichhorn[8] found patients with newly diagnosed cardiac disease to be less compliant than those with established disease. In a study by Charney et al.[14] of children taking oral penicillin, compliance was related to the mother's perception of severity of the disease rather than to the doctor's. This was also demonstrated in a recent report by Gordis and Markowitz.[10]

Type of Regimen

Most studies agree that compliance is related to the nature of the regimen prescribed. Restriction in behavior or changes in personal habits have been shown to be more difficult to comply with than prescriptions for medicine,[12] yet patients with ulcers, in one study, were found to be as compliant in following a diet as in taking the prescribed medications.[15] Another study showed that penicillin was taken better in tablet form than when liquid was ordered.[16] Davis and Eichhorn[8] suggested that patients probably comply with two-thirds of the total medical regimen prescribed and tend to choose the part that is least difficult for them.

Doctor-Patient Relation

Fewer studies have dealt with exactly how the doctor-patient relation affects compliance. It has been stated that barriers in the communication could not account for noncompliance.[9,12] One study showed that a formal type of interaction with the doctor was more likely to

Table 1
Research design.

Doctor	Patient's Mother	Postvisit Interview	Follow-up Interview	
Interaction	Mother's perceptions of visit		Outcome	$\left\{\begin{array}{l}\text{Compliance}\\\text{Reassurance}\\\text{Satisfaction}\end{array}\right.$
Independent Variable			Dependent Variable	

result in compliance than a friendly one[8]; however, Charney et al.[14] found that a long-standing warm relation with a pediatrician correlated with better follow-through on medical advice. Others are studying how cooperation between doctor and nurse, health aide, or associate health workers may improve communication and patient cooperation.[17-19] The present study, although it deals with all the variables reviewed above, focuses specifically on the effect of doctor-patient communication on outcome in terms of satisfaction and compliance.

Method

Eight hundred patient visits[20] were studied by means of tape recording of the medical interview, by chart review, and by follow-up interviews (table 1). The interviews were semistructured and designed for verbatim recording. Information was obtained concerning the following points: the mother's perceptions of her child's illness, her subjective experience with the illness, her expectations from the medical visit, her perceptions of her interaction with the physician, her satisfaction with the visit, and her compliance with the advice given by the physician.[21]

There were three groups of patient visits in the sample. All data-collection procedures were carried out on Group 1 cases. The interview immediately after the visit (the postvisit interview) was omitted from Group 2. Tape recording was omitted from Group 3 because of the general belief that the presence of a tape recorder in the examining room might alter the physician's behavior and the patient's responses.

The basic hypothesis for the study was that attributes of the interaction between the physician and the patient (in pediatrics, the parent) influence the outcome of the consultation as measured in terms of satisfaction, reassurance, and compliance.

The study differs from most compliance studies in that it dealt with acute, often short-term, sometimes self-limited illnesses. Also, follow-up interviews were held 7–14 days after the initial medical visit, and, for the most part, the duration of the regimen to be followed did not exceed 10 days.

The extent to which the mothers followed through on the physicians' advice—that is, the degree of compliance—was determined primarily on the basis of responses to follow-up interviews. In view of the often-expressed skepticism concerning the reliability of compliance data obtained from interview responses, every care was taken to facilitate the reporting of noncompliance. The questions regarding compliance were planned on the basis of many unstructured exploratory interviews with clinic patients. The questions, which were designed to be open-ended, nonthreatening, and nonjudgmental, were pretested during a year of pilot study for their acceptability and ease of comprehension and to ascertain whether they made it possible for patients to admit failures to comply. Typical questions were: "How long did you feel Johnny needed the medicine?" and "Parents often find it hard to remember about medicine. What happened when you forgot?" To document compliance more objectively, inquiries were also directed at such information as the cost of the medication and the pharmacy where it was purchased.

Responses to compliance questions were tabulated and compared to the doctor's notations in the chart and to the tape-recorded verbal instructions given to the patient. Group 3 visits were excluded from this phase of the analysis because these were not tape-recorded and precise information was therefore unavailable. Return-appointment compliance, however, was calculated on all 800 visits, and no difference was found between the three study groups. Advice concerning aspects of therapy other than prescriptions for medicine was also documented, so that the final rating constituted a combination of compliance with medicines, treatment, diet, return appointment, and other advice concerning daily activity and routines. Also, the interviewers made a subjective estimate of overall compliance that was considered in the ultimate compliance rating. When possible, the medicine bottles were checked to ascertain whether the medicine had indeed been obtained and the extent to which it had been used. Bottle checks were attempted for the 330 patients who had prescriptions for oral medication. In the 129 documented bottle checks, there were only 11 cases in which noncompliance could be inferred from the amount of medicine remaining in the bottle when interview responses

Table 2
Distribution of compliance ratings.

Rating of Compliance	No. of Visits	Percentage
High	247	42.1
Moderate	224	38.2
Low	67	11.4
No regimen	49	8.3
Totals	587	100.0

had implied compliance. All these observations confirmed that compliance was being reported with honesty and reasonable accuracy.

Derivation of Compliance Rating

Patients were placed in four categories: "high compliance," "moderate compliance," "low compliance," and "no regimen." Those who carried out all the doctor's instructions were considered highly compliant; those who carried out few or none were labeled noncompliant. Patients who followed the medical regimen in part were regarded as moderately compliant. This included patients who were given medications for less than the stated period, patients who were given some but not all of the prescribed medicines, and patients who followed the doctor's advice faithfully, but failed to keep the return appointment.

Since this report includes the relation of compliance to satisfaction, it seems appropriate to explain briefly how satisfaction ratings were derived. These were evolved from responses to the questions in the interview that directly addressed the patient's satisfaction (such as "How did your visit go?"), responses to other questions that indirectly addressed patient satisfaction (such as "What were some of the things that you did not like about your visit with the doctor?"), and "global" satisfaction ratings by experienced interviewers in the field.[1]

Results

In the sample of 587 patient visits for which compliance was calculated, 42.1 percent resulted in high compliance, 38.2 percent in moderate compliance, and 11.4 percent in noncompliance, as shown in table 2. Eight and three-tenths percent of the patients were offered no therapy.

Table 3
Social class and compliance.

Social Class*	No. of Patients	High Compliance (%)
I and II	131	44.8
III	270	46.3
IV and V	186	31.5[†]

* As defined by Hollingshead, A. de B., and Redlich, F. C. *Social Class and Mental Illness: A Community Study.* New York: Wiley, 1958.
[†] When reduction in compliance was checked by chi-square calculations (with use of absolute numbers of patients and only extremes in compliance), the difference of this group of patients from remainder of sample was not statistically significant.

Table 4
Mothers' education and compliance.

Education	No. of Mothers	High Compliance (%)
1–3 yr high school	168	44.6
4 yr high school	226	38.1
1–3 yr college	110	43.6
Other	303	38.5

To test the widely held hypothesis that patients' socioeconomic status, their educational level, and their ethnic background influence follow-through on medical advice, a systematic attempt was made to estimate the relation of these attributes of the patient population to compliance. None were found to relate significantly to the outcome of the consultation in terms of patient satisfaction or compliance with medical advice. Tables 3 and 4 illustrate that neither educational level nor social class influenced patient responses in this study to a significant degree, although compliance was reduced for the lower socioeconomic group. Attributes such as family size, number of siblings, and patient's age were also found to be unrelated to the level of patient cooperation.

Patient Expectations

It is generally accepted, and it was documented in this investigation, that the extent to which a patient's expectations from the doctor are met will influence satisfaction with a medical visit.[1] When analysis was directed at the relation of unmet expectations to compliance with medical advice, the findings bore out the same general trends.

Two methods were used in this study to determine the extent to which a specific patient's expectations remained unmet: The interviews provided repeated opportunities for the mother to tell to what extent she *perceived* that her expectations had been met, and content analysis of the recorded interaction showed which of the expectations enumerated by the mother on interview were dealt with by the doctor during the interaction. Results of both approaches yielded internally consistent findings for individual mothers. Consequently, in the final analysis the mother's own perceptions concerning unmet expectations were used.

Regarding patient satisfaction, mothers who expected to learn the causation and the nature of their child's illness and failed to do so were less likely to be satisfied than any other group of patients.[1] Similarly, there was a significant decline in follow-through on medical advice in the patients who had this expectation unmet ($p < 0.01$). Noncompliance increased from 11 percent to 24 percent when the hoped-for explanation of causation had not been offered by the doctor. Also, the patients who expected "shots," laboratory tests, or x-ray studies and did not receive them were somewhat less compliant than the remainder of the sample.

When all patients with unmet expectations were analyzed as a group, the decrease in cooperation with medical advice was not statistically significant. However, for those who perceived that none of their expectations were met, there was a significant reduction in compliance as well as satisfaction. In this group of 216 patients, noncompliance constituted 17 percent of the sample.

Doctor-Patient Relations

It has been shown in this study, as well as in other investigations, that the personality and manner of a physician as well as the quality of the doctor-patient relation (the "expressive role" of the physician) influenced patient satisfaction.[1] Other studies have also suggested that compliance is influenced by these factors. In the present study, it was found that friendliness or warmth on the part of the doctor as perceived by the patient did not in itself result in increased compliance. However, in the cases in which the mother stated that the doctor did not *seem* friendly, there was a significant reduction in compliant behavior as compared to the remainder of this sample ($p < 0.01$). Similarly, if the mother thought that the doctor did not understand

Table 5
Mother's perception of doctor in relation to compliance.

Mother's Perception	No. of Mothers	High Compliance (%)
Doctor was friendly	236	46
Doctor was businesslike	140	31
Doctor did understand concern	467	44
Doctor did not understand concern	54	37
Total sample	587	42

her concern over the child's illness, compliance was apt to be diminished. Table 5 shows the extent to which compliance was reduced in this group of patients.

All pediatricians who participated in the study had satisfied and dissatisfied patients, and all treated some patients who followed the medical advice given and others who failed to do so. However, there were a few doctors whose patients showed significantly more satisfaction with their visits, and a few other individual physicians whose patients were significantly more highly compliant.

It must be remembered that the present study dealt with new, short-term relations between a physician and a patient. Hence, the rather limited findings concerning the quality of the doctor-patient relation as it affects outcome of a consultation must be interpreted with caution.

Satisfaction and Compliance

The current investigation was concerned only with initial encounters between physicians and patients. In spite of the need to relate to a new physician, 76 percent of the visits studied resulted in patient satisfaction and 24 percent of the patients were dissatisfied.[1] It is a general assumption that satisfied patients will be likely to cooperate with the advice they receive. The data resulting from this study indicate that the relation between satisfaction and compliance is not a simple one. As shown in table 6, there were compliant and noncompliant patients in each satisfaction group. The correlation between satisfaction and compliance was most marked at the extremes of the satisfaction scale, and it can be seen that the highly satisfied patients were significantly more compliant than those who were grossly dissatisfied with their clinic visit. Still, there were a large number of patients

Table 6
Satisfaction and compliance.

Rating of Satisfaction	No. of Visits	High Compliance (%)
High satisfaction	238	53.4
Moderate satisfaction	197	42.6
Moderate dissatisfaction	68	32.4
High dissatisfaction	84	16.7
Total sample	587	42

who, although high satisfied with their visit, failed to follow through on any of the recommendations, and others who were highly dissatisfied with their visit and yet followed all the doctor's instructions.

Type and Severity of Illness and Compliance

In the current study the type of illness could not be shown to influence patient cooperation in general, yet there was a tendency for patients with gastrointestinal complaints to be less cooperative. The fact that they also tended to be dissatisfied may be the reason for the finding and since they were a small group the statistical significance could not be established. On the other hand, there was a slight increase in overall patient compliance in response to the illnesses that the mother perceived to be "very serious." The increase in the proportion of patients who kept their appointment for follow-up visits was even more marked ($p < 0.001$), as shown in table 7.

Type and Complexity of the Medical Regimen and Compliance

Two factors could be shown to correlate statistically with noncompliance. One was that when three or more medicines were prescribed, compliance was significantly lower ($p < 0.01$). Also, when both medicines and treatments were prescribed for the same patient, overall compliance decreased to 25 percent. It was thought that antibiotics might be prescribed with more conviction on the part of the doctor and taken with more enthusiasm by the patients than would symptomatic medication. When antibiotic prescriptions were analyzed separately, however, the compliance was no higher than for other medicines prescribed. It was also noted that there was non-

Table 7
Compliance when mothers perceived a child's illness as "very serious."

Nature of Cooperation	No. of Visits	High Compliance (%)
Overall compliance	68	47
Appointment compliance	59*	73
Total sample	587	42

* Compliance calculated only for patients who had return appointments.

compliance in a larger proportion of the patients whose follow-up interview occurred after a course of more than seven days of treatment than in those with a shorter follow-up period.

Descriptive Data Regarding the Noncompliant Patients

A more intensive scrutiny of the individual patients who had presented noncompliant behavior was undertaken. This group of 67 patients did not differ in demographic or other background data from the remainder of the sample. The medical diagnoses were distributed within the sample in the usual fashion, except that 25 percent of the 67 presented gastrointestinal disturbances, versus only 14 percent of the total sample of 800.

Since one feature of the compliance scale was concerned with failure to keep return appointments, a question on the follow-up interview asked the reasons for breaking return appointments to the clinic. When these responses were inspected, the three most common explanations offered by the patients were the lack of transportation, the lack of money (these two were often interrelated), and problems at home with the family, such as sickness in the household. Although completely unrelated to satisfaction with the clinic visit, these and a few other explanations that occurred less frequently seemed to explain the failure to comply.

The patients who were noncompliant were also examined to ascertain the extent to which their expectations had been met. It was found that 38 of the 67 patients, or 56 percent, had none of their stated expectations fulfilled at the time of their clinic visit. This proportion is significantly higher ($p < 0.001$) than the proportion of patients who had all their expectations unmet in the remainder of the sample.

In this context, it was also relevant to inspect individual case histories of noncompliant patients for explanation of their behavior.

One theme that recurred was the tendency for the doctor, especially when faced with a child with gastrointestinal disturbance, to prescribe a fairly complex, graded feeding regimen with different strengths of formula at different points in time, with variously restricted menus, and with detailed instructions about how to prepare one-half skim-milk formula or jello water or the like. Some of these were so complex that the research workers found them hard to interpret and were not surprised to learn that parents had floundered.

There were other cases in which the doctor ordered a formula or other foodstuff that the child refused to take, or took but then vomited—either course resulting in noncompliance with the doctor's orders. Similarly, if the prescribed regimen left the baby hungry and unsatisfied, or actually made the baby appear worse, the mother usually changed the regimen. Occasionally, the physician prescribed a medicine that had previously been used by the same patient without the desired effects, or else a home remedy had worked better. A few cases of noncompliant behavior appeared to be explicable on the basis of failure to perceive the instructions, and others on the basis of failure to understand the rationale of the treatment.

Discussion

The short time span, the acute (often mild) nature of the illnesses involved, and the kind of doctor-patient relation that prevailed in the walk-in clinic all limit the degree to which the present study can be used to explain noncompliant behavior as it reflects the nature of the doctor-patient interaction. Still, a number of conclusions can be drawn from the available data for all medical consultations. Also, with the changing pattern of delivering medical care, with increasing specialization leading to the need for patients to relate to a galaxy of different health workers, there will be more need to understand the type of relation that was investigated in this study.

A crucial finding is the extent to which compliance is correlated with and perhaps influenced by patient satisfaction. Although high satisfaction does not necessarily imply good follow-through on medical advice, there was certainly an impressive association between the two. A critical observer might doubt the causal relation and also postulate that high satisfaction might be the result rather than the cause of high compliance. It has been suggested that a patient who cooperates has a feeling of satisfaction with himself that may be reflected onto the doctor and the medical consultation. However, although it is unprovable, the much more probable, commonsense explanation seems to be that a patient who is satisfied with the physician would be more apt to carry out the medical advice than one who was unimpressed with the doctor and thought his needs were not met by the medical visit.

The present study indicates that the seriousness of the illness as perceived by the mother, the complexity of the instructions offered, and the practical circumstances in which the patient finds himself all have considerable influences on the degree to which medical advice will be followed, regardless of what takes place in the communication with the doctor. That compliance reflects the measurable attributes of the doctor-patient interaction less sensitively and less accurately than patient satisfaction might have been anticipated. This finding emphasizes the fact that there are many forces that motivate health behavior and patient cooperation besides exactly what is done or what is said by the physician.

The doctor's show of concern, friendliness, and personality attributes as perceived by the patient, which have previously been shown to be strong determinants of the outcome of a consultation in terms of patient satisfaction, are also reflected less directly in patient cooperation. Apparently, an actively unpleasant manner on the part of the doctor affects cooperation adversely, whereas extra warmth and friendliness lead to increased satisfaction but have no measurable effects on follow-through with medical advice. In view of the fact that some investigators have proposed that increased social distance makes for greater compliance, it is worth noting that lack of warmth, to the extent that it affected follow-through at all, did so in a negative direction.[8] It can be speculated that in long-lasting warm relations between doctors and individual patients, attributes of the doctor-patient·interaction might be found that do affect the compliance more than any that could be documented in the present study. The report by Charney et al.[14] certainly suggests that a long-lasting relation in itself makes for increased compliance in private pediatric practices.

It had seemed likely that the kind of illness and the doctor's actual diagnosis would be strong determinants of follow-through on medical advice. However, it was found that, although the mother's ideas concerning the seriousness of her child's ailment were significantly related to outcome of consultation, the doctor's diagnosis and the kind of illness were not. Apparently, the doctor's ideas concerning the presenting problem and the health threat that it posed did not influence the mother's motivation as much as her own perceptions of the illness. This may again have been due in part to the fact that most of the illnesses studied were of an acute, relatively short-term nature.

It has been suggested that certain patients are simply more apt to be cooperative because of their personality makeup.[5] The data from this study had no bearing on this idea.

Other factors that have previously been linked with failure of patients to follow medical advice, such as social disorganization in the home, the number of siblings, and the parents' education, although not significant in the present study, might be more important in a different research situation. It is conceivable that certain families can muster sufficient resources, organization, and motivation to comply with short-term, relatively simple courses of treatment; however, if long-term cooperation with penicillin prophylaxis, anticonvulsive medication, or treatment of chronic tuberculosis were required in the same disorganized family situation, with all its social stresses, the disorganization might interfere seriously with cooperation. Similarly, if the health behavior required involved a preventive measure, such as vaccination, prophylactic treatment, or health supervision, it might be that the patient's educational level and understanding of the reasons for the measures could be shown to be of stronger influence than in this study.

Acknowledgments

This work was supported by Grant H-10 from the United States Children's Bureau. Dr. Korsch was the recipient of a research career-development award (5-K3-HO-28, 297) from the National Institutes of Health.

We are indebted to Milton Davis for continued consultations, to the staff of Childrens Hospital of Los Angeles for cooperation, to the research team for assistance, and to Ray Mickey and Coralee Yale for collaboration in data processing. Computing assistance was obtained from the Health Science Computing Facility, University of California, Los Angeles, sponsored by National Institutes of Health Grant FR-3.

References

1. Korsch, B. M., Gozzi, E. K., and Francis, V. Gaps in doctor-patient communication. 1. Doctor-patient interaction and patient satisfaction. *Pediatrics* 42: 855–871, 1968.

2. Burns, J. L. Why do some parents object to diphtheria immunization? *Health Educ. J.* 9: 70–73, 1951.

3. Deasy, L. C. Socio-economic status and participation in poliomyelitis vaccine trial. *Am. Sociol. Rev.* 21: 185–191, 1956.

4. Riffenburgh, R. S. Doctor-patient relationship in glaucoma therapy. *Arch. Ophth.* 75: 204–206, 1966.

5. Davis, M. S. Physiologic, psychological and demographic factors in patient compliance with doctors' orders. *M. Care* 6: 115–122, 1968.

6. Glasser, M. A Study of public's acceptance of Salk vaccine program. *Am. J. Pub. Health* 48: 141–146, 1958.

7. Elling, R., Wittemore, R., and Green, M. Patient participation in pediatric program. *J. Health & Human Behav.* 1: 183–191, 1960.

8. Davis, M. S., and Eichhorn, R. L. Compliance with medical regimens: panel study. *J. Health & Human Behav.* 4: 240–249, 1963.

9. Johnson, W. L. Conformity to medical recommendations in coronary heart disease. Presented at annual meeting of American Sociological Association. Chicago, September 2, 1965. (Mimeographed.)

10. Gordis, L., and Markowitz, M. Factors related to patients' failure to follow long-term medical recommendations. Presented at eighth annual meeting of Association for Ambulatory Pediatric Services, Atlantic City, April 30, 1968.

11. Davis, M. S. Variations in patients' compliance with doctors' advice: empirical analysis of patterns of communication. *Am. J. Pub. Health* 58: 274–288, 1968.

12. Berkowitz, N. H., Malone, M. F., Klein, M. W., and Eaton, A. Patient follow-through in outpatient department. *Nursing Research* 12: 16–22, 1963.

13. Donabedian, A., and Rosenfeld, L. S. Follow-up study of chronically ill patients discharged from hospital. Presented at ninety-first annual meeting of American Public Health Association, Kansas City, 1963. (Mimeographed.)

14. Charney, E., et al. How well do patients take oral penicillin? Collaborative study in private practice. *Pediatrics* 40: 188–195, 1967.

15. Ellis, R. Relationship between psychological factors and remission of duodenal ulcer. Doctoral dissertation, University of Chicago.

16. Bergman, A. B., and Werner, R. J. Failure of children to receive penicillin by mouth. *New Eng. J. Med.* 268: 1334–1338, 1963.

17. Mallory, M. J., et al. Effective patient care in pediatric ambulatory setting: study of acute care clinic. Read by title, Association for Ambulatory Pediatric Services, Atlantic City, New Jersey, April 30, 1968.

18. Wingert, W. A., et al. Utilization of health aide in pediatric emergency room: motivation to complete immunizations. Read by title, Association for Ambulatory Pediatric Services, Atlantic City, New Jersey, April 30, 1968.

19. Wingert, W. A., Larson, W., and Friedman, D. Utilization of indigenous health aide in pediatric emergency room: educating parents in nutrition. Read by title, Association for Ambulatory Pediatric Services, Atlantic City, New Jersey, April 30, 1968.

20. These were initial visits concerning a new illness. The pediatricians involved were usually unknown to the patients and were members of the house staff with one to four years' pediatric experience.

21. A detailed description of methodology used in the study and results of patient satisfaction is given in reference 1.

9

Explanatory Models in Health-Care Relationships: A Conceptual Frame for Research on Family-Based Health-Care Activities in Relation to Folk and Professional Forms of Clinical Care

Arthur Kleinman

Cross cultural and social studies in the health field by social scientists, epidemiologists and other public-health workers, psychiatrists, and physicians[1-7] are radically altering our conceptions about health care. We are now confronting a view of health-care systems in which the medical profession is but one of several quite distinct and interconnected components.

Health-Care Systems: Professional, Folk, and Popular Sectors

Health care systems can be defined broadly as the entire realm of health-related events, in which institutions, roles, beliefs, and practices are linked to the social and physical (even physiological) environment.[3] These systems can be studied in terms of how they are shaped by "external" factors (such as geography, disease prevalence, economics, social structure and development, cultural values and beliefs, and political ideology); they can also be examined for the influence of "internal" factors (such as individual, family, and community beliefs and practices). From this ecological perspective, health-care systems are conceived of as local entities containing three major sectors: professional medical care, folk care, and popular culture.

In sociocultural terms, these sectors are separate but interconnected domains, each of which is concerned with definitions of illness, the patterning of its experience, and particular values about health

Adapted, with the permission of the author, from a paper that appeared in *Health and Family* (Washington, D.C.: National Council for International Health, 1975).

and illness, modes of diagnosis, and treatment. Each sector relates to five basic tasks of clinical care:

(1) the construction of a hierarchy of health values, including criteria for using and evaluating resources for care and treatment,

(2) the construction of *illness* as a psychosocial and psycho-cultural experience of *disease* (disease being defined here as maladaptive physiological-psychological processes),

(3) the cognitive and communicative procedures for managing the individual's illness experience, including its labeling, classification, and explanation,

(4) therapeutic and preventive practices per se, ranging from medical and surgical interventions to healing rituals, the "laying on of hands," psychotherapeutic techniques, and self-treatment, and

(5) the management of treatment outcomes, including the cure of acute and chronic states, as well as the control of chronic illness, disability, and death.

In short, the health-care systems are interrelated not only on the levels of beliefs, behavior, and institutions, but also in terms of the tasks of clinical care.

Explanatory Models, Illness Behavior, and Clinical Care

Of all the various "external" and "internal" factors of health care systems, the explanation of illness is one "internal" factor that shares all systems and is central to clinical care.[8,9] Explanatory models allow us to relate the patient's illness and clinical care to social and cultural factors, offer a means for studying what impedes or facilitates clinical care, and substantially increase our understanding of the often crucial roles of the family and indigenous practitioners in health care.

All attempts to understand illness and treatment can be thought of as explanatory models. Although they may differ considerably in explanatory capacity and power,[10] folk and popular beliefs[11-13] can be compared as explanatory models that have been patterned by particular social and cultural determinants. Explanatory models can be objectively elicited as coherent accounts of reality, though they often are ambiguous, changing, and contradictory and contain various degrees of logical development.[14,15] As sociologists have shown,[16-18] the different sectors of health systems employ distinct explanatory models, which complement, compete with, conflict with, or distort one another. Interactions between such sectors involve negotiations between these different explanatory models.

These interactions are perhaps best understood as translations between different languages of health care.[19] In terms of this language metaphor, the translation processes of elicitation and analysis of the explanatory model, its transfer from one language to another, and its restructuring into the other language are important, as are the levels of language itself (for example, the professional languages of specialization and the popular languages of laypersons). Between these two is a wide range of explanatory models which appear with still different levels of language: technical, formal, informal, casual, intimate.[19] Failure in the processes of translation, especially in elicitation and transfer, is often a major obstacle to optimal clinical care.

The Doctor-Patient Relationship

Health care involves exchanges between the users of these models, who perceive, interpret, evaluate, and respond to illness and treatment in terms of particular, often different, explanatory models. The doctor-patient relationship is an obvious arena for fruitful study using explanatory models. Patient-family, family-doctor, patient-folk, and paraprofessional-practitioner interactions are other arenas in which to examine explanatory models in health care. We might use a simple paradigm to study these interactions. Clinical care involves the translation of scientific explanatory models to the explanatory models of clinical practice; these, in turn, are transferred to patients and patients' families. This process involves an interaction between clinical explanatory models and those of popular-culture health care (idiosyncratic, family-based, and cultural). The outcome of such interactions may be several: acceptance, rejection, or distortion of clinical explanatory models, perhaps their misinterpretation (mistranslation), and even varying degrees of assimilation and change. Clearly, however, the explanatory models of folk practitioners and families are often closely related, drawing on a similar cultural framework of beliefs and values,[20,21] whereas those of practitioners of modern medical science tend to be considerably different from both.[22] This holds important implications for facilitating or impeding clinical communication. Thus, Horton[22] argues that traditional medical systems and popular health care employ explanations oriented toward the personal and social meaning of illness, whereas modern scientific medicine uses explanations oriented toward technological and nonpersonal realities.

From cross-cultural experiences, I have observed the tremendous impact of explanatory models on clinical care and illness behavior in our own culture. Several case descriptions illustrate the general significance of explanatory models in health care and their specific relevance for understanding illness behavior and performing clinical work.

Case 1

Mr. W. is a 33-year-old Chinese male (Cantonese-speaking) who presented at the medical clinic at Massachusetts General Hospital with tiredness, dizziness, general weakness, pains in the upper back described as rheumatism, a sensation of heaviness in the feet, 20-1b weight loss, and insomnia. Past medical history was noncontributory.

Medical workup was unrevealing, except that the patient seemed anxious and looked depressed. Mr. W. refused to acknowledge either, however. He initially refused psychotherapy, stating that talk therapy would not help him. He finally accepted psychiatric care only after it was agreed that he would be given some kind of medication. During the course of his care, Mr. W. never accepted the idea that he was suffering from a mental illness. He described his problem, as did his family, as due to "wind" (*fung*) and "not enough blood" (*m-kra huet*).

Pertinent history included the following: Mr. W. was born into a family of educated farmers and teachers in a village in Kwantung Province. He and his family moved to Canton when he was a young child. His father died during the war with Japan, and Mr. W. remembered recurrent feelings of grief and loneliness throughout his childhood and adolescence. At age 10 he accompanied his family to Hong Kong; 10 years later they moved to the U.S. Mr. W. denied any family history of mental illness. He reported that his health problem began two years before when he returned to Hong Kong to find a wife. He acquired the "wind" disease, he believes in retrospect, after having overindulged in sexual relations with prostitutes, which resulted in loss of *huet-hei* (blood and vital breath), causing him to suffer from "cold" (*leung*) and "not enough blood." His symptoms worsened over the past 6 months, following his wife's second miscarriage (they have no children) and shortly after he had lost most of his savings in the stock market and in a failing restaurant business. However, he denied feeling depressed at that time, though he admitted being anxious, fearful, irritable, and worried about his financial situation. These feelings he also attributed to "not enough blood."

Mr. W. first began treating himself for his symptoms with traditional Chinese herbs and diet therapy. This involved both the use of tonics to "increase blood" (*po-huet*) and treatment with symbolically "hot" (*it*) food to correct his underlying state of humoral imbalance. He did this only after seeking advice from his family and friends in Boston's Chinatown. They concurred that he was suffering from a "wind" and "cold" disorder. They prescribed other herbal medicines when he failed to improve. They suggested that he return to Hong Kong to consult traditional Chinese practitioners there. While the patient was seen at Massachusetts General Hospital's medical clinic, he continued to use Chinese drugs and to seek out consultation in the local Chinese community. He was frequently told that his problem could not be helped by Western medicine. At the time of receiving psychiatric care, Mr. W. was also planning to visit a well-known traditional Chinese doctor in New York's Chinatown, and he was also considering acupuncture treatment locally. He continued taking Chinese drugs throughout his illness, and never told his family or friends about receiving psychiatric care. He expressed gratitude, however, that the psychiatrist listened to his views about his problem and explained to him in detail psychiatric ideas about depression, etc. He remembered feeling bad about his care in the medical clinic, where after the lengthy workup almost nothing was explained to him and no treatment was given him. He had decided not to return to the clinic.

Mr. W. responded to a course of antidepressant medication with complete remission of all symptoms. He thanked the psychiatrist for his help, but confided that (1) he remained confident that he was not suffering from a mental illness, (2) talk therapy had not been of help, (3) antidepressants perhaps were effective against "wind" disorders, and (4) since he had concurrently taken a number of Chinese herbs, it was uncertain what had been effective, and perhaps the combination of Chinese and Western drugs had been responsible for his cure.

This case illustrates the usefulness of the concept of explanatory models as a way of understanding illness behavior and clinical care.

First, it demonstrates the wide boundaries and multiple components of the pluralistic health-care system of which Mr. W. was part. This patient's initial health-care resource was self-treatment; when this failed, he turned pragmatically to the family- and community-based beliefs and practices available to Chinese-Americans, which in large part reflect traditional Chinese medicine but which also include elements of the mainstream American popular-cultural health domain. When he again failed to receive relief, Mr. W. resorted to professional medical care.

Second, Mr. W. was unhappy with the care he received in the medical clinic because he failed to receive medication and because he was not given a meaningful explanation of his problem. This dissatisfaction occurred in part because he and his physician held very different expectations of the communicative process in the doctor-patient relationship. Fortunately, Mr. W. was acculturated to a sufficient degree to enable him to shift his expectations and to accept referral and use antidepressant medication.

Third, this case illustrates what is meant by the psychocultural experience of illness. Mr. W., his family, his friends, and local community "experts" defined his problem in terms of the local popular understanding of the classificatory system of traditional Chinese medicine.[23,24] Their expectations and actions were based on their belief that he was suffering from a "wind" disorder owing to an underlying "cold" imbalance and "not enough blood." Mr. W. reinterpreted his past behavior in light of this diagnosis, since it is thought that this disorder is brought on by the loss of the body's vital essence—especially owing to excessive semen loss through masturbation or frequent intercourse. The characteristic symptoms believed to be associated with this disorder—tiredness, general weakness, nonspecific arthritic complaints, insomnia, and various emotional complaints, from anxiety and irritability to anger and loneliness, felt to be secondary to the physical disturbance—accounted for his complaints; the belief that it is very difficult to cure and can remain for a long period of time again fits with his actual experience. Mr. W. turned to modern scientific medicine and sought treatment for a physical illness because this problem is not regarded by the Chinese as a mental illness.

Fourth, from what is already known about psycho-cultural aspects of illness among Chinese, this case can be viewed as an illustration of their tendency to express emotional problems via somatic complaints and of the cultural patterning of symptoms.[25–27] Because of the phenomenon of somatization, along with the stigma they attach to mental illness, it is not unusual for Chinese patients with mental illness to present symptoms of, and demand the label of, physical illness. Even very disturbing and frankly bizarre behavior will be tolerated by the family, who prefer to label it eccentric rather than sick. Chinese culture encourages the labeling of many forms of deviance, most mental illnesses included, as physical illness. The sick role has usually been employed in the narrow context of physical illness to legitimate psychological and interpersonal problems.

It is important to stress the fact that Mr. W.'s evaluation of health-care practices involved both a pragmatic concern for effective symptom control and culturally based expectations about the proper doctor-patient relationship and appropriate treatment approaches. Though successfully treated for his depression and its accompanying somatic complaints, Mr.W. did not interpret this as empirical documentation of the efficacy of modern psychiatric care. Not unlike Navaho patients who, though successfully treated for tuberculosis with modern drugs, still demand traditional religious ceremonies to "complete" their cure,[28] Mr. W. remained uncertain as to what was actually curative in his case and continued taking Chinese herbs after completing his course of psychotropic-drug treatment. He concluded that both Chinese and Western medicines had been helpful, but his framework for understanding and responding to illness remained centered in the explanatory system peculiar to the hybrid of Chinese-American popular health beliefs.

Unfortunately, using an example from a non-Western culture suggests that these issues are esoteric. The vignettes that follow are intended to provide evidence from ordinary Western patients on the significance of explanatory models and the implications of this framework for clinical practice.

Case 2

Mrs. F. is a 60-year-old white Protestant grandmother who is recovering from pulmonary edema secondary to atherosclerotic cardiovascular disease and chronic congestive heart failure on one of the medical wards at Massachusetts General Hospital. Her behavior is described as strange and annoying by the house staff and nurses. While her cardiac status has greatly improved and she has become virtually asymptomatic, she induces vomiting and urinates frequently into her bed. She becomes angry when told to stop these behaviors. As a result, psychiatric consultation is requested.

Review of the lengthy medical record reveals nothing as to the personal significance of the patient's behavior. When queried about this behavior and asked to explain why she engages in it and what meaning it has for her, the patient's response is most revealing. Describing herself as the wife and daughter of plumbers, the patient notes that she was informed by the medical team responsible for her care that she has "water in the lungs." She further reports that to her mind the physiology of the human body has the chest hooked up to two pipes, the mouth and the urethra. The patient explains that she has been trying to be helpful by helping to remove as much water from her chest as possible through self-induced vomiting and frequent urination. She analogized the latter to the work of the "water pills" she is taking, which she has been told are getting rid of the water on her chest. She concludes: "I can't understand why people are angry at me." After appropriate explanations, along with diagrams, she acknowledges that the "plumbing" of the body is remarkable and quite different from what she had believed. Her unusual behavior ended at that time.

This amusing but actual case study is a very striking example of the important role played by alternative explanatory models in health care. I use it because it derives from the still poorly understood and inadequately studied popular-culture health-care domain rather than from the far better appreciated and researched folk-medical domain. Yet it is the former—family- and community-centered beliefs and practices—that have the greatest impact on all forms of health-care-related behavior (especially in technologically advanced societies, where the folk sector may be less extensive than in more traditional societies). It is precisely here in our own system of health care that we can "locate" American cultural orientations at work. And it is the interaction of popular-culture explanatory models with the explanatory models of medical science and clinical practice that is responsible for communicative problems in the doctor-patient interaction.

Many other encounters could be cited that would illustrate the importance of popular and folk explanatory models for health care. Unfortunately, only the systematic study of such individual cases within the total context of specific health-care systems can fully develop the ideas that have been discussed. Yet in the period of a few months I collected a surprisingly large number of illustrative encounters at Massachusetts General Hospital, of which the following is another example.

Case 3

A 38-year-old university professor presented with chest pain diagnosed in a cardiology clinic as angina based on coronary artery disease. He has refused to accept this diagnosis, and has demanded that his cardiologist also reject it and instead relate the problem to an imagined pulmonary embolus. The psychiatric consultant uncovers not a disease phobia as part of a neurotic disorder, but a popular explanatory model: the belief, shared by his wife and friends, that the development of angina signals the end of an active lifestyle and the development of invalidism. This patient is trying to prove that his cardiologist has made a mistake and that he has been mislabeled. Unfortunately, his cardiologist did not appreciate this hidden explanatory model and therefore could not attempt to correct it or negotiate with it.

This case, which describes problems resulting from unappreciated alternative explanatory models and which represents not idiosyncratic behavior or psychopathology but socially and culturally constructed health belief systems, is quite common. Such beliefs frequently lead to noncompliance, failure to use health facilities, and, in consequence, poor medical care. Physicians usually do not examine their patients' understanding of the explanations they give them, let alone inquire into their patients' own explanations of illness and treatment. When alternative beliefs and unexpected attitudes are uncovered, rarely do modern physicians attempt to negotiate with the patient seriously over these alternative views. This represents professional medicine's disregard for the often very different cognitive orientations of the folk and popular sectors of health-care systems.[16,29,30] In our society, these professional, folk, and popular sectors—along with their explanatory models—coexist, compete, and cooperate. The interactions that occur between these models, though of little concern thus far to practitioners, are of considerable importance to their patients and help determine the real quality of health care. From family-based health beliefs come the use of therapies, criteria for choosing between health-care alternatives, and values for evaluating treatment practices.

The Doctor's Explanatory Models

It can be shown, further, that in the explanatory process itself physicians begin by translating scientific explanatory models into clinical ones. Thus, the hemodynamic basis of congestive heart failure may be explained in terms of a dammed-up lake leading to flooding, or a blocked pipe overloading a boiler. But it also may be explained in a complex and confusing technical idiom. There is clearly a wide variance in clinical explanations and explanatory skills, and yet, as with patients' beliefs, there are a limited number of explanatory models of heart disease.

Patients and their families respond to these models by translating them into their own explanatory frameworks. This often involves systematic distortion and failure to recall significant amounts of very relevant information. This process of recall and distortion can be quantified. Over time, the explanatory material acquired by patients and their families is assimilated and changed, and it often comes to resemble their original beliefs. Usually without their doctors' awareness, they work with explanatory models that are substantially different from those their doctors hold.

Future research into this largely unexplored area will, one hopes, eventually facilitate clinical communication, diminish gaps in understanding, and encourage the practice and teaching of more personally responsive and socially appropriate health care. In order to accomplish these goals, research into explanatory models must become considerably more than superficially descriptive, as these few case studies have necessarily been. Such research should work out formal methods for describing in full and analyzing the structure and functions of these models and relating them to specific social and cultural factors.

Acknowledgments

The work reported in this paper was supported by awards from the Foundations' Fund for Research in Psychiatry, the Social Science Research Council, and the Dupont-Warren Fund of Harvard University.

References

1. Fabrega, H. *Disease and Social Behavior*. Cambridge, Mass.: MIT Press, 1974.

2. Field, M. Comparative sociological perspectives on health systems. In *Medicine in Chinese Cultures*, ed. A Kleinman et al. Washington, D.C.: Fogarty International Center, 1974.

3. Kleinman, A. Toward a comparative study of medical systems: An integrated approach to the study of the relationship of medicine and culture. *Science, Medicine and Man* 1: 55–65, 1973.

4. Leslie, C. (ed.). *Toward the Comparative Study of Asian Medical Systems*. Berkeley: University of California Press, 1974.

5. Litman, T., and Robins, L. Comparative analysis of health care systems: A sociopolitical approach. *Soc. Sci. and Med.* 5: 573, 1971.

6. Nader, L., and Maretzki, T. (eds.). *Cultural Illness and Health*. Washington, D.C.: American Anthropological Association, 1973.

7. Yap, P. M. *Comparative Psychiatry*. University of Toronto Press, 1974.

8. Fabrega, H. An integrated theory of disease: Latino-Mestizo views of disease in the Chiapas Highlands. *Psychosom. Med.* 35: 223, 1973.

9. Kleinman, A., et al. (eds.). *Medicine in Chinese Cultures*. Washington, D.C.: Fogarty International Center, 1974.

10. Engelhardt, H.T. Explanatory models in medicine: Facts, theories, and values. *Tex. Reports on Biol. and Med.* 32: 225–239, 1974.

11. Jahoda, G. *The Psychology of Superstition*. Baltimore: Penguin, 1969.

12. Snow, L. Folk medicine beliefs and their implications for care of patients. *Annals of Int. Med.* 81: 82–96, 1974.

13. Yap. P. M. *Comparative Psychiatry*. University of Toronto Press, 1974.

14. Cancian, F. New methods of describing what people think. *Sociol. Inquiry* 41: 85, 1971.

15. Metzger, D., and Williams, G. Tenejapa medicine: The curer. *Southwestern J. of Anthrop.* 19: 216–234, 1963.

16. Freidson, E. *Profession of Medicine: A Study of the Sociology of Applied Knowledge*. New York: Dodd, Mead, 1970.

17. McKinlay, J. Social networks, lay consultation and help-seeking behavior. *Soical Forces* 51: 275, 1961.

18. Twaddle, A. The concept of health status. *Soc. Sci. and Med.* 8: 29–38, 1974.

19. Nida, E., and Taber, C. *The Theory and Practice of Translating*. Leiden: Brill, 1969.

20. McCorkle, T. Chiropractic: A deviant theory of treatment in contemporary Western culture. *Hum. Org.* 20: 20, 1961.

21. Harwood, A. The hot-cold theory of disease: Implications for treatment of Puerto Rican patients. *JAMA* 216: 1153, 1971.

22. Horton, R. African traditional thought and Western science. *Africa* 37: 50, 1967.

23. Ahern, E. Sacred and secular medicine in a Taiwan village: A study of cosmolog-

ical disorder. In *Medicine in Chinese Cultures*, ed. A. Kleinman et al. Washington, D.C.: Fogarty International Center, 1974.

24. Topley, M. Chinese and Western medicine in Hong Kong: Some social and cultural determinants of variation, interaction and change. In *Medicine in Chinese Cultures*, ed. A. Kleinman et al. Washington, D.C.: Fogarty International Center, 1974.

25. Lin, T. Y. Anthropological study of the incidence of mental disorder in Chinese and other cultures. *Psychiatry* 16: 313, 1953.

26. Rin, H., et al. Psychophysiological reactions of rural and suburban populations in Taiwan. *Acta Psychiatrica Scandinavica* 42: 420, 1966.

27. Solomon, R. *Mao's Revolution and the Chinese Political Culture*. Berkeley: University of California Press, 1971.

28. Adair, J., and Deuschle, K. *The People's Health: Medicine and Anthropology in a Navajo Community*. New York: Appleton-Century-Crofts, 1970.

29. *Symposium on the Greater Medical Profession*, 1973. New York: Josiah Macy, Jr. Foundation.

30. Suchman, E. Social patterns of illness and medical care. *J. Health and Hum. Behav.* 6: 2, 1965.

IV

Barriers to Communication: Why Care Differs

Barriers to communication that interfere with the establishment, management, and outcomes of doctor-patient relations are probably the most popular topics in the patient-care literature. These studies are popular because remedies to their findings do not require a reorganization of practice, only a reeducation of the participants (a much safer and easier strategy).

The beliefs and attitudes of both participants are most frequently examined. As previously noted, attitudes of patients may be related to such behaviors as their failure to keep appointments and take medicines; in turn, explanations of such attitudes are usually sought in the patient's social class and ethnic, educational, and psychological background. For the most part, these numerous studies have been conducted in public clinics, where the staff members are available only on a part-time basis and where the opportunities for long-term attachments between patients and doctors are thus limited. In these study settings, one examines, instead, discontinuous encounters under conditions almost certain to guarantee "bad" behavior by both participants. Although practices reorganized for full-time work would change the relation and remedy many communication barriers, this structural remedy often seems to be politically and economically difficult. Thus, easier "solutions" that educate patients or doctors are undertaken instead. Yet, even when the easier reeducation solutions are undertaken, these may not get full support since the relation is not always a priority in medical education, nor is the change necessarily supported by treatment institutions.

Putting the organizational setting and context aside, the following papers discuss communication barriers that may be viewed, on one hand, as insurmountable obstacles or, on the other, as challenges to the educational reform of doctors or patients. Charles Kadushin ("Social Distance between Client and Professions," *Am. J. Sociol.* 62 [1967]: 517) has written about the general problem of distance between help-seeker and healer, and this problem is echoed in other medical writings, such as Margaret Hegarty and Leon Robertson's "'Slave Doctors' and 'Free Doctors'" (*New Engl. J. Med.* 284 [1971]: 646). Hegarty and Robertson are concerned with the reluctance of the profession to serve poor populations. Kadushin notes that doctor-patient distance is not all bad—it may in fact stabilize relations—and that there are consequences to removing it. J. L. Walsh and R. H. Elling, in "Professionalism and the Poor" (*J. Health and Soc. Behav.* 9 [1968]: 16) cite a particular example: The higher one goes on the professional ladder, the more limited is one's communication with poor patients. Jay Katz has argued in *The Silent World of Doctors and Patients* (Free Press, 1984) that doctors' failure to communicate meaningfully with patients is rooted in their professional ideas of uncertainty, authority, and autonomy. In "Who Is Really Ignorant—Physician or Patient?," reprinted below, John B. McKinlay notes how the words doctors choose may fail to convey the meanings they intend, and that these words are not redefined for patients in simpler terms even when staff members recognize that the doctor is using overtechnical language. Others, including Charles Boyle ("Differences between Patients' and Doctors' Interpretation of Some Common Medical Terms," *Brit. Med. J.* 2 [1970]: 286) have written on the same theme. Language-communication misunderstandings may involve—in addition to knowledge—acoustics, phonology, syntax, lexicon, conceptions, intent, and credence (E. J. Cassell, L. Skopek, and B. Fraser, "A Preliminary Model for the Examination of Doctor-Patient Communication," *Language Sciences* 10 [1976]: 43; E. Cassell, *Talking with Patients*, volume 1 [MIT Press, 1985]). These elements of doctor-patient communication have become of interest to linguists (see A. R. Bennett, ed., *Communications between Doctors and Patients* [Oxford University Press, 1976]), who argue that words and their uses contain essential meanings that are poorly understood by doctors.

Looking at the outcomes of communication in such behavior as compliance with medical advice, Milton Davis, in "Variations in Patients' Compliance with Doctors' Advice" illustrates the analysis that can be made of the doctor-patient communication and its impact. Irving K. Zola's "Problems of Communication, Diagnosis, and Patient Care" represents one of the few attempts to look at organization and communication together rather than separately, as they are often examined.

10

Who Is Really Ignorant—Physician or Patient?
John B. McKinlay

Since the ability of the patient to cooperate with the physician appears dependent both on the patient's understanding and definition of his condition and on the physician's knowledge and definition of the patient and his problem, the nature of information communicated, when it should be given, and by whom are factors obviously related to the benefit derived from medical care. Recent literature in medical sociology and medical education is replete with discussions of information exchange in the doctor-patient relationship. However, a clear majority of such reports are based on impressionistic material rather than on scientific data from reputable and replicable studies.

A few attempts have been made to isolate so-called "barriers" to communication between physicians and patients, most tending to ascribe culpability to patients. For example, the barriers listed in the well-known paper by Samora et al. (1961) consist in the main of patients' deficiencies. They include the following: physical inability of the patient to hear information, psychological unwillingness to receive unpleasant information, anxieties and inhibitions stemming from perceived status differences, problems of memory recall, differences in what patients and physicians know about disease, factors associated with social-class or ethnic-group membership, differing role expectations that patients and physicians may have of each other, and differences in the ability to comprehend terms commonly used in medical discourse. Perhaps, with the exceptions of the studies by Dodge (1961) and Skipper et al. (1964), there are few reports that focus on physician culpability and the possibility that limited communication may, in various ways, serve the professional interests and needs of physicians. A chronological review of studies in this area

Reprinted, with permission, from *Journal of Health and Social Behavior* 16, no. 1 (1975): 3–11. Copyright 1975 by American Sociological Association.

provides an indicting illustration of the failure of researchers to take adequate account of earlier omissions and deficiencies, with the result that knowledge seldom seems to advance cumulatively.

A pioneering study by Redlich (1945) concerned a small sample ($N = 25$) of neuropsychiatric patients (none of whom had more than a high-school education) who were asked to define 60 medical terms occurring frequently in discourse with their physicians. Understanding was scored on a four-point scale by two physicians, with recourse to a dictionary for contradictions. It is not clear from the report whether the physicians' ratings were made independently. In a later study, Collins (1955) surveyed a group of 100 women attending a public-welfare antenatal clinic in order to assess their understanding of words relating to nutrition that were frequently used in bulletins and by health personnel. A final list of 20 words was reviewed by nutritionist/nurses and physicians for typicality and was presented in an interview format to the women, each word being used in the context of a sentence to assist understanding. In rating replies, "any reasonable definition" was accepted (presumably by the author), and no rating scale was used.

A more sophisticated study (Seligman et al. 1957; Pratt et al. 1957) focused on general comprehension of ten common diagnosable conditions. A sizable randomly selected sample ($N = 214$) of hospital outpatients were presented a self-administered multiple-choice test in an attempt to assess the level of information in a patient population. Apart from the use of a relatively large sample, a further innovative aspect of this study was the inclusion in the survey of 89 physicians from the same clinic. These physicians were asked to assess what the patients' level of information should ideally be and what they thought the patients' actual level of information was. These two assessments were then compared with the precoded responses of the patients themselves. Another departure (of questionable value) from the two earlier studies was the inclusion of diseases which the patients may not have encountered in their own life experiences. Differences in understanding, according to experience of the disease (in self or other), were found.

More recently, Samora et al (1961) reported an investigation of word understanding along the lines of earlier studies, with some methodological improvements. Although from predominantly lower socio-economic groups, the target population was more heterogeneous than those in the previously cited studies (including gynecological, general medical, and surgical patients of varying sex and race). A list of words in common use with all patients was selected.

Each word was placed in the context of a sentence during an interview, as in the earlier survey by Collins (1955), and the level of comprehension was rated on a four-point scale corresponding to that employed by Redlich (1945). However, the rating procedure involved immediate scoring by the interviewer without recording the actual response, thus precluding the possibility of checking the consistency of the scores assigned. The same authors, in a further study, replicated the work of Seligman, Pratt, and co-workers (Samora et al. 1962).

One of the most recently reported studies in the area of patient comprehension presents for the first time data collected outside the United States (Plaja et al. 1968). In three outpatient clinics in Colombia, two tasks were considered. The first was an adaptation of the earlier hospital study by Samora et al. (1961) to an outpatient population; the second involved analysis of tape-recorded interviews between physicians and patients, with emphasis on the possible effects of social-class distance on communication. Fifty-nine patients attending the clinics for the first time (43 female, 16 male) were involved, mainly in the age group 20–45 years. All were classified as of lower-class status and of both urban and rural origin. The 17 physicians involved in the interviews represented three different levels of training. Immediately following the tape-recorded interview, physician and patient were interviewed separately, and at this time the word-study questionnaire was presented to the patients. Scoring was carried out by the researcher after the interview, using a four-point scale similar to that employed in earlier studies.

Of all these studies, only the earliest (Redlich 1945) used physicians to assess patients' replies, but these scores were not compared with an independent physician's knowledge. In the only large-scale study of comprehension (Seligman et al. 1957; Pratt et al. 1957), an attempt was made to compare patients' scores with independent physicians' assessments—a comparison not made in any of the other studies reported. Yet even here, the patients' scores were precoded. If the scores had been assigned independently by physicians, a more realistic comparison could have been made between the physicians' direct assessment of patient comprehension and their hypothetical assessment of understanding.

Methodology

The data for the present report were obtained as a part of an intensive exploratory study of the organization of health and social-welfare services and their utilization by lower-working-class families in Aberdeen, Scotland. Eighty-seven unskilled working-class families—consisting of two subsamples of respondents closely defined as utilizers and underutilizers—were interviewed four times over a period of roughly 1½ years. The sampling strategy employed in this study was essentially random, assuming that the composition of the population of childbearing women visiting the prenatal clinic did not alter appreciably over time. The present data were collected during a fourth interview with respondents that was, in every case, conducted in the home. Additional aspects of the design and execution of this research have been reported in detail elsewhere (McKinlay 1970a, 1970b, 1973; McKinlay and McKinlay 1972).

For a period of one month during the early stages of the field work I attended morning and afternoon rounds of the obstetrics and gynecology wards on a regular basis. At the request of the medical staff, I donned a white coat and joined the six to twelve people (mostly physicians and medical students) who attended these rounds. A list was compiled of some 57 words that were employed with patients by more than six different physicians repeatedly during the rounds, or that appeared in the literature routinely distributed to mothers when they attended the clinics.

A letter accompanying this list of words was then sent to each physician in the department of obstetrics and gynecology who was serving the maternity hospital and having regular contact with patients, to remind them of the study and inform them of my interest in how much lower-working-class patients understand about what they are asked and have explained to them. The physicians were requested to strike out any word on the list that they would not normally employ when questioning or explaining something to a patient. For some words, a majority of the physicians (13 or more) indicated that they would not use them (struck them off the list), while for other words a majority of physicians indicated that they would use them by retaining them on the list. Assuming extreme frequencies indicated that the physicians considered such words either in common usage among the patients or quite incomprehensible to patients; words with these frequencies were excluded from the study. With such reasoning I hoped to retain those words at risk to some misunderstanding by the patients—those in the "gray zone" of verbal comprehension.

The resulting list of 13 words was inserted in an interview schedule and presented to the respondents in the study. Because of the importance of not allowing the respondents to feel that they were ignorant of certain topics through fostering a school-test situation, the section of the interview concerning medical vocabulary knowledge was preceded with a cautious introduction (see appendix below). Each word was first sounded out and then used in the context of a sentence. Responses were recorded verbatim on a standard form. Two of the participating physicians (one of each sex) who had expressed interest in the study were asked to undertake scoring. To ensure objectivity in the scoring, patients were assigned numbers for purposes of identification, and the scoring was done independently by each physician on separate scoring sheets. In other words, the scoring was blind, the physicians having no knowledge about either the social characteristics or the utilization behavior of the respondents.

On the completion of the field work (over a year after the initial word selection), the current group of physicians having regular contact with patients (excluding the two raters) was presented with the 13 words and asked to indicate for each word whether they would expect the average lower-working-class women to (A) not understand at all and say so, (B) get the meaning quite wrong, (C) have an incomplete or vague understanding, or (D) understand pretty well. (See end of appendix for details of scoring procedure.) Given the deliberate time lapse of over one year, there had been changes and an increase in the physician staffing of the maternity hospital. Despite these changes, twelve of the original panel (eighteen) were included in the followup. Such a technique permitted a comparison between the actual level of comprehension of the respondents (as rated by physicians) and the level of comprehension expected by the physicians.

Analysis

In rating respondents' comprehension, agreement between the ratings of the two physicians was very good for the majority of words. Only one or two discrepancies of the type A,B occurred; these were classed as A. Differences of the type C,D, which were somewhat more numerous, were classed as D on the assumption that some understanding was clearly indicated by both physicians. Of the remaining irreconcilable discrepancies, almost all were of type B,C or B,D. The male physician consistently assigned the lower rating (less evidence of comprehension), thus crediting the women respondents with less understanding than his female colleague.

The principal results of this investigation are presented in table 1. The two middle ratings, B (wrong understanding) and C (incomplete understanding), were combined, as these constituted the majority of

Table 1
The distribution of comprehension of thirteen words by two groups of lower-class women and the comprehension expected by eighteen physicians. Given as percentages of the number of respondents, for each word.

	Underutilizers			Utilizers			Physicians		
	A: No Knowledge	B/C: Wrong or Vague	D: Adequate	A: No Knowledge	B/C: Wrong or Vague	D: Adequate	A: No Knowledge	B/C: Wrong or Vague	D: Adequate
Antibiotic	11.1	60.0	28.9	13.9	44.4	41.7	27.8	68.7	5.6
Breech	8.9	6.7	84.4	0.0	0.0	100.0	11.1	66.7	22.2
Enamel	8.9	40.0	51.1	8.3	30.6	61.1	27.8	44.4	27.8
Glucose	17.8	44.4	37.8	19.4	36.1	44.4	11.1	61.1	27.8
Membranes	24.4	31.1	44.4	11.1	25.0	63.9	50.0	50.0	0.0
Mucus	33.3	33.3	33.3	30.6	22.2	47.2	38.9	50.0	11.1
Navel	4.4	15.6	80.0	11.1	33.3	55.6	0.0	27.8	72.2
Protein	37.8	62.2	0.0	30.6	58.3	11.1	27.8	55.6	16.7
Purgative	57.8	28.9	13.3	72.2	13.9	13.9	16.7	44.4	38.9
Rhesus	13.3	75.6	11.1	11.1	86.1	2.8	55.6	38.9	5.6
Scanning	13.3	35.6	51.1	8.3	30.6	61.1	66.7	33.3	0.0
Sutures	48.9	6.7	44.4	50.0	11.1	38.9	61.1	33.3	5.6
Umbilicus	84.4	15.6	0.0	83.3	5.6	11.1	50.0	38.9	11.1
Total respondents	45 (100.0%)			36 (100.0%)			18 (100.0%)		

disagreements between the ratings assigned by the two physicians to the actual responses obtained. Moreover, this combination would be partly consistent with the mode of analysis reported by Samora et al. (1961). Two comparisons are presented in this table: between the understanding of two groups of respondents (divided according to their utilization of prenatal services) and between the results for the respondents and the comprehension ratings assigned hypothetically by the physicians.

The first comparison indicates a consistently higher word comprehension among the utilizers, as rated blind and independently by the two physicians. Only two words appeared to be understood less clearly by the utilizers ("navel" and "rhesus"), and both these differences were due partly to a higher proportion of disagreements between the physicians in rating the replies of mainly utilizers. With the exception of "membranes," "protein," "purgative," "scanning," and "sutures," the remaining words showed a difference between utilizers and underutilizers that was largely a difference between incomplete or incorrect understanding and adequate understanding. More underutilizers either possessed an inadequate understanding of these words or expressed their understanding less clearly than the utilizers.

The results for these two groups were also examined for any evidence of differences between primiparous and multiparous women, which may indicate increased understanding with greater experience. The 37 multiparae and the 8 primiparae among the underutilizers exhibited no differences in understanding. The 14 primiparous utilizers, on the other hand, showed evidence of greater disagreement in the physicians' ratings of replies than their multiparous counterparts, perhaps indicating an increase in understanding with experience. The difference is not marked, however, and would, of course, require confirmation from larger samples.

When these two sets of results are compared with the hypothetical ratings of the physicians, the discrepancies are marked. For the first six words listed, as well as for the terms "scanning" and "sutures," the understanding of the lower-working-class respondents was well above expectation, particularly for "breech" (22 percent of the physicians considered understanding would be adequate, while 84 and 100 percent of respondents' actual replies were rated as showing adequate comprehension), "membranes," and "scanning" (for each of the latter, about half the respondents showed understanding—a result anticipated by none of the physicians). Only for the word "purgative" were the physicians' ratings markedly more optimistic, a 39 percent expected comprehension being matched with actual percentages of 14 and 13 among respondents.

Given the low percentages of respondents showing adequate understanding of the words "protein," "rhesus," and "umbilicus" (predicted by the physicians), as well as of "purgative," the replies for these four words were examined in some detail in order to ascertain the types of misunderstandings evident. For "protein" the major source of misunderstanding appeared to be confusion between tests for sugar and albumin levels. Many respondents in both groups equated this word with sugar, starch, vitamins, or, more vaguely, with "food" or "eating too much." of those attempting a definition, about one-third of the underutilizers and one-sixth of the utilizers classified "protein" as a germ or an infection.

With regard to "rhesus," it was clear that the physicians' concept of adequate understanding (rating D) included a judgment as to the blood type's desirability; for example: "That's your blood. People have different blood groups. Rhesus positive is good." A reply of "your blood" or "your blood group" without such a qualification was consistently rated as "incomplete understanding" (rating C). Most respondents did not know the meaning of "umbilicus" and said so (about 84 percent), although a considerable number described "navel" in such terms as "the place where your cord used to be." Of the few who did attempt a definition, the underutilizers were generally vague (for example, "the shape of her stomach," "something in your stomach"), while most utilizers identified it correctly as the "cord," or incompletely as "your navel" or "tummy-button." "Purgative" was probably confused in the minds of many women with an enema of soapy water administered in a syringe, as it was described vaguely as a "needle" or "injection" in the majority of incorrect answers of both utilizers and underutilizers.

Clearly, these confusions in actual patient understanding were not anticipated by the majority of the physicians who expected adequate understanding of these somewhat technical terms ("protein," "rhesus," and "umbilicus").

Given the overwhelming underestimation by the 18 physicians in the study of the level of respondents' word comprehension (with the exception of the three words noted above), the possible effect of seniority (experience) on this difference was considered. Of the 18 anonymous replies received, 15 were identifiable (through an accompanying letter, the handwriting, or the envelope) to the extent that they could be rated as from either senior or junior staff. Although the numbers were too small to indicate any clear differences, there was

Table 2
The relationship between physicians' reported word use and assessment of patient comprehension.

	Percentage hypothetical adequate understanding	Percentage using word
Antibiotic	5.6	44.4
Breech	22.2	38.9
Enamel	27.8	50.0
Glucose	27.8	66.7
Membranes	0.0	44.4
Mucus	11.1	61.1
Navel	72.2	61.1
Protein	16.7	55.6
Purgative	38.9	50.0
Rhesus	5.6	61.1
Scanning	0.0	38.9
Sutures	5.6	33.3
Umbilicus	11.1	44.4
Total physicians*	18 (100.0%)	18 (100.0%)

* These totals each include six physicians not present in the other. The equality of the totals is coincidental.

evidence of an assumption of greater knowledge among the junior staff on all words except "mucus," "navel," "purgative," and "umbilicus." For these terms, senior staff appeared to expect greater understanding. This possibly negative association of imputed understanding with physician seniority could be a subject for further study with more adequate samples.

A further interesting comparison is that between the physicians' reported word usage, obtained during the word-selection process, and their hypothetical assessment of patient comprehension. The relevant data, presented in table 2, indicate a clear tendency among physicians to employ words without expecting patients to understand their meaning.

Discussion

The findings from this exploratory British study are, despite limited numbers, consistent with those from studies in the United States. First, there was a consistently higher level of word comprehension among the utilizers, as rated blind and independently by the two rating physicians. Second, some differences emerged by parity among the utilizers: The multiparae had a slightly higher level of comprehension than the primiparae. Such differences were not apparent among the underutilizers. Third, there is clear evidence that the physicians consistently and markedly underestimated the level of word comprehension of all the lower-working-class respondents.

It should be emphasized that the patient populations for this and earlier studies were predominantly or exclusively of low socio-economic status. The consistently low expectation of word comprehension by physicians in all these studies may, therefore, be a function of social distance—ignorance being imputed to lower socio-economic groups. Two major questions remain for further investigation: Given the apparently high level of comprehension among lower-class patients, how does this actual level compare with that among patients of higher socio-economic status? A further independent question is whether physicians impute the same degree of ignorance to patients of higher socio-economic status as they appear to assume exists among lower-class patients.

Perhaps the most vivid way of highlighting these findings is through the following comment by one of my respondents regarding the sources of information on her condition while in the hospital:

Well, I ask the nurses about the blood pressure and if they don't tell me, I go to my chart and look at it. It's six of one and half-a-dozen of the other. When the doctor comes by, I listen to him. I get some information from him when he's speaking about me to the students, although he doesn't know he's giving it to me.

I have already alluded to the presence of a body of literature on the breakdown of patient-physician communication, which, in the main, ascribes culpability to the patient. The results presented in this report may, of course, be explained by reference to this literature and, in particular, to a combination of some or all of the factors listed in the paper by Samora et al. (1961). In departing from this predominant "blaming the victim" or patient-culpability tradition, I wish to present several alternative reasons for the imputation of patient ignorance by physicians, and to argue that responsibility may be more correctly attributed to physicians and to aspects of professionalism than to patients.

Skipper et al (1964), in a much neglected departure from the patient-culpability tradition, considered the meaning and function of communication to hospitalized patients and some barriers to effective communication. They presented the following four reasons: (1)

Limited communication has the anticipated result of keeping interaction with patients on a strictly instrumental basis and geared toward the main ends of the hospital. (2) Not informing the patient about his illness protects health-care personnel from encountering unmanageable reactions from those patients who would "not understand" and might cause difficulty for personnel. (3) It also tends to guarantee that there will be no emotional reactions to the knowledge of illness which might hamper the patient's chances of getting well. (4) Limited communication serves to safeguard health-care personnel from the possibility that patients will discover errors of neglect and incompetence in their work. One could perhaps add to these reasons the finding by Dodge (1961) that willingness to keep patients medically informed is related to certain aspects of the health provider's emotional makeup—in particular, to his self-conception and his feeling of personal adequacy and psychological strength. Clearly, these fairly specific reasons have little to do with the characterological features of patients; rather, they have to do with the routine behavior and emotional needs of health professionals.

An additional reason incorporates directly the findings of this and previous papers regarding physician underestimation of patient comprehension. Pratt et al. (1957) rather vividly outlined the possible dynamics of the situation:

When a doctor perceives the patient as rather poorly informed, he considers the tremendous difficulties of translating his knowledge into language the patient can understand along with the dangers of frightening the patient. Therefore, he avoids involving himself in an elaborate discussion with the patient; the patient, in turn, reacts dully to this limited information, either asking uninspired questions, or refraining from questioning the doctor at all, thus reinforcing the doctor's view that the patient is ill-equipped to comprehend his problem. This further reinforces the doctor's tendency to skirt discussions of the problem. Lacking guidance by the doctor, the patient performs at a low level; hence, the doctor rates his capacities as even lower than they are.

This paper has considered two important aspects of research into patient-physician communication. First, the bias toward physician imputation of patient ignorance and the discontinuity in research methods have been noted. Second, a possible research design, which overcomes a number of previous shortcomings, has been described in some detail. Although the present study is only exploratory and clearly suffers from restricted numbers, I would suggest that a comparable methodology could be used in the design of a larger investigation. It would perhaps be fruitful if such a study could also incorporate other types of professional-client encounters (e.g. those of lawyers, accountants, clergy, social workers), and could include client populations of varying socio-economic status to determine whether client ignorance is similarly imputed in these relationships. Indeed, in a subsequent paper, I plan to explore, on a more theoretical level, why this imputation of ignorance may in fact be a necessary structural ingredient in all professional-client encounters and, following some of the suggestions of Moore and Tumin (1950), the various functions it appears to serve.

Acknowledgments

This paper reports some results from an intensive exploratory study, supported by the Nuffield Provincial Hospitals Trust, of the utilization behavior of a lower-working-class subculture in Aberdeen, Scotland. I would like to thank Howard Becker (Northwestern University), Eliot Freidson (New York University), and S. M. Miller (Boston University) for very helpful comments. As always, I particularly acknowledge the encouragement and advice of Sonja McKinlay (Boston University).

Appendix: Research Instrument Concerning Medical Vocabulary Knowledge

INTRODUCTION: I would like to read you some words, some of them you may have come across before. I'd like you to tell me what you think each of them means. If you're not sure, just say what you think it might mean. This is not a test. We are trying to find out if doctors use words that patients can't understand, so it's really a test of them. (Score A, B, C, or D—see below.)

ANTIBIOTIC: If a doctor told a patient that he's going to put her on antibiotics, what's he going to do?

BREECH: If a doctor told a patient that she's going to have a breech, what do you think is going to happen?

ENAMEL: If a doctor looked in a patient's mouth and said her enamel was bad, what is he talking about?

GLUCOSE: If a nurse tells a patient that she is going to have a glucose test, what do you think they are going to test?

MEMBRANES: If a doctor says to a patient that he is going to break her membranes, what is he going to do?

MUCUS: If a patient is told that she has a lot of mucus, what has she got a lot of?

NAVEL: If a doctor, while examining a patient, mentions the word "navel," what is he talking about?

PROTEIN: If a patient is told that she has protein in her water, what is it she has in her water?

PURGATIVE: If a nurse tells a patient that she is going to give her a purgative, what is she going to give her?

RHESUS: Doctors sometimes, while examining a woman who is expecting, say she's "rhesus positive." What are they talking about?

SCANNING: If a patient is told that she has an appointment for a scanning, what is it she is going to get?

SUTURES: If a nurse tells a patient that she is going to take her sutures out, what is she going to take out?

UMBILICUS: If a doctor, while examining a patient, mentions the word "umbilicus," what is he talking about?

SCORING: The scoring procedure was adapted from that developed by Samora et al. (1961) and took the following form:

Score A when you think that a patient would not recognize the word and would not know any meaning for it. This score will usually be given when you think that a respondent will actually say that she does not know the word or when she will most likely be unable to say anything that might be construed as a definition.

Score B when you think that a patient would have an erroneous understanding of the meaning of the term (e.g. the uterus is something to do with urine), or when you think that a respondent's answer would be vague incomplete, superficial, or ambiguous but contain enough of an element or error to lead you to the conclusion that the patient is "on the wrong track" in the definition or explanation she might attempt (e.g. "breech" means to turn the mother upside down).

Score C when you think that a patient would recognize the word but would give such a vague, incomplete, superficial, or ambiguous explanation that it could be reasonably doubted that she understands the term well enough for a clear or full communication in the clinic or hospital situation (e.g. an abortion is a kind of childbirth).

Score D when you think that a patient would have a fairly clear idea of the meaning of the term and would be likely to understand it when it is used in context in the hospital or clinic situation.

References

Collins, G. E. 1955. Do we really advise the patient? *Journal of Florida Medical Association* 42 (August): 111–115.

Dodge, J. S. 1961. Nurses' sense of adequacy and attitudes toward keeping patients informed. *Journal of Health and Human Behavior* 2 (fall): 213–216.

McKinlay, J. B. 1970. Some Aspects of Lower Working-Class Utilization Behavior. Doctoral dissertation, Aberdeen University.

McKinlay, J. B. 1970b. A brief description of a study on the utilization of maternity and child welfare services by a lower working-class subculture. *Social Science and Medicine* 4: 551–556.

McKinlay, J. B. 1973. Social networks, lay consultation and help-seeking behavior. *Social Forces* 51 (March): 275–292.

McKinlay, J. B., and S. M. McKinlay. 1972. Some social characteristics of lower working-class utilizers and underutilizers of maternity care services. *Journal of Health and Social Behavior* 13 (December): 369–382.

Moore, W. E., and M. M. Tumin. 1949. Some social functions of ignorance. *American Sociological Review* 14 (December): 787–795.

Plaja, A. O., L. M. Cohen, and J. Samora. 1968. Communication between physicians and patients in out-patient clinics. *Milbank Memorial Fund Quarterly* 46 (April): 161–213.

Pratt, L. A., W. Seligman, and G. Reader. 1957. Physicians' views on the level of medical information among patients. *American Journal of Public Health* 47 (October): 1277–1283.

Redlich, F. 1945. The patients' language. *Yale Journal of Biology and Medicine* 17, no. 3: 427–453.

Samora, J., L. Saunders, and R. F. Larson. 1961. Medical vocabulary knowledge among hospital patients. *Journal of Health and Human Behavior* 2 (summer): 83–92.

Samora, J., L. Saunders, and R. F. Larson. 1962. Knowledge about specific diseases in four selected samples. *Journal of Health and Human Behavior* 3 (fall): 176–185.

Seligman, A. W., N. E. McGrath, and L. Pratt. 1957. Level of information among clinic patients. *Journal of Chronic Disease* 6 (November): 497–509.

Skipper, J. K., D. L. Tagliacozzo, and H. O. Mauksch. 1964. Some possible consequences of limited communication between patients and hospital functionaries. *Journal of Health and Human Behavior* 5 (spring): 34–40.

11

Variations in Patients' Compliance with Doctors' Advice: An Empirical Analysis of Patterns of Communication
Milton S. Davis

Introduction

This paper stems from a larger study of the major social, psychological, and physical factors that account for variations in patients' compliance with doctors' orders. The investigation considered the extent of patient noncompliance and the range and nature of factors that may lead to or help explain these variations. The factors reported in this paper represent a continuation of the analysis of dimensions that characterize doctor-patient interaction.[1]

In principle, the range of factors that may account for variations in patients' compliance is immense. The following set of assumptions, however, guided the larger investigation from which this report stems.

• Individuals who go to a doctor have in common the fact that something is troubling them, but differ more or less in their *personal characteristics.*

• In some measure, these personal characteristics are taken into account by the doctor so that variations occur in the nature of the *regimen* prescribed for each patient.

• After being told their regimens, patients may discuss and assess the doctors' advice with paramedical and other *influential persons,* i.e., relatives, friends, and associates, whose opinions on the matter they value.

• Such influences interact with the personal characteristics a patient brings to the situation, the nature of the regimen, and the nature of the *doctor-patient relationship* to produce patterns of compliance with the doctor's orders.

Reprinted, with permission, from *American Journal of Public Health* 58 (1968): 274–288.

Patterns of Compliance

To label patients compliant or noncompliant without elaboration is misleading. The medical regimen is ordinarily a composite of recommendations, and a patient may comply with all, some, or none of the advice. Different degrees of compliance also characterize each regimen, and, assuming that the patient complies at all, it is clear that he may do so consistently or intermittently through time. A review of the literature demonstrates a range from 15 to 93 percent of patients reportedly noncompliant. [2] This wide range is not surprising when the variety of populations, the various methods of data collection, and the different medical problems investigated are considered. Nevertheless, a pattern emerges when these studies are examined as a whole. Regardless of the differences, at least a third of the patients in most studies failed to comply with doctors' orders.

Patient Characteristics

A review of the literature on noncompliance evidences conflicting conclusions regarding what demographic attributes characterize a noncompliant patient. Although many factors have been investigated, they are not dealt with consistently in each study, and the results are inconclusive. Therefore, it is only possible to cull some impressions about what patient characteristics influence noncompliant behavior. It seems that females are somewhat more likely to default than males,[3] and that older people,[4] patients in lower socioeconomic status groups,[5] and patients with little education[6] are least likely to follow doctors' orders.

One might expect that physical characteristics of patients would affect variations in patient compliance. Most studies, however, focus on a population with a particular diagnosis, and comparative findings are few. Patients with long-term illnesses are reportedly more compliant if they are given careful instruction,[7] and the urgency of an acute illness has been related to compliance.[8]

Studies concerned with psychological characteristics of patients have shown that noncompliant patients can be identified by examining coping mechanisms,[9] dependency,[10] and defensiveness and externalization.[11] One author suggests that fear arousal is necessary for acceptance of medical advice.[12]

Regimen

A suggested medical regimen usually combines prescriptions (behavior to be initiated) and proscriptions (behavior to be prohibited).[13] Most patients, however, choose to comply with two out of three regimens and select those that are the least difficult.[14] Restrictions that necessitate relinquishing personal habits are the most difficult to follow; medications are the easiest. Compliance with one specific regimen appears to affect adherence to others.[15] However, no relationship was found between follow-through with regimens requiring patient self-care and compliance with advice involving the patient in clinic procedures.[16] The former, (regimens requiring patient judgment) are more closely associated with noncompliance. There is also agreement that the more complex regimens affect increased noncompliance.[17] These findings evidence a need for more explanation and presentation of advice in the least complex manner.

Personal Influence
It is possible that influence from family members, friends, and associates may conflict with the medical advice and counteract the doctor's potential authority. But there is also the possibility that these extramedical influences will reinforce the doctors' recommendations. Family discord is closely associated with noncompliance[18]; availability of local help and family cohesiveness during crises are associated with increased levels of compliance.[19] The more stable home situation is perhaps associated with positive reinforcement of medical advice.[20] Such positive reinforcement is particularly functional when one considers that the patient is not able to relate to his doctor with the same frequency and intensity as he does with family, friends, and co-workers.

Doctor-Patient Relationship
Few empirical investigations have dealt with the way in which interaction between patient and doctor influences patient compliance. Those who have studied this factor empirically have been concerned with perceptions of doctors and patients and have not considered objective measurement of the doctor-patient interaction or how this might influence the patient's decision regarding compliance.[21] This may account for incongruent findings. For example, in one report, barriers in doctor-patient communication could not account for patient noncompliance.[22] Another study shows that communication between doctor and patient is less important than the psychological readiness of the patient.[23] However, when doctors fail to clearly convey the significance of a regimen to the patient, there is a reciprocal failure on the part of the patient to comply.[24] Reciprocity seems to affect compliance, whether between a very docile approval-seeking patient and a nurturant doctor or between a pseudo-

independent patient and an aloof doctor.[25] Although there is not complete agreement on exactly how the doctor-patient relationship affects compliance, most investigations do recognize the importance of communication and explanation.[26]

Hypothesis and Design of the Study

Although a full range of factors affecting compliance are recognized and were investigated in the larger study, this paper is particularly concerned with the ways in which dimensions of doctor-patient interaction relate to patient compliance. It is hypothesized that patterns of communication that deviate from the normative doctor-patient relationship will be associated with the patient's failure to comply with the doctor's advice.

Study Group

The study group consists of 154 new patients seen by 76 junior physicians (fourth-year medical students), who regularly care for patients in the clinics, and 78 senior (attending) physicians assigned to the general medical clinic of a large general voluntary teaching hospital. A new patient either had never been to the general medical clinic before or had not attended the clinic for at least one year. Patients were excluded from the sample who had a chief complaint that indicated that they would probably be sent to another clinic after one visit, who came regularly to one or more other hospital clinics (although they were considered new to the general medical clinic), who sought follow-up care of a condition already diagnosed and well known to the patient, or who had a language or hearing problem.[27]

Survey data were collected on a random sample of clinic patients prior to this investigation to describe and characterize patient experiences in the general medical clinic. The composition of the present study population compares favorably with the estimated clinic population based on that survey.[28]

Data Collection and Analysis

Prior to the initiation of the present study, exploratory data were collected from doctors and patients over successive patient visits to the general medical clinic to evaluate the relative merits of various technics for studying doctor-patient interaction.[29] On the basis of this exploratory work, it was decided that data could most feasibly be collected by a combination of tape recordings, survey methods (in-

Table 1
Bales's categories for interaction process analysis.

1. Shows solidarity; raises other's status; gives help, reward.
2. Shows tension release, jokes, laughs; shows satisfaction.
3. Agrees, shows passive acceptance, understands, concurs, complies.
4. Gives suggestion, direction, implying autonomy for others.
5. Gives opinion, evaluation, analysis; expresses feeling, wish.
6. Gives orientation, information; repeats, clarifies, confirms.
7. Asks for orientation, information, repetition, confirmation.
8. Asks for opinion, evaluation, analysis, expression of feeling.
9. Asks for suggestion, direction, possible ways of action.
10. Disagrees; shows passive rejection, formality; withholds help.
11. Shows tension, asks for help, withdraws out of the field.
12. Shows antagonism, deflates other's status, defends or asserts self.

cluding interviews and questionnaires), and a content analysis of patients' medical records.

Tape Recording of Interaction
A method developed by Robert F. Bales, interaction process analysis, was adapted for this research.[30] With this method, all doctors' and patients' verbal communication is coded into 12 categories of action (table 1). Scores representing the amount of activity devoted to each of the 12 categories were computed separately for each doctor and patient and transferred onto code sheets, from with IBM cards were punched. Data analysis involved correlating an independent measure of patient compliance with four types of data derived from the interaction process analysis. First, the relative volume of participation by doctor and patient was determined; second, communication profiles for doctor and patient were compared; third, by manipulating category scores, indexes of difficulties encountered in the interaction were measured; and fourth, a factor analysis was performed. Although the latter analysis was not in Bales's original formulation, it was employed here to discover what additional dimensions in the doctor-patient relationship might account for variations in patients' compliance. This paper is primarily concerned with the factor-analysis data.

Interaction process analysis is an expensive method requiring extensive time for tape-recording, transcribing, coding, and analyzing data.[31] Consequently, only two crucial periods of interaction were recorded: first, the doctor's formulation (presentation of medical regimen and diagnosis to the patient) during the primary visit; and second, the entire interaction between doctor and patient at the time of the patient's revisit. The latter was recorded to examine changes in the doctor-patient relationship.

A total of 223 doctor-patient interactions were subsequently coded. Of the 154 doctor-patient pairs in the study group, 80 had both visits taped, 39 only the first visit, 24 only the second, and 11 neither visit. Reliability in coding averaged 85 percent—rather good, considering the subjective nature of the material.[32]

Survey Methods
Personal interviews and a self-administered questionnaire were used to study the perceptions of doctors and patients with reference to their own specific role obligations and the role expectations of the other.

During the exploratory phase of the study, a series of questionnaires and interview schedules were developed and pretested. Data were subsequently collected from the patient study group by means of four interviews: one before the primary visit, one after that visit, and one each after the second and third clinic visits. However, because of variations in patients' illnesses, the number of appointments, and the formulation of medical regimens on any specific visit, it was necessary to allow the interviewers a certain amount of leeway in the administration of the various interview schedules. In addition, a self-administered questionnaire was completed by each physician treating a study patient.

Content Analysis of Patients' Medical Records
Some months after the survey data were collected, a chart review was designed to collect demographic data, a listing of all regimens recorded by the doctor, and a record of the proportion of broken appointments during a six-month period.

Index of Compliance
A variety of indexes have been employed in other studies to measure compliance, some based on subjective reports and others on objective physical measurements.[33] In this study, the composite index of compliance includes patients' perceptions of their compliant behavior, doctors' perceptions of the patients' compliant behavior, and an independent review of patients' medical records. The inclusion of these three types of data to measure noncompliant behavior overcomes many of the difficulties inherent in accepting the patients'

word, the doctors' word, or the medical records as the sole source of information.

The compliance score is a weighted average of patient follow-through with two types of recommendations ordered by the doctor. First, recommendations may involve patient initiative at home or at work. This category includes prescription and nonprescription medications, recommended diets, changes in rest habits and worrying, limitation of smoking and alcohol consumption, and changes in work activities. Second, recommendations may also require patient participation in the hospital organization. Here we examined diagnostic procedures, specific treatments, referrals to specialty clinics, and revisits to the clinic. Medical records were used to ascertain a list of specific regimens. In addition, patients were asked if any other regimens were recommended by the doctor. Some patients reported advice which the doctor did not list in the medical record.[34]

After it was discovered which orders were recalled, the patient was asked how closely he followed these recommendations. The responses were coded for each regimen as follows: (0) none of the time, (1) very seldom, (2) less than half the time, (3) most of the time, and (4) all of the time. The physicians were also asked how closely the patient followed the advice, and these responses were coded similarly. When the responses of the physician and the patient were not in agreement, an average was taken of the two. A patient was categorized as not at all compliant with regard to those regimens reported by the physician but not recalled by the patient. We assumed that patients who did not recall a recommendation when asked were not following the advice. The proportions of broken appointments for revisits, referrals, and diagnostic tests were also coded according to congruent categories and included in the composite index. For each type of recommendation, a weight was assigned indicating the relative importance of the regimen.[35]

Results

Extent of Noncompliance and Demographic Differences

In this study group, 37 percent of the patients were classified as noncompliant and 63 percent as compliant. This rate of compliance, in accordance with the findings of the literature review, indicates that, although the majority of patients follow their doctors' advice, over one-third of patients simply do not do what they are told.

The data from the present study show, contradictory to many reports, that there is no significant relationship between compliance and any of the demographic characteristics investigated. This finding is, nevertheless, noteworthy. No variations in patient compliance can be attributed to demographic characteristics peculiar to the patient, e.g. age, sex, marital status, religion, education, or occupation. This supports the contention that dimensions in the doctor-patient relationship are more fruitful avenues for explaining variations in patient compliance.[36]

Interaction between Doctor and Patient

Presumably, all doctors and patients have certain ideas about the kind of relationship they should have and the kind of roles they are expected to play.[37] The way in which doctors and patients initially behaved and whether or not they continued to conform to expected ways of behavior was examined in an earlier paper.[38] Failure to adhere to medical advice *after* the doctor visit was related to deviant communication *in* the doctor-patient relationship. There was a reversal in roles over successive doctor visits. Though the doctor was directive and emotionally neutral in the primary visit and the patient passively conformed with his role, data from the revisit suggest that this conformity was only momentary. In the second visit, many doctors passively accepted the patient, whose participation was increasingly active. Noncompliant behavior was further explained by increased difficulty of communication and attempts by doctors and patients to control each other.[39]

Factor-Analyzed Dimensions of Doctor-Patient Interaction

The 12 categories of interaction (table 1), in and of themselves, have a theoretical significance which describes the structure and process of group interaction.[40] The doctor-patient profiles and the indexes suggested by Bales represent only a few ways of combining the 12 categories. Furthermore, they did not account for much noncompliance. In order to discover some other dimensions, a factor analysis on the interaction categories was completed. The method of factor analysis was selected for its advantage in permitting the grouping of interaction categories in a way independent of any a priori thought. It was expected that discovery of such factors would further our knowledge of dimensions of the doctor-patient interaction which ultimately could be related to variations in patient compliance.

The rates for the 12 interaction categories for doctor and patient were correlated to form a 21 × 24 product moment correlation matrix. Principle factors were extracted, with unity as the diagonal value. Ten factors, judged salient on the basis of the magnitude of factor loadings, were rotated to oblique simple structure by the Promax procedure.[41] Each of the ten factors is defined by a particular group of categories. A list of the factors with the loadings and weights for each category appears in table 2.

Seven of the 24 categories were heavily loaded on more than one factor and consequently were differentially weighted for each dimension. To compute scores, the weight of the factor loading was multiplied times the rate of doctor-patient activity which fell into the categories.

The ten factors represent empirically determined dimensions of doctor-patient communication. The label for each factor is an arbitrary name intended to summarize the interaction categories defining that dimension.

Factor I, *malintegrative behavior*, characterizes the type of doctor-patient communication that exhibits negative social-emotional interaction. Both participants appear to be formal, show passive rejection, and withhold help from the other. The patient shows antagonism toward the doctor and simultaneously withdraws from the situation. What we find here is a dimension measuring deviant interaction.

Factor II, *active patient–permissive doctor*, represents a pattern of communication between an authoritative patient and a doctor who passively accepts the authoritative position taken by the patient. The patient is likely to present his own evaluation and analysis of the situation and shows little acceptance of what the doctor says. It is assumed that a doctor-patient relationship which exhibits a high score on this factor is deviant from the normative doctor-patient interaction.

Factor III, *solidary relationship*, is indicative of communication characterized by friendly behavior on the part of both doctor and patient. Positive social-emotional interaction reckons high in this factor. The patient is able to show satisfaction with the interaction and to release much of the tension that arises from the situation.

The communication in which factor IV, *nondirective antagonism*, is high suggests an antagonistic doctor who neglects to give the patient information, explanation, or orientation. He confines his activity to expressing opinions and feelings about the situation.

Factor V, *informative nonevaluativeness*, typifies the doctor who gives a great deal of direction to the patient but does not present any diagnosis or evaluation.

Items defining factor VI, *nonreciprocal informativeness*, reflect the way in which doctors collect information in order to make a diagnosis. The doctor asks for information from the patient, and the patient coopera-

Table 2
Primary loadings and weights for categories defining factors in doctor-patient interaction ($N = 152$).

Factor I: Malintegrative behavior

Loading	Weight	
0.72	0.58	Patient: Shows antagonism, deflates other's status, defends or asserts self.
0.66	0.50	Doctor: Disagrees; shows passive rejection, formality; withholds help.
0.52	0.36	Patient: Disagrees; shows passive rejection, formality; withholds help.
0.36	0.11	Patient: Shows tension, asks for help, withdraws out of field.

Factor II: Active patient—permissive doctor

Loading	Weight	
0.80	0.37	Doctor: Agrees, shows passive acceptance, understands, concurs, complies.
−0.72	0.39	Patient: Agrees, shows passive acceptance, understands, concurs, complies.
0.63	0.36	Patient: Gives orientation, information, repetition, confirmation.
0.46	0.23	Patient: Gives opinion, evaluation, analysis; expresses feeling, wish.

Factor III: Solidary relationship

Loading	Weight	
0.95	0.79	Patient: Shows solidarity; raises other's status; gives help, reward.
0.53	0.28	Patient: Shows tension release, jokes, laughs, shows satisfaction.
0.36	0.11	Doctor: Shows solidarity; raises other's status; gives help, reward.

Factor IV: Nondirective antagonism

Loading	Weight	
0.84	0.65	Doctor: Gives opinion, evaluation, analysis; expresses feeling, wish.
0.52	0.28	Doctor: Shows antagonism, deflates other's status, defends or asserts self.
−0.49	0.40	Doctor: Gives orientation, information, repetition; confirms, clarifies.

Factor V: Informative nonevaluativeness

Loading	Weight	
0.99	0.82	Doctor: Gives suggestion, direction, implying autonomy for others.
−0.48	0.24	Doctor: Gives orientation, information; repeats, clarifies, confirms.

Table 2 (continued)

Factor VI: Nonreciprocal informativeness

Loading	Weight	
0.85	0.68	Doctor: Asks for orientation, information, repetition, confirmation.
−0.63	0.49	Doctor: Gives orientation, information; repeats, clarifies, confirms.
0.36	0.12	Patient: Gives orientation, information; repeats, clarifies, confirms.

Factor VII: Evaluative congruence

Loading	Weight	
0.49	0.59	Patient: Agrees, shows passive acceptance, understands, concurs, complies.
−0.45	0.46	Patient: Asks for opinion, evaluation, analysis, expression of feeling.
0.41	0.42	Doctor: Agrees, shows passive acceptance, understands, concurs, complies.
−0.35	0.34	Doctor: Asks for opinion, evaluation, analysis, expression of feeling.

Factor VIII: Entreative inquiry

Loading	Weight	
0.69	0.77	Patient: Asks for orientation, information, repetition, confirmation.
0.51	0.52	Patient: Asks for suggestion, direction, possible ways of action.

Factor IX: Tension buildup

Loading	Weight	
0.68	0.73	Doctor: Shows solidarity; raises other's status; gives help, reward.
0.54	0.52	Patient: Shows tension, asks for help, withdraws out of the field.
0.41	0.42	Doctor: Shows tension, asks for help, withdraws out of the field.

Factor X: Tension release

Loading	Weight	
0.54	0.58	Doctor: Shows tension release, jokes, laughs, shows satisfaction.
0.51	0.43	Patient: Shows tension release, jokes, laughs, shows satisfaction.

---

tively orients the doctor. In this case, however, the doctor also withholds information from the patient. There is no feedback.

Factor VII, *evaluative congruence*, measures the successful solution of the problems introduced by lack of agreement on values and expectations. The doctor and the patient agree on what they consider important and beneficial for their relationship.

An encounter scoring high on *entreative inquiry*, factor VIII, illustrates how a patient who desires information communicates in order to determine what the problem is and how he can resolve it. This type of patient does not wish the doctor to withhold any information. He asks for orientation, information, and analysis.

Factor IX presents one way doctors manage interaction saturated with tension. High scores on the factor *tension buildup* indicate that both doctor and patient show a great deal of tension regardless of the doctor's attempts to achieve reintegration by communicating in a friendly manner.

Factor X, *tension release*, is a corollary of factor IX. Here the doctor and the patient exhibit tension release through joking, laughing, and showing some satisfaction with the relationship.

Compliance and Factors of Doctor-Patient Communication

It was hypothesized that patterns of communication deviant from prescribed institutional doctor-patient relationships will result in patients' failure to comply with doctors' advice. Scores for the ten factors for each doctor-patient pair were computed for the first visit and the revisit, and subsequently correlated with patients' compliance.

First, there is very little association between what occurs in the primary visit and later compliance. In the first visit, not one of the factors was significantly associated with later patient compliance. In the revisit, however, five of the ten factors were associated with patients' compliance. Table 3 shows a significant correlation between compliance and malintegrative behavior (factor I). The greater the malintegrative behavior in the interaction, the less likely is the patient to follow the doctor's orders after he leaves the doctor's office.

There is also a negative correlation between compliance and factor II, active patient–permissive doctor. When a patient acts in a authoritative manner with a permissive doctor, the doctor's position is threatened and the patient is unlikely to comply. Similarly, factor IV, measuring the extent to which a doctor is nondirective in an antagonistic way, is also negatively correlated with compliance. When a doctor confines his activity to analysis of the situation and ex-

Table 3.
Product moment correlations and levels of significance for doctor-patient interaction factors and compliance behavior.

Interaction factors	Primary visit ($N = 119$)		Revisit ($N = 104$)	
	r	p	r	p
I. Malintegrative behavior	−0.141	>0.05	−0.260	<0.01
II. Active patient—permissive doctor	−0.132	>0.05	−0.304	<0.01
III. Solidary relationship	0.072	>0.05	0.173	>0.05
IV. Nondirective antagonism	−0.040	>0.05	−0.236	<0.01
V. Informative nonevaluativeness	−0.070	>0.05	0.040	>0.05
VI. Nonreciprocal informativeness	−0.029	>0.05	−0.315	<0.01
VII. Evaluative congruence	0.102	>0.05	0.123	>0.05
VIII. Entreative inquiry	−0.031	>0.05	−0.053	>0.05
IX. Tension buildup	−0.081	>0.05	−0.060	>0.05
X. Tension release	0.108	>0.05	0.223	<0.05

pression of his opinions, he is likely to promote noncompliance. The opposite type of behavior, however, does not ensure compliance. Factor V, indicative of a minimum of analysis and evaluation and a maximum of direction on the doctor's part, is not significantly related to compliance. These data suggest that compliance is a function of a delicate balance of direction and evaluation presented in a manner acceptable to the patient.

Compliance is also a function of reciprocal interaction.[42] Noncompliance was significantly associated with factor VI, nonreciprocal informativeness. Apparently it makes little difference how much information the patient requests (factor VIII), but when the doctor takes time to collect information without giving any feedback the patient will probably react in a reciprocal deviant or noncompliant way.

It is interesting to note that only three of the ten dimensions iterated in the factor analysis measure positive rapport in the interaction (solidary relationship, evaluative congruence, and tension release), and only one of these (tension release) is significantly related to patient compliance. When tension is built up it effects malintegration, but if it is released through joking or laughing the possibility of patient adherence to the medical regimen is increased.

Factor III, measuring the amount of friendly rapport in the relationship, is not significantly correlated with patient compliance. As the relationship between the doctor and patient becomes friendly, strains are created which interfere with their role functions. It may be easier then for a patient to ignore the advice of a friendly physician than that of one who is formal and authoritative. If the friendly doctor's authority is undermined, the patient may be as likely to accept the advice of a friend as to accept that of the doctor.

This is also evident when factor VII, evaluative congruence, is examined. Doctors and patients who are on the same wavelength, who agree on what they consider desirable, right, and proper, may communicate more effectively, but this activity is unrelated to the patient's later compliance.

In sum, the hypothesis relating patient noncompliance and deviant patterns of communication is supported by these data. Caution, however, is recommended when interpreting the findings. The nature of each factor is such that a negative correlation between compliance and any factor does not imply that the absence or reverse of that factor is positively correlated with compliance. For example, although malintegrative behavior is negatively correlated with compliance, the absence of such behavior does not necessarily affect compliance. As indicated above, compliance is not affected by the extent to which the interaction is characterized as a solidary relationship. One should also note that, although these data evidence some statistically significant correlations, the associations are relatively small. Furthermore, the factors iterated in this particular investigation have not been standardized. Consequently, there are descriptive characteristics of this particular population of doctor-patient relationships. The significance of this research would be increased greatly if, in further studies, these factors were to be employed as independent variables to investigate compliance in medical as well as other settings.

Summary and Discussion

Communication between doctor and patient ideally necessitates a certain degree of reciprocity. Each person has certain rights and obligations. When the doctor performs a service, the patient is obligated to reciprocate—first, by cooperating with the doctor in their interaction; and second, by complying with the medical recommendations once he leaves the doctor's office. We have seen, however, that there are deviations from these norms. The data reported in this study, collected by means of tape recordings of doctor-patient interactions and supplemented with a series of patient interviews, a self-administered questionnaire completed by physicians, and a content analysis of patients' medical records, were analyzed to determine the extent of deviant patient behavior within and outside the doctor-patient relationship.

Thirty-seven percent of the patients disregarded what their doctors advised. A factor analysis suggested some patterns of communication that help explain noncompliance. Although interaction in the primary doctor visit was not associated with later compliance, the data suggest that revisits between an authoritative patient and a physician who passively accepts such patient participation may promote patient noncompliance. Effective communication is impeded when doctors and patients evidence tension in their relationship. Unless this tension is released, noncompliance may result, regardless of the doctor's efforts to achieve solidarity. And when the doctor seeks information from a patient without giving any feedback, the patient is unlikely to follow the doctor's orders once they are formulated.

Implicit in this discussion of noncompliance is the problem of controlling patient behavior. In the doctor-patient relationship, whether in private practice, in a hospital clinic, or on a ward, the doctor must rely on his ability to establish good rapport in order to inculcate in his patient a positive orientation and a commitment to the relationship so that ultimately the patient will follow his advice. In order to do this, it becomes necessary for the doctor continually to explore and diagnose the social and psychological facets of his interaction with his patients as well as the manifest medical problem.

Acknowledgment

For criticism and suggestions in the research plan and in preparing this paper the author is grateful to Mary E. W. Goss. Thanks also to Joan Z. Cohen and Jean Como, whose work as assistants on this project has benefited it greatly. The author would also like to acknowledge the help of Jane Germer, Herman Freeman, and Joseph Reed in programing and statistical analysis of the data.

This paper was presented before the Medical Care Section of the American Public Health Association at the Annual Meeting in San Francisco, Calif., November 3, 1966.

The research reported here is part of a larger investigation of variations in patients' compliance with doctors' orders carried out as part of a program in patient-care research at Cornell University Medical College, Comprehensive Care and Teaching Program,

George G. Reader, director, with the support of U.S. Public Health
Service Program Grant CH00103 01.

Notes and References

1. Preliminary findings relating compliance to dimensions of the doctor-patient
interaction were reported in M. S. Davis, Deviant Interaction in an Institutionalized
Relationship: Variation in Patients' Compliance with Doctors' Orders, paper presented before Medical Sociology session, Sixth World Congress of Sociology, Evian,
France, 1966.

2. A systematic review of compliance literature may be found in M. S. Davis,
"Variation in patients' compliance with doctors' orders: Analysis of congruence
between survey responses and results of empirical investigations," *J. Med. Educ.* 41
(1966): 1037–1048.

3. W. M. Dixon, P. Stradling, and I. Wooton, "Outpatient PAS therapy," *Lancet* 273
(1957): 871–873; G. R. Luntz and R. Austin, "New stick test for PAS in urine," *Brit.
J. Med.* 1 (1960): 1679–1683; R. Morrow and D. L. Rabin, "Reliability in self-
medication with isoniazid," *Clin. Research* 14, no. 2 (1966): 362; N. Wynn-Williams
and M. Arris, "On omitting PAS," *Tubercle* 39 (1958): 138–142.

4. B. Cobb, R. L. Clark, C. McGuire, and C. D. Howe, "Patient-responsible delay of
treatment in cancer," *Cancer* 7 (1954): 920–925; M. S. Davis and R. L. Eichhorn,
"Compliance with medical regimens: A panel study," *J. Health and Human Behavior* 4
(1963): 240–249; D. Schwartz, M. Wong, L. Zeitz, and M. E. Goss, "Medication
errors made by elderly, chronically ill patients," *AJPH* 52 (1962): 2018–2029.

5. Cobb et al., op. cit.; A. Donabedian and L. S. Rosenfeld, "A follow-up study of
chronically ill patients discharged from hospital," *Pub. Health Rep.* 79 (1964): 228;
M. C. Hardy, "Psychologic aspects of pediatrics: Parent resistance to need for remedial
and preventive services," *J. Pediat.* 48 (1956): 104–114; W. J. Johannsen, G. A.
Hellmuth, and T. Sorauf, "On accepting medical recommendations," *Arch. Environ.
Health* 12 (1966): 63–69; M. E. MacDonald, K. L. Hagverg, and B. J. Grossman,
"Social factors in relation to participation in follow-up care of rheumatic fever,"
J. Pediat. 62 (1963): 503–513; W. Mather, "Social and economic factors related to
correction of school discovered medical and dental defects," *Pennsylvania Med. J.* 62
(1954): 983–988; H. Pragoff, "Adjustment of tuberculosis patients one year after
hospital discharge," *Pub. Health Rep.* 77 (1962): 671–679; D. D. Watts, "Factors
related to the acceptance of modern medicine," *AJPH* 56 (1966): 1205–1212.

6. F. E. Bates and I. M. Ariel, "Delay in treatment of cancer," *Illinois Med. J.* 49
(December 1948): 361–365; Davis and Eichhorn, op. cit.; W. L. Johnson, Conformity to Medical Recommendations in Coronary Heart Disease, paper presented
at annual meeting of American Sociological Association, Chicago, 1965; Pragoff,
op. cit.

7. J. H. Abrahamson, F. G. Mayet, and C. C. Majola, "What is wrong with me? A
study of the views of African and Indian patients in a Durban hospital," *South African
Med. J.* 35 (1961): 690–694.

8. J. P. Ambuel, J. Cebulla, N. Watt, and D. Crowne, "Doctor-mother communications," *Midwest Society Pediat. Res.* 65 (1964): 113–114.

9. Cobb et al., op. cit.

10. R. Ellis, The Relationship between Psychological Factors and Remission of Duodenal Cancer, doctoral dissertation, University of Chicago, 1964.

11. G. A. Hellmuth, W. J. Johannsen, and T. Worauf, "Psychological factors in cardiac patients," *Arch. Environ. Health* 12 (1966): 771–780.

12. H. Leventhal, "Fear communications in the acceptance of preventive health practices," *Bull. New York Acad. Med.* 41 (1965): 1144–1168.

13. For a discussion of the content of normative prescriptions and proscriptions, see E. Mizruchi and R. Perrucci, "Norm qualities and differential effects of deviant behavior: An exploratory analysis," *Am. Sociol. Rev.* 27 (1962): 391–399. See also M. Hollander, *The Psychology of Medical Practice* (Philadelphia: Saunders, 1958).

14. Davis and Eichhorn, op. cit.

15. M. S. Davis, "Predicting non-compliant behavior," *J. Health and Social Behav.* 8 (1967): 265–271; Johannsen et al., op. cit.

16. N. H. Berkowitz, M. F. Malone, M. W. Klein, and A. Eaton, "Patient follow-through in the out-patient department," *Nursing Res.* 12 (1963): 16–22; "Patient care as a criterion problem," *J. Health and Human Behav.* 3 (1962): 171–176.

17. Davis, ref. 2 above; P. Ley and M. S. Spelman, "Communications in an out-patient setting," *Brit. J. Social and Clinical Psychol.* 4 (1965): 114–116; C. S. Riley, "Patients' understanding of doctors' instructions," *Med. Care* 4, no. 1 (1966): 34–37.

18. R. Elling, R. Whittemore, and M. Green, "Patient participation in a pediatric program," *J. Health and Human Behav.* 1 (1960): 183–191; R. Ku and G. Jordan, A Study of Self-Administration of Isoniazid in Children (Health Research Training Program, New York City Department of Health, 1964), pp. 1–11; H. M. Wallace et al., "Study of follow-up of children recommended for rheumatic fever prophylaxis," *AJPH* 46 (1956): 1563–1570.

19. R. L. Eichhorn, D. C. Reidel, and W. H. M. Morris, "Compliance to perceived therapeutic advice," in Proceedings of the Purdue Farm Cardiac Seminar, ed. W. H. M. Morris (Lafayette, Indiana: Agricultural Experiment Station, 1958), pp. 65–68; Pragoff, op. cit.

20. Abramson et al., op. cit.; Davis and Eichhorn, op. cit.; Watts, op. cit.

21. The single exception here is the doctoral dissertation of Ellis (op. cit.).

22. Berkowitz et al., op. cit.; Johnson, op. cit.

23. Johannsen et al., op. cit.

24. M. S. Davis and R. P. von der Lippe, "Discharge from hospital against medical advice: A study of reciprocity in the doctor-patient relationship," *Social Sci. and Med.* 1 (1968): 336–342; R. Hoffman, The Doctor's Role: A Study of Consensus, Congruence, and Change, doctoral dissertation, University of Nebraska, 1958; A. Sapolsky, "Relationship between doctor-patient compatability, mutual perception, and outcome of treatment," *J. Abnorm. Psychol.* 70, no. 1 (1965): 70–76; R. Sobel and A. Igalls, "Resistance to treatment, explorations of the patient's sick role," *Am. J. Psychotherapy* 18 (1964): 562–573.

25. Ellis, op. cit.

26. Abramson et al., op. cit.; Ambuel et al., op. cit.; Cobb et al., op. cit.; Davis and Eichhorn, op. cit.; Elling et al., op. cit.; Leventhal, op. cit.; Ley and Spelman, op. cit.;

D. N. Mohler, D. G. Wallin, and E. G. Dreyfus, "Studies in the home treatment of streptococcal disease," *New Engl. J. Med.* 252 (1955): 1116–1118; Riley, op. cit.; G. F. Robbins, A. J. Conte, J. E. Leach, and M. MacDonald, "Delay in diagnosis and treatment of cancer," *JAMA* 143 (1950): 346–348; A. Ullmann and M. S. Davis, "Assessing the medical patient's motivation and ability to work," *Social Casework* 46 (1965): 195–202; Watts, op. cit.

27. Interviewers were instructed to drop patients judged to be noninterviewable. Because of insufficient numbers of suitable new patients coming to the clinic at certain times, an interviewer occasionally attempted to administer the first interview schedule to someone he hoped would be suitable but who, in fact, was not. Ten such patients were eliminated because of language barriers, hearing difficulties, and inappropriate medical problems. Another five patients were dropped from the study at the request of the physician, two because of the sensitive nature of their problems and one because her doctor felt that the study was too distracting for her. (He insisted that she had been so fascinated by the tape recorder that she had ignored him completely.) A number of doctors and patients expressed reservations about the tape recorders, but only one patient and one doctor refused to be taped. Three others were dropped from the study because they refused to be interviewed. Finally, ten patients were eliminated from the study group because the interviewer assigned to the case either failed to or was unable to follow them properly. Altogether, 32 patients were dropped from the study population.

28. L. Turgeon and D. Long, A Study of New Patients in the General Medical Clinic, research memorandum, Comprehensive Care and Teaching Program, New York Hospital–Cornell University Medical Center, 1965. The sample included patients seen in October 1962; the present report is based on a sample of patients seen between November 1964 and June 1965. Data comparing demographic characteristics of the study population with the estimated composition of the clinic population on the basis of the 1962 survey are available on request.

29. The exploratory phase of the research was supported by U.S. Public Health Service Grant MH08458-01 and was entitled Dimensions of Compliant Doctor-Patient Relationships.

30. R. F. Bales, *Interaction Process Analysis* (Addison-Wesley, 1951). Although interaction process analysis has been employed experimentally and to study the interaction between doctor and patient in a psychotherapeutic situation, it has not been used in an investigation of interaction in a medical situation. On other methods of recording interaction, see the following: L. M. Adler, A Scale to Measure Psychotherapy Interactions, mimeo, School of Medicine, University of Southern California, 1964; L. F. Carter, "Recording and evaluating the performance of individuals as members of small groups," *Personal Psychol.* 7 (1954): 477–484; L. Carter, W. Haythorn, B. Meirowitz, and J. Lanzetta, "A note on a new technique of interaction," *J. Abnormal and Social Psychol.* 46 (1951): 258–260; E. D. Chapple, "The interaction chronograph: Its evolution and present application," *Personnel* 25 (1949): 295–307; A. T. Dittman, "The interpersonal process in psychotherapy: Development of a research method," *J. Abnormal and Social Psychol.* 47 (1952): 236–244; J. Dollard, "A method of measuring tension in written documents," *J. Abnormal and Social Psychol.* 42 (1947): 3–32; M. B. Freedman, T. F. Leary, A. G. Ossonio, and H. S. Coffey, "The interpersonal dimension of personality," *J. Personality* 20 (1951): 143–161; H. Guetzkow, "Unitizing and categorizing problems in coding qualitative data," *J. Clin. Psychol.* 6 (1950):

47–58; R. W. Heyns and R. Lippitt, "Systematic observational techniques," in *The Handbook of Social Psychology*, ed. G. Lindzey (Addison-Wesley, 1954); H. L. Lennard and A. Bernstein, *The Anatomy of Psychotherapy* (Columbia University Press, 1960), chapter 2; J. D. Matarazzo, G. Saslow, and R. G. Matarazzo, "The interaction chronograph as an instrument for objective measurement of interaction patterns during interviews," *J. Psychol.* 41 (1956): 347–367; M. Melbin, "Field methods and techniques: The action-interaction chart," *Human Organization* 12 (1953): 34–35; H. Murray, "A content analysis method for studying psychotherapy," *Psychol. Monogr.* 70 (1956): 13; G. Psathas, "Problems and prospects in the use of a computer system of content analysis," *Sociol. Q.* 7 (1966): 449–468; J. Ruesch, J. Block, and L. Bennett, "The assessment of communication. I. A method for the analysis of social interaction," *J. Psychiatr.* 35 (1953): 59–80; B. Stenzar, "The development and evaluation of a measure of social interaction," *Am Psychol.* 3 (1948): 266; P. J. Stone, D. C. Dunphy, M. S. Smith, and D. M. Ogilvie, *The General Inquirer: A Computer Approach to Content Analysis* (MIT Press, 1966).

31. Four coders worked in pairs, each pair coding together for a week. Every week partners were changed to produce the greatest uniformity in coding and to minimize the chance of developing rigid coding idiosyncracies. The coders listened to each recording, unitizing the dialogue on transcripts and indicating statements of affect. This was done individually and then pairs were compared. Any disagreements were resolved through discussion or, if necessary, by relistening to the tape. Coding was then done individually and the two code sheets compared. Again differences were resolved through discussion and relistening to the interaction. Any disagreements that could not be resolved were referred to the other two coders during the period set aside for that purpose each day. When the coding was completed, there was some concern that increased familiarity with the code might cause some significant differences in coding between tapes done at the beginning and at the end of the coding period. A random sample of visits from the early tapes was recorded and 4 percent of the answers were changed. However, when a random sample from all the other tapes was taken and recorded, 3 percent of the codes were changed from one category to another. It was concluded, therefore, that a certain insignificant percentage of codes would be changed regardless of how many times the interactions were recoded.

32. Bales, op. cit., chapter 4. By coding after the observation of doctor-patient interaction, many of the difficulties of reliability of categorizing were eliminated. The problem of reliability of attribution and unitizing was nonexistent because the transcription was utilized and interaction was unitized and attributed to doctor or patient prior to the coding.

33. For a comparison of indices of compliance see Davis and Eichhorn, op. cit., and Davis, *J. Health and Social Behav.*, op. cit.

34. Several patients were administered specific regimen and compliance sections of the interview when regimens were not recorded by the doctor either in the patient's medical record or the doctor's questionnaire. Occasionally, the physician made a suggestion, e.g., "Don't worry about yourself," "Maybe you should lose some weight," and so on, which was not meant as a specific recommendation.

35. For example, consider a patient who was advised to make six clinic visits during the period he received medical care, received a prescription for a single medication, was told to cut down on his smoking, and was advised to eliminate alcoholic beverages.

According to the chart review, the patient kept only three of his appointments (50 percent broken appointment rate). The patient reported that he had cut down on his smoking as recommended and took the medication most of the time. He did not recall the doctor telling him anything about alcoholic beverages. The doctor reported in the questionnaire that the patient did not take his medications at all but had cut down on his smoking. According to the doctor, the patient had not curbed his drinking habits at all.

With regard to the clinic visits, the patient was given a score of 3—compliant most of the time. (Each patient was allowed a proportion of broken appointments before he was considered deviant.) For the medication regimen, he was given a score of 1.5, the average of the disagreement 3 + 0. The doctor agreed that the patient had indeed complied with the smoking regimen, and the patient was given a score of 4—compliant all the time. With regard to the alcohol regimen, the patient was scored as 0—not at all compliant. Accordingly, the compliant profile for the patient is as follows:

Regimen	Compliance score	×	Weight	=	Weighted score
Clinic visits	3		1		3
Medication	1.5		2		3
Smoking	4		2		8
Alcohol	0		1		0
			6		14

The composite index of compliance is the sum of the weighted scores divided by the sum of the weights. In this case, the index is equal to 14/6, or 2.3—compliant less than half the time.

36. More detailed data relating extent of compliance and demographic variables can be found in the paper delivered by Davis at the Sixth World Congress of Sociology, at Evian, France (op. cit.).

37. R. L. Coser, *Life on the Ward* (Michigan State University Press, 1962); S. V. Kasl and S. Cobb, "Health behavior, illness behavior, and sick role behavior," *Arch. Environ. Health* 12 (February 1966): 246–266; H. O. Mauksch and D. M. Tagliacozzo, The Patient's View of the Patient Role, Publication 2, Department of Patient Care Research, Presbyterian–St. Luke's Hospital, Chicago, 1962; D. Mechanic and E. H. Volkart, "Illness behavior and medical diagnoses," *J. Health and Human Behav.* 1 (1960): 86–94; T. Parsons, *The Social System* (Free Press, 1951), chapter 10.

38. Davis, Sixth World Congress of Sociology, Evian (op. cit.).

39. Ibid.

40. Bales, op. cit., chapter 2.

41. A. E. Hendrickson and D. O. White, "Promax: A quick method for rotation to oblique simple structure," *Brit. J. Statistical Psychol.* 17 (May 1964): 65. The relations among the factors of the oblique solution range from 0.22 to −0.29. Most of the items have a high loading on one factor and a low loading on the remaining factors. Only items with factor loadings of 0.30 or greater were used to define factors.

42. A. W. Gouldner. "The norm of reciprocity: A preliminary statement," *Am. Sociol. Rev.* 25 (April 1960): 161–178. A paradigm of types of doctor-patient reciprocity can be found in Davis and von der Lippe, op. cit.

12

Problems of Communication, Diagnosis, and Patient Care: The Interplay of Patient, Physician, and Clinic Organization

Irving Kenneth Zola

As every beginning medical student learns, history taking is a major diagnostic tool. Such interviewing requires a great deal of skill and understanding, and when there are reasons for reticence and fear, such as in an initial medical visit, even greater demands are placed on the doctor and the patient in their attempt to communicate with one another.[1,2] The nature of this communication, moreover, is determined by a number of nonmedical factors, three of which will be delineated in this paper: the patient's ethnic background, the physician's medical specialty orientation, and the clinic's spatial design and organization. An attempt will be made to demonstrate how each of these may operate to prevent or limit communication between patient and doctor and thus affect ultimate diagnosis and treatment.

The Patient's Ethnic Background

A number of studies have noted that both the diagnoses and the treatments received by a psychiatric patient were related to the patient's social class. [3-6] There has, however, been little speculation about the effect of social background on the diagnosis and the treatment of medical patients and their physical disorders.[7] In a study on the decisions of lower-class Italian-, Irish-, and Anglo-Saxon-Americans to seek aid at the medical, eye, and ENT (ear, nose, and throat) clinics of a large urban hospital, proportionately more Italian-Americans [hereafter referred to as Italians] were found to be labeled "psychiatric problems" by their physicians, despite the fact that there was no evidence that psycho-social problems were more frequent among them. On three general ratings of such problems, there were

Reprinted, with permission, from *Journal of Medical Education* 38 (1963): 829–838 no statistically significant differences among the ethnic groups, and thus there was no objective reason to expect a greater frequency of "psychiatric diagnosis" in one group. [In obtaining a measure of the amount and the nature of psycho-social problems in the study population, all the patients were rated on three categories: (1) Note was made of the spontaneous mention by the patient that he was "very nervous" or that "nerves" was one of his greatest problems. (2) Note was made of the spontaneous mention of very pressing and difficult vocational, personal, or interpersonal situations (e.g., being in the process of a divorce, having to care for a mentally ill husband or child, hating his present work and life). (3) A clinical psychologist rated the patient's interview responses for "presence of obvious psychological problems interfering with adequate functioning."]

Such differences in diagnosis might, however, be related to how the patients presented themselves and thus how they were perceived and ultimately diagnosed and treated. In the larger study, basic differences were found between the Italians and the Irish (the Anglo-Saxons occupied a middle position but more often resembled the Irish) in the way they presented their chief complaints and illnesses and in the specific circumstances surrounding the decision to come to a doctor. The overall study is reported elsewhere,[8,9] but some specific findings on the Italians are pertinent here: They tended to show more diffuse reactions to being sick. They reported more symptoms and stated more often that the symptoms made them irritable and difficult to get along with. In describing the specific circumstances bringing them to a doctor, they more often felt that their symptoms interfered with social and personal relations, or mentioned the presence of an interpersonal crisis. In another study of Italians, Zborowski[10] felt that their "uninhibited display of reactions" to pain and their over-involvement with symptoms would tend to provoke distrust in the doctors treating them. Since the Italians in our sample might also be perceived as "overacting," we speculated that this might have influenced the high number of psychiatric diagnoses.

The hypothesis that the patient's social background (i.e., ethnicity) and thus the way he presented himself influenced his diagnosis was tested by examining a group of cases where no medical basis for the symptoms had been found. It was felt that in these cases the operation of nonmedical factors would be most clear. So that we might err on the side of conservatism, a number of diagnoses that did little more than describe the patient's symptoms were excluded. (For example, "vitreous opacities" referred to the fact that the patient saw spots in

Table 1
Physicians' diagnoses of female patients with no organic basis for symptoms.

	Italian	Irish	Anglo-Saxon
Psychogenesis implied	11	2	2
No psychogenesis implied	1	9	4
Total	12	11	6

Italian vs. Irish $\chi^2 = 10.60$ (corrected for continuity); $P < 0.01$.

front of his eyes, and "tinnitus" meant he heard hums, rings, buzzing, etc. It is interesting to note, however, that these "descriptive" diagnoses were attributed primarily to the Anglo-Saxon and Irish patients.) Because the number of males fitting these criteria was too small for statistical comparisons, the hypothesis was tested only on a subsample of women: 10 Italians, 13 Irish, and 6 Anglo-Saxons.

When the previously mentioned ratings of psycho-social problems were applied to the above three groups, no statistically significant differences were found. Each of these three groups was then further subdivided by the implied etiology of their symptoms. The first category, "psychogenesis implied," included patients with one of three diagnoses: tension headache, functional complaint (e.g., functional pain in the left arm), and emotional disorder (e.g., anxiety, depression, neurosis). The second category consisted of patients where no explicit psychogenesis was implied. It included only those women in whose cases the physician had explicitly stated there was "no pathology" and a few cases of asthenopia (tired eyes). Table 1 shows how the doctors diagnosed patients where no organic basis for their complaints had been found. It is worth noting that the two "psychogenesis" cases of the Anglo-Saxons had the most obvious psychopathology in the entire sample of 200. One of these presented herself as being "mentally ill" and had been referred by the local Mental Health Association. The second entered the interview reeling and unsteady, accompanied by the distinct aroma of liquor, and was subsequently diagnosed by her physician as "alcoholic."

In short, when no medical disease was found, the Italians were diagnosed as having a psychological problem but the Anglo-Saxons and the Irish were not. Since psychosocial problems were equally present in all groups, there was no reason to expect one of the three ethnic groups to have more diagnoses in the "psychogenesis implied" category. Thus, one can only conclude that a patient's ethnic background, which influenced the way she presented herself and her complaint, may have inordinately and inappropriately influenced the diagnosis by the examining physician.

The Physician's Specialty Orientation

The forces that affect doctor-patient communication stem from attributes of the doctor as well as the patient. What the patient tells the doctor is influenced, for example, by what cues and interests he perceives and thus what he thinks the doctor wants to hear. What the doctor wants to hear is, in turn, the product of his background, training, and speciality orientation.

When attention was focused on the doctor's recognition of the concerns directly related to the patient's symptoms and his decision to seek aid, evidence was found of a barrier in doctor-patient communication. Our material indicated that not only were there many instances where such concerns were not considered, but also that recognition, or lack of recognition, of these concerns was more marked at one clinic that another. More patients with psycho-social problems appeared in the medical-clinic population; proportionately fewer were acknowledged at either the eye or the ENT clinic. (Incidentally, the tendency toward giving the Italians, rather than the Anglo-Saxons or Irish, diagnoses which implied a psychogenic basis was most evident at the eye clinic and least evident at the medical, with the ENT intermediate.) Thus, a person, regardless of the nature of her presenting complaint, had the best chance of having her personal and psychosocial problems recognized if she was first seen by a doctor in the medical clinic, and the worst chance if seen by a doctor in the eye clinic. This seemed to imply that there was a differential tendency on the part of specialty orientations to be aware of the present personal concerns of the patient.

Unfortunately, no objective statistics were collected on what transpired between patient and doctor. The research situation, however, often permitted the author to speak with both the doctor and the patient after the latter was seen. By systematic record review, it was also possible to check the nature of the treatment (including mention of reassurance, guidance, etc.) and the medical progress. From this information and from the more systematically collected interview data, it was possible to create a fairly complete picture of the concerns, both medical and otherwise, surrounding the patient's decision to seek aid. The following cases are illustrative of instances where the psycho-social concerns of the patient were not recognized.

No Organic Pathology

Mary B. was 23, married, and in her seventh month of pregnancy with her first child. She felt that she was nearsighted and that it had been too long since her last checkup (3 years). In recent months she had suffered from headaches in and around her eyes and some dizziness. On examination, the doctor found "no visible problem" and told her to return *pro re nata*. Since she was pregnant, the doctor explained to the author, he did not think it necessary to check her glasses; the prescription would change once she delivered. "I told her to return then if she was still bothered by [the headaches]. Her vision was 20/20 with glasses." Why then did this patient come in with such minor problems? The research interview revealed that she was extremely embarrassed about her appearance and felt that this was affecting all her relationships. About 3 months earlier, she had broken her glasses (they were now taped together), but "we didn't have the money with my husband out on strike." "The other day my cousin was over at the house and I was talking about being ashamed of the glasses and how I look 'cause we were going to a wedding." When asked about the general effects of her symptoms (headache, etc.), she responded: "Well, I might have stayed home when I could have gone out.... I couldn't go to a movie or anything like that (the way I looked), and so my husband had to go with his brothers." Again and again she told, somewhat defensively, how much her husband had opposed her coming to the clinic; however, she had felt that she could not wait any longer, and so she had gone against his wishes.

In understanding this case, it is irrelevant whether the patient's embarrassment and her anxiety really stemmed from the taped glasses or were related more to her pregnancy; the point is that she went to the doctor. Although he examined her and correctly dismissed her ocular symptoms as minor and inconsequential, he did not recognize her more pressing concerns. Knowledge of these might have led to a discussion, a prescription for a new pair of eyeglass frames, or a referral elsewhere. The patient, however, returned empty-handed and discouraged to her husband, who had told her not to go in the first place.

Minor Organic Pathology

Carol C. was a 45-year-old single bookkeeper. Within the preceding year her mother had died, and shortly thereafter her relatives had begun insisting that she move in with them, quit her job, work in their variety store, and nurse their mother. With her vacation approaching, they had stepped up their efforts to persuade her to try this arrangement. Although she had a number of minor aches and pains, her chief complaint was a small cyst on her eyelid (diagnosis: fibroma). She feared that it might be growing or that it could lead to something more serious, and so she felt that it should be checked (on the second day of her vacation) before it was too late. It was only in a somewhat mumbled response to the question of what she expected or would like the doctor to do that she made a connection between the stress she was undergoing with her family and her present insistence on taking care of the cyst. From a list of possible outcomes to her examination, she chose "maybe a hospital (ization).... Rest would be all right ... [and then in a barely audible tone] just so they [family] would stop bothering me." The examining physician acceded to her request for removal of the fibroma and referred her to the outpatient operating room. The cyst, however, was only her calling card, and its removal only temporarily alleviated her difficult and threatening interpersonal situation. Her subsequent pattern of medical care bore this out.

Within two weeks after recovery from the operation, she returned to the eye clinic claiming that something was still wrong with her eyes. She was sent to refraction, but the tests revealed that glasses were unnecessary. Four months later, she returned again to the eye clinic, this time presenting headaches in and around her eyes as the chief complaint. Once again she was examined by an opthalmologist, and once again she was refracted. This time, the doctor noted in the record: "Headaches not thought to be on an ocular basis." He did, however, prescribe Collyrium 26 and tell her to see her local medical doctor for a more complete examination. (According to her replies in the research interview, she did not really have one.) Seven months later, she appeared at the emergency ward with "terrific headaches." She was examined by the attending physicians and given a skull series. The final report states there was no pathology, "though possibly increased intracranial pressure." Several weeks later, she turned to still another avenue of help and asked for an appointment at the medical clinic. Here again she presented chiefly the complaint of headaches but this time accompanied by a great deal of bloating and belching. After a series of tests, there appeared in the record the first documented awareness of an underlying psychogenic problem. The final diagnosis was functional headache and epigastric distress. In the course of two years, this woman has presented herself at the clinics of the hospital on five separate occasions, involving some ten visits, with as many doctors and technicians and countless tests and examinations.

Major Organic Pathology

Paul W. was 39, married, a college graduate, and between assign-
ments as a waiter. A week prior to this visit, his face had become
chapped when he had gone for a long walk on a windy, rainy day. He
applied cold cream and almost immediately his face began to swell.
At about the same time he noticed a loss of vision in his right eye, but
he decided to wait awhile before doing anything. As he put it, "I like
to feel self-sufficient." When asked when he considered himself
sick enough to go to a doctor, he replied: "I don't know ... something obviously calling for medical aid, like appendicitis.... I feel
most people go too frequently, magnify their symptoms out of
proportion.... If they had greater knowledge of self and physical
functions, they wouldn't go as often.... I only go when I can't help
myself." As an example, he cited a recent incident: "Last summer I
cut my foot and allowed it to become poisoned ... It became pretty
bad.... When the glands in my groin started to swell and pain, it was
time to see a doctor ... and that was the first time in years." When
asked what made him come now, he replied: "Every man has a dream
... and this affected mine. You see, I do some writing, and that's why
we follow the resorts. In between jobs I'm able to do this [writing],
but if my eyes go, I couldn't drive to the resorts.... My worry reached
a peak last night. I was the first time that it became so prominent
that it affected my continuity, my ability to concentrate and do my
work." The physician, however, did not recognize his concern about
self-reliance and independence, which was reflected both in his
general pattern of medical care and in his delay in seeking help for
his current visual problem. Instead he told him that it was necessary
to come back for further tests. Paul W. took the appointment slips and
never returned. The probably major diagnosis of optic neuritis or
multiple sclerosis only emphasizes the implications of this break in
treatment.

While it is expected that there would be instances where the
patient's psycho-social concerns would go unnoticed, two conclusions
may nevertheless be drawn: that the lack of recognition was in large
part due to the doctor's orientation and communication (or lack
thereof) with his patient, and that this lack of attention was more
frequent among the practitioners of one specialty rather than another
(eye and ENT vs. medical). Perhaps the clinician cannot be concerned with the patient's psycho-social problems in their global and
general dimensions. It nevertheless seems apparent from these cases
that he must at least be concerned with those problems that pertain to

the patient's presenting complaint and his decision to seek aid. If he does not recognize these concerns, the examining physician may lose an opportunity to treat his patients effectively.

The Clinic's Spatial Design and the Organization of Work

While the physical structure of a clinic is often thought to be determined by the nature of the disorders, the number of patients, and the most efficient mode of treatment, this very structure can also contribute to the dilemma of the physician in attempting to deal with the patient's "problems."

The clinics, for example, differed in physical structure. At the time of this study, each patient in the medical clinic was led by his doctor into a private examination room, in most instances a room not visible to the other patients. In the ENT clinic, only a curtain and a partition (open at the top) closed off the world of the doctor and the patient from the world of "waiting." The other patients were relatively near, sitting on benches only a yard or two away. The eye clinic, both in the screening room and in the clinic proper, was the most open of all. No doors, screen, or walls—only 6 feet of space—separated the patient being seen from those who were waiting.

An innovation at the medical clinic indicates that the physical setting of a clinic has more to do with a basic philosophy of patient care than with the limitations set by the disease under treatment. Though the medical examination rooms ensured physical privacy, the new chief felt that they did not ensure psychological privacy and so had the walls extended to the ceilings. He felt that it was essential to better medical treatment to facilitate communication between the doctor and the patient, and that by ensuring complete privacy he was removing one of the barriers.

The flow of patients and thus the demands on a doctor determine, in part, the amount of time he can spend with each individual. In the medical clinic, a modified block appointment system was in operation and limited numbers of patients were assigned to the staff. On the other hand, in both the ENT and the eye clinic a sizable portion of patients were seen without appointments. The majority of these "walk-in" patients were not strictly emergency cases, a fact well known to the staff.

Another organizational feature worthy of mention, which was peculiar to the eye clinic, was the utilization of paramedical personnel. The pattern of this was especially crucial in the case of the patients who came in for such complaints as headaches, blurriness of vision, or difficulty in reading or seeing objects and whose final diagnosis indicated that nothing was physically wrong. Initially, they were seen in the screening room or in the clinic proper. Upon examination, no ocular disease was detected. The doctor, however, felt that their eyes should be tested more thoroughly or that their glasses should be checked, and so referred them to the refraction clinic. There they were seen by an optometrist and told that there was nothing wrong with their vision or that there was no need to change the prescription of their glasses. Unless the patients requested it (they rarely if ever did), they were not referred back to their examining physician but were sent along, still with their headache, their blurriness, their difficulty in seeing. The last person to see these patients was an optometrist, who by training and organizational role in this clinic functioned primarily as a technician and thus was perhaps the one least likely to be in a position to help them, as well as the one least likely to be asked by these patients for further help.

Thus, the utilization of paramedical personnel, the flow of patients, and the use of physical space served to make the medical clinic best suited to the recognition of the patient's psycho-social concerns and the eye clinic least suited. More important, these features illustrate how the differing spatial structures and organizations of the clinics implicitly supported the differing orientations of their physicians.

Discussion

Originally, clinics were dispensaries to screen patients for hospital admission, and therefore they were not conceived as treatment centers.[11] The increasing number of chronically ill patients and the nature of their medical problems make it evident, however, that more and more patients will be treated in outpatient facilities. In one sense, then, this paper is an extension of previous studies that have called attention to the presence and importance of psycho-social problems in outpatient or ambulatory populations.[12-15]

The major observations of this study suggest that recognition of and attention to such problems are influenced by an interplay of several nonmedical factors: the patient's ethnic-group membership and the way he presents himself and communicates to the doctor; the examining physician's specialty orientation as it is reflected in his tendency to overlook the patient's psycho-social concerns; and the clinic's spatial design and organization, which can be either a stimulant or a barrier to communication. Particularly in cases where the medical condition is not clear-cut, these factors will influence the diagnosis and treatment a patient receives.

None of these factors are immutable. The physical and spatial structure can be changed to ensure more communication. Organizational changes are also possible. For example, in the eye clinic, refraction might routinely precede the regular examination, or some arrangement might be devised whereby a patient is referred back to the examining physician, especially when nothing organic is found to account for his symptoms. All clinics could, without sacrificing emergency coverage, regulate the intake and flow of patients and thus allow more time for physician-patient contact. If an individual's condition goes untreated and therefore worsens or becomes more difficult to manage, or if, though untreated, he continues to seek a solution through different avenues, the total costs in time and money would certainly outweigh the costs of an extended or more thorough initial visit.

Physical and organizational changes are, however, only part of the story. Regardless of the degree of privacy, the patient may be unwilling to talk. Findings of the larger study[8] indicated that patients differed in the way they presented themselves to the doctor. It may also be inferred that they differed in what they thought relevant to their illness and what they deemed necessary to tell the doctor. In this paper, it has been demonstrated that, in reality, patients of all three ethnic groups studied had major psycho-social problems and concerns which either caused or exacerbated their conditions or interfered with effective treatment. Yet, in part because of the way the patient initially presented his complaint (which differed by ethnic groups), the recognition of such problems was confined inordinately to one ethnic group. Thus, greater attention must be given to the fact that illness or disease is not a purely physical and isolated problem but arises, is perceived, and is treated within a social context; this, in turn, will affect the nature of all communication about it.

Doctor-patient communication is, however, a two-way street, and evidence has been presented showing that physicians were often unwilling to listen to or probe the patient. Moreover, it seems evident that doctors' clinical training is at least partly responsible for their difficulty in recognizing and treating such problems, and that the training for some specialties prepares one less well for these tasks. This last observation assumes greater importance as we realize that, with the increasing sophistication of the lay population (as well as the increasing specialization of medical personnel), more and more people go directly to specialists or are referred to them at their own request.[16] While the specialist is necessarily concerned with the treatment of a specific organ or disease, the dilemma arises over what his responsibility is to the patient. In an ever growing number of cases, there simply is no "family doctor"[17] to whom he can return the patient who has pressing psycho-social problems.

Conclusion

The question now becomes this: Should all medical practitioners be capable of recognizing and treating the psycho-social concerns and complaints of the patient? Some feel that this should be the task of other professionals or of a special group of medical specialists. To emphasize this point, Churchill[18] cited the following example:

> ... a conscientious doctor responded to the call (re: a sick child) but found that the real reason for the vomiting and pain was an angry dispute between the child's parents. After a long day he (the doctor) has to stay until long past midnight in an effort to straighten matters out. An experienced visiting nurse or trained social worker or even the wise neighbor next door might have handled this situation.

While it is problematical to speculate who could best have helped these parents, it is completely unreasonable to expect that any professional or semiprofessional other than the physician would have been called in under any circumstances where the immediate problem was a child's vomiting and pain. A similar situation often confronts the specialist. With increasing sophistication, and regardless of the "true" or underlying concerns of the patient or the etiology of his specific condition, patients with visual symptoms are more likely to consult an eye specialist, those with a nasal condition an ENT man, those with a limb or back ailment an orthopedist, etc. This has led Balint,[19] Magraw,[20] and Yudkin[21] to claim that psycho-social concerns and problems are part of most illnesses and that attention to them is integral to the effective practice of any medical specialty. Thus, while we cannot expect all specialties to be equally interested in the global and general concerns of the patient, we should expect the physician to be aware of those concerns that affect the patient's presenting complaint, his decision to come, and his subsequent willingness to continue in treatment.

If (as Coleman contends) the emotional distance and the barrier to patient-doctor communication is "not a necessary or inevitable result, nor the price the physician must pay for calling" but "merely the price he pays for the neglect of this aspect of his training,"[22] then it is within the realm of medical education that a solution will have to be found. Certainly, there is ample evidence, both in this paper and in other investigations, that the vast majority of patients are reticent, anxious, and even fearful of consulting a doctor. In other words, there is probably a general tendency toward delay. Cognizant of this phenomenon, physicians in general, regardless of the seriousness of the patient's presenting complaint, could acknowledge this anxiety and attempt to reinforce his openness as well as the very fact of his coming at all. There is too little awareness of the two-sidedness of the doctor-patient relationship.

> The roles of the doctor and patient are complementary, and it would be most unusual if ideas in role behavior held by patients were not interlocked with and reinforced by expectations of patients which are held by doctors.[23]

Perhaps the major step toward such awareness is the not-so-simple realization that the doctor can block or reject the patient's communication by his very reaction, or lack of reaction, to the patient's concerns, and that this will have profound effects on how much he can help and treat the patient's medical condition.

While the comments in this paper have relevance for the handling of all disorders, they seem to have particular relevance for the treatment and management of chronic illness. With the overwhelming majority of such disorders, there is at present no instant cure, no miracle drug, no medical surgical procedure, and yet there are continual requests and demands for help and support made by the patient. Treatment has become a question of controlling, maintaining, and rehabilitating—processes in which the patients themselves play the major role. With awareness of himself as well as of the patient, the doctor would be in a position to more intelligently intervene and support the patient's own efforts to cope with his disorder.

Acknowledgments

This paper is part of a larger project sponsored by the departments of psychiatry (Dr. Erich Lindemann) and medicine (Dr. Walter Bauer) of Massachusetts General Hospital. I also wish to acknowledge the criticisms and suggestions of Dr. John D. Stoeckle, Mrs. Leonora Zola, and Dr. Bernard Bergen.

References

1. Kahn, R. L., and Cannell, C. F. *The Dynamics of Interviewing*. Wiley, 1957.

2. Magraw, R. M., and Dulit, E. P. The patient's presenting complaint—Signpost or goal? *Univ. Minn Med. Bull.* 29: 329–340, 1958.

3. Hollingshead, A. B., and Redlich, F. C. *Social Class and Mental Illness*. Wiley, 1958.

4. Kahn, R. L., Pollack, M., and Fink, M. Social factors in selection of therapy in a voluntary hospital. *J. Hillside Hospital* 6: 216–218, 1957.

5. Kahn, R. L. Pollack, M., and Fink, M. Socio-psychologic aspects of psychiatric treatment in a voluntary mental hospital. *A.M.A. Arch. Gen. Psychiat.* 1: 565–574, 1959.

6. Siegel, N. H., Pollack, M., Kahn, R. L., and Fink, M. Social Class, Diagnosis, and Treatment in Three Psychiatric Hospitals. Paper presented at the Annual Meeting of the American Sociological Association, St. Louis, 1961.

7. Ruesch, J., Jacobson, A., and Loeb, M. B. Acculturation and illness. *Psych. Monog.* 62: 292, 1948.

8. Zola, I. K. Socio-cultural Factors in the Seeking of Medical Aid. Ph.D. thesis, Harvard University, 1962.

9. Zola, I. K. Socio-cultural factors in the seeking of medical aid: A progress report. *Transcultural Psychiatric Research* 14: 62–65, 1963.

10. Zborowski, M. Cultural components in response to pain. In *Patients, Physicians, and Illness*, ed. E. G. Jaco. Free Press, 1958.

11. Washburn, F. A. The out-patient department and emergency ward. In *The Massachusetts General Hospital*. Houghton Mifflin, 1939.

12. Grobin, W. Personal experience in the practice of internal medicine. *Canad. Med. Assoc. J.* 79: 259–265, 1958.

13. Mannucio, M., Friedman, S. M., and Kaufman, M. R. Survey of patients who have been attending non-psychiatric outpatient department services for ten years or longer. *J. Mt. Sinai Hosp.* 18: 32–52, 1961.

14. Shepherd, M., Fisher, M., Stein, L., and Kessel, W. N. N. Psychiatric morbidity in an urban group practice. *Proc. Roy. Soc. Med.* 52: 269, 1959.

15. Tyler, S. H. On the nature of private practice and the need for psychotherapy. *Amer. Practit.* 1: 1303–1308, 1950.

16. Williams, T. F., White, K. L., Andrews, L. P., Diamond, E., Greenberg, B. G., Hamrick, A. A., and Hunter, E. A. Patient referral to university clinic. Patterns in rural state. *Amer. J. Public Health* 50: 1493–1507, 1960.

17. Geiger, H. J. The Choice and Use of Physicians by Families: Physician Quality and Family Choice. Paper presented at American Sociological Association Meetings, Washington, D.C., August 29–September 2, 1962.

18. Churchill, E. D. Medical wants and needs in mature and developing nations. *Medical Times*, November 1961.

19. Balint, M. *The Doctor, the Patient, and His Illness*. Homan, 1957.

20. Magraw, R. M. Psychosomatic medicine and the diagnostic process. *Postgrad. Med.* 25: 639–645, 1959.

21. Yudkin, S. Six children with coughs, the second diagnosis. *Lancet* 2: 561–563, 1961.

22. Coleman, J. V. Mental health, patient care, and medical practice. In Integration of Mental Health Concepts with the Human Relations Professions. Proceedings of a lecture series sponsored by Bank Street College of Education as a memorial to Ruth Kotinsky, 1962.

23. Apple, D. How laymen define illness. *J. Health and Human Behav.* 1: 219–225, 1960.

V

Studying the Relation: Can It Be Researched?

In this era of mega-medical research, do the public, the profession, and the patients view the doctor-patient relation as a useful subject for investigation? Probably not. One reason, already mentioned, is that medicine has been more interested in medical technique than in the process of care itself, assuming that it is only technique that can modify care and the outcome of illness. Fortunately or not, with the growing numbers of chronically ill, dependent, and handicapped persons and their need for care outside the hospital, medicine's traditional focus may be changing a little. As a result, care in society has become a public concern. While the focus of the concern is economic, eventually the quality of care, including the relations among practitioners and patients, may become a topic for research and of public concern for what care their money buys.

Two other reasons partake of the mystique of technique. One is simply the nature of the relation as a research problem. Studies of the doctor-patient relation involve interpersonal behaviors and communication, phenomena that do not fit the paradigm of so much laboratory and clinical medical research that has been the traditional activity of medical schools. The other is that research on the relation holds a promise quite different than research on, say, disease. The latter promises better understanding of its biochemical-and-immune basis and the possibility of new treatment technologies. Research on the doctor-patient relation promises few new techniques for ready diffusion into medical practice; rather, it can only promise changes in behavior and organizational action that are often disruptive of the status quo.

In the papers that follow, several research perspectives on the relation are illustrated. Howard Waitzkin and John D. Stoeckle, in "Information Control and the Micropolitics of Health Care," as well as in "Communication of Information about Illness" (in *Advances in Psychosomatic Medicine*, volume 8, ed. Z. Lipowski [Karger]) have summarized the methods that can be used in the study of communication; see also H. Waitzkin, "Information Giving in Medical Care," *J. Health and Social Behav.* 26 (1985): 81. They recognized that the transmittal of information can enhance the autonomy of the patient or the power of the doctor. Alvin Shapiro, J. Myers, M. E. Reiser, and E. B. Ferris, Jr., illustrated in "Comparison of Blood Pressure Response to Veriloid and to the Doctor" (*Psychosom. Med.* 16 [1954]: 478) how the doctor-patient relation may influence physiological responses favorably or unfavorably; this phenomenon was also noted by G. Mancia, G. Bertiniere, G. Grossi, G. Parati, G. Pomidossi, A. Ferrari, L. Gregorini, and A. Zanchetti ("Effects of Blood Pressure Measured by the Doctor on Patient's Blood Pressure and Heart Rate," *Lancet* 2 [1983]: 695) and by J. J. Lynch (*The Language of the Heart* [Basic Books, 1985]). Other physiological studies of the interaction have been carried out in psychotherapy (A. Demascio, R. W. Boyd, and M. Greenblatt, "Physiological Correlates of Tension and Antagonism during Psychotherapy: A Study of 'Interpersonal Physiology,'" *Psychosom. Med.* 19 [1957]: 99; D. Shapiro and A. Crider, "Psychophysiological Approaches in Social Psychology," in *Handbook of Social Psychology*, volume 3, ed. G. Lindzey and E. Aronson [Addison-Wesley, 1969]). Similar responses to the doctor are reported in the large literature on placebo effects; see R. Liberman, "An Analysis of the Placebo Phenomenon," *J. Chronic Dis.* 15 (1961): 761; H. Brody, *Placebos and the Philosophy of Medicine: Clinical, Conceptual, and Ethical Issues* (University of Chicago Press, 1977).

From a cross-cultural perspective, Emily Ahern ("Chinese-Style and Western-Style Doctors in Northern Taiwan," reprinted here) looks at differences in the nature of the relation and in what it holds for patients. She reports that the Chinese-style doctors and their patients may hold the same set of ideas about disease, whereas Western-style doctors and their Chinese patients may not. The point is important both for the individual and for the organization of health services. Shared beliefs about illness facilitate communication and support. Continued public-health promotion of Chinese-style doctors may ensure less "distance" between doctor and patient and so effect care that is more supportive. Yet such promotion of alternative medical practices may not be needed. On their own, patients may simultaneously seek help from practitioners of different systems, from Western science and from folk medicine presumably selecting the elements of cure and care that they need from each.

Distinctive verbal and nonverbal aspects of the relation have been illustrated by S. Milmoe, R. Rosenthal, H. T. Blane, M. E. Chafetz, and I. Wolf ("The Doctor's Voice: Postdictor of Successful Referral of Alcoholic Patients," *J. Alc. Psychol.* 72 [1967]: 78, a paper that suggests that voice was critical in successful referral of alcoholic patients for continuing care) and by P. Ekman and W. Friesen ("Nonverbal Leakage and Clues to Deception," *Psychiatry* 32 [1969]: 88, a paper that reports the usefulness of observing movement of extremities as a sign of deception in communication from the patient). Deception is not found on only one side of the relation; Sisela Bok (*Lying*: *Moral Choice in Public and Private Life* [Pantheon, 1978]) has noted how doctors rationalize deceptive communication with patients in everyday practice. Research on nonverbal clues and self-analysis might lead to helpful recognition of repressed affect and to more effective communication by health workers concerned with their own behaviors, some of which are nontherapeutic and less than truthful.

Much research on the relation has come out of the disciplines of social psychology, linguistics, communication, and ethnology. Videotaping has facilitated the visual and auditory analysis of the doctor-patient interaction. Ethnological studies observe and describe our "everydayness"—the mundane tactile, verbal, and nonverbal interaction of doctor and patient—from tapes or participant observation of the interview and the examination. Recent observational studies are numerous, and examples should be mentioned. Taped interviews of British general practitioners have been examined by P. S. Byrne and B. E. L. Long (*Doctors Talking to Patients*: *A Study of the Verbal Behavior of General Practitioners Consulting in Their Surgeries* [HMSO, 1976]), who have classified the elements of the consultation—from the greeting to the closure—in terms of styles such as "doctor-centered," "patient-centered," and "negative." William Stiles, S. M. Putnam, M. H. Wolf, and S. A. James ("Verbal Response Mode Profiles of Patients and Physicians in Medical Screening Interviews," *J. Med. Ed.* 54 [1979]: 81) examined eight categories of the interview behaviors of doctors and patients—disclosure, questions, edification, acknowledgment, advisement, interpretation, confirmation, and reflection—to look at patient satisfaction in interviews as well as to typify the encounter. David Pendleton has gone beyond such descriptions of the office encounter to suggest a model for its study and improvement ("Communication in the Doctor's Office: A Model and a Strategy for Health Communication Research," in *Straight Talk*: *Explorations in Provider and Patient Interaction*, ed. L. S. Pettegrew [Humana, 1982]; see also D. A. Pendleton and J. Hasler, *Doctor-Patient Communication* [Academic, 1983]).

Other studies deal with linguistics, the use and measurement of words and interruptions, and their sequences; interaction analysis focuses on these patterns and meanings of the exchange. In such research, behavioral scientists are looking for systematic regularities in verbal and nonverbal behaviors and their correlates to explain what is going on. H. S. Friedman, in "Non-Verbal Communication between Patients and Medical Practitioners" (*J. Social Issues* 35 [1979]: 82), reviews these studies—in particular, those on the effects of voice, olfaction, gaze, facial expression (see P. Ekman and W. V. Friesen, "Felt, False and Miserable Smiles," *J. Nonverbal Behav.* 6 [1982]: 238), and touch. Richard Frankel, with his interests in linguistics, ethnography, and medical instruction, has sought patients' perspectives on the medical encounter by having them review videotapes, and has (along with others) described the verbal and nonverbal processes of the interview; see R. M. Frankel and H. B. Beckman, "Impact: An Interaction-Based Method for Preserving and Analyzing Clinical Transactions," in *Straight Talk*, ed. L. S. Pettegrew (Humana, 1982); R. M. Frankel, "Talking in Interviews: A dispreference for Patient-Initiated Questions in Physician-Patient Encounters," in *Interactional Competence* (Irvington, 1983); C. West, *Routine Complications: Troubles with Talk between Doctors and Patients* (Indiana University Press, 1984); P. A. Rowland-Morin, "Physician Behaviors that Affect Patient Satisfaction" (abstract), *Soc. Res. and Ed. in Primary Care Int. Med.*, 1982; M. Coulthard and M. Ashby, "A Linguistic Description of Doctor-Patient Interviews," in *Studies in Everyday Medical Life*, ed. M. Wadsworth and D. Robinson (Martin Robertson, 1976). In the field of social psychology, the importance of the communication of affect in doctor-patient encounters has been noted by Robin DiMatteo ("A Social Psychological Analysis of Physician-Patient Rapport: Towards a Science of the Art of Medicine," *J. Soc. Issues* 35 [1979]: 12), by J. Hall, D. L. Roter, and C. S. Rand ("Communication of Affect between Patient and Physician," *J. Health and Soc. Behav.* 22 [1981]: 18), and by Debra Roter ("Patient Participation in Patient-Provider Interaction: The Effects of Patient Question Asking on the Quality of Interaction, Satisfaction, and Compliance," *Health Education Monographs* 5 [1977]: 281). Despite the growth and the explanatory value of such studies (R. J. DiPietro, *Linguistics and the Professions* [Ablex, 1982]), by themselves they offer few specific instructional aids to the practitioner interested in effective behavior or new norms for the improvement of physician-patient communication. However, it should be said that they explicitly and implicitly call for more patient communication and participation, as with patient questions, and more physician attention to the patient's perspective (Health Education Studies Unit, *The Patient Project* [Health Education Council, 1982]). To become useful, such research needs to be integrated into clinical practice and instruction, which is a special effort itself. After identifying the meanings of patient behaviors, new, more appropriate responses by the doctor might then be learned, whether by making the meanings a topic for discussion, by responding to them in the encounter, or by changing the doctor's responses in practice sessions with simulated patients.

13

Information Control and the Micropolitics of Health Care
Howard Waitzkin in association with
John D. Stoeckle

Introduction

Investigators in health-care research recently have tended to shift
their attention away from the doctor-patient relationship, using
instead a more "macro" approach to study structural and organizational problems in the medical care system. (I [H.W.] have used the
macro approach myself in several previous studies of the U.S. and
other national health systems.) But still, this change in emphasis is
surprising, in view of continuing widespread dissatisfaction with the
quality of the doctor-patient relationship. For example the doctor's
communication of information about illness to the patient—to
consider only one element of their relationship—continues to be a
troublesome problem. Several studies have demonstrated that patients tend to be more dissatisfied about the information they receive
from their doctors than about any other aspect of medical care.[1-6]

It is difficult to believe that policy changes suggested by macro
research ultimately will succeed in improving the effectiveness and
efficiency of the health-care system while critical gaps and misunderstandings persist at the "micro" level of the doctor-patient
relationship.

Background
For several years I have been engaged in a study of the informative
process in medical care. The broader orientation of the research,
however, transcends doctor-patient relationships alone and views the
informative process in medical care as one example of communication
between professionals and clients generally.

Perhaps it is appropriate to say a few words about how I became

Reprinted, with permission, from *Social Science and Medicine* 10 (1976):
263–276.

interested in this topic. During medical school, before we began to see patients on our own, our first lecture on cancer included a presentation of three young people who indeed had cancer. Our professor, an esteemed physician and chief of the department of medicine at a prestigious teaching hospital, gave the class a warning before the patients entered the room. None of the patients, he said, knew that he or she had cancer. He continued that it was very important for the patients' morale—as with most cancer patients—that they not find out their diagnoses, at least not yet. Therefore, we medical students should be sure not to say anything or to ask any questions that might indicate the patients' true problem. Each of the patients entered the amphitheater, exchanged a few words with the professor, and then departed. After the last patient left, the professor again emphasized the need for discretion and asked that we not talk about the patients after the session.

Later in medical school I became struck that other of my teachers approached this problem in quite a different way. Rather than withholding information from patients with cancer, these doctors were open about the patients' diagnosis and prognosis. In these situations, I could not detect a worsening of the patients' morale; often the bond between doctor and patient seemed to grow stronger with greater candor.

In short, I became aware of the variability in the process of information transmittal. What a doctor told a patient seemed to depend on what kind of person the doctor was, as well as the characteristics of the particular patient. In addition, I noticed that the situation in which doctors and patients interact—private practice, outpatient departments, emergency rooms, etc.—seemed to make a difference in the nature of their communication. This variability also seemed to occur for problems that were much less serious than cancer. Some patients with relatively minor disorders seemed to receive little information from their doctors, while other patients obtained more.

On a deeper level, I began to feel that the nature of information transmittal between doctors and patients showed something about society more generally. It seemed to show how some people—that is, experts or professionals—maintain power over other people—clients, patients, etc.—by controlling the information that is communicated. Information control seemed to be one structural basis of stratified relations between doctors and patients, between other professionals and their clients, and among people generally in everyday life.

Later I reviewed the literature on communication between doctors and patients. I was quickly struck by the classic distinction between positive and normative statements. Positive statements describe "what is"; normative statements describe "what ought to be." Normative statements abound in writings about the communication of information in treating sick people. They usually reflect the ethical position or evaluative judgment of the writer, but are seldom clearly deducible from positive statements describing empirical observations.[7]

For example, a leading textbook of medicine offers a normative statement which indicates that a physician should decide what information to convey on the basis of patient characteristics:

There should be no iron-clad, inflexible rule that the patient must be told "everything," even if he is an adult and the head of his family. How much the patient is told will depend upon his own desires and character, the wishes of his family, the state of his affairs, and perhaps his religious convictions.[8]

Many other writers agree with this approach, claiming that in the transmission of information physicians should respond differently to the needs of different patients rather than adopting a single standardized approach.[9-12] A second set of opinions seems to reflect Kant's categorical imperative,[13] calling for complete truthfulness under all circumstances, irrespective of patients' individual needs.[14-21] A third viewpoint, applied mainly to patients with fatal illness, essentially calls for falsehood under all circumstances, with embellishment or modification of the truth to preserve the patient's hope.[22-26]

Although these normative propositions may be based partly on impressions of clinical practice, for the most part they are not deduced from experiments comparing the effects of different informative techniques. The main conclusion from this voluminous literature on what the doctor *should* say is that such normative statements reflect an author's personal values much more than actual tests of clinical efficacy. While recognizing the importance of values in clinical practice, I came to believe that more enlightened normative principles to guide communication might be suggested by detailed observation of actual communicative patterns.

I then began a small pretest of a research project. This involved the direct recording and analysis of interaction between two doctors and ten patients. Some of the results were frankly astonishing to me. During an average interaction of about 20 minutes, the doctor's average time spent in communicating information about illness to the patient was less than a minute; the range was 2–85 seconds over the 10 patients. When asked in an interview, doctors thought they were spending 10–15 minutes per patient on information transmittal. The information that was communicated was at a very low technical level. Less than 10 percent of informative statements could be considered "scientific" rather than "common-sense." Qualitatively, doctors seemed to use a variety of mechanisms to avoid answering patients' direct questions about their conditions.

There were many methodological problems in the pretest. Still, the results strengthened the impressions that information transmittal is a variable phenomenon and that its variability probably is related to variability in physician characteristics, patient characteristics, and the concrete situations in which doctors and patients interact. In addition, the pretest results seemed to support the theoretical notion that information control is a basis of power and of hierarchies based on expertise.

Research Goals

The pretest motivated me, along with several co-workers, to begin a more formal research project. To do a manageable study, we decided to narrow the questions we were asking. Therefore, we undoubtedly are missing many of the nuances of the doctor-patient relationship. The particular questions under investigation are: What attributes of physicians, patients, and the organizational settings in which they interact are associated with communicated information? What criteria do physicians use in determining the information about illness they convey to patients? Based on the pretest, my co-workers and I have operationalized a multivariate model to study these problems. An association is hypothesized between transmitted information— the dependent variable—and several independent variables, which are classified under the headings of physician characteristics, patient characteristics, and situational characteristics.

In our previous work we have presented a review of the literature on this subject, emphasizing the clinical, sociological, and methodological issues involved in the study of the informative process and developing our own theoretical approach.[27] We also have analyzed restricted communication as one basis of stratification within medicine, both between health workers and patients and among health workers.[28] We are viewing the doctor-patient relationship (or the professional-client relationship, more generally) as a micropolitical situation. In this situation, information control is used, at least in part, to maintain patterns of dominance and subordination.

This paper briefly summarizes some of the clinical and sociological considerations guiding our research on the informative process in the doctor-patient relationship and describes our methodological approach.

Clinical Considerations

Prior investigations have shown that the *process* of information transmittal is particularly important because it is closely related to severe crucial *outcomes* of health care. The transmission of information affects the quality of care and the course of treatment. The doctor's success in transmitting accurate information about illness may "feed back" to the same doctor, or to other doctors, through the patient's later ability in subsequent contacts to provide a meaningful history.[27] Notes concerning transmitted information increase the usefulness of medical records.[29] As several recent studies have confirmed, patients' compliance with medical instructions is closely related to the extent that their desire for information is met.[30-36] Similarly, patients' dissatisfaction with medical care is tied to insufficient, contradictory, or confusing information.[37,38] Physiologic studies indicate that a patient's postoperative course is improved by providing detailed information prior to surgery.[39-41] Recently it has been postulated that patient delay in reporting symptoms of cancer may be related to incomplete information communicated by practitioners, and that this informative gap may have a differential impact in different social classes.[42]

In general, patients respond enthusiastically to attempts to communicate information about illness in simple language; such attempts appear to enhance patients' response to treatment.[43-46] The advantages of increasing transmitted information by giving patients their own medical records have been reviewed.[47] Increasingly, information transmittal has been placed in the clinical context of heightened concern for informed consent and patients' rights.[48-53] In summary, many studies indicate the clinical importance of information transmittal, but few examine the many factors that affect information transmittal in actual clinical practice.

The research to be reported assumes an association between the process of information transmittal and the above health-care outcomes. We do not examine this association in detail. Our purpose is to study systematically the informative process. The research design is analytic rather than descriptive; the methods that are used should permit a detailed assessment of variability an information transmittal within different health settings, and should yield reliable and generalizable conclusions.

Sociological Background

Before presenting the research methods, it is appropriate to review briefly the project's theoretical background. (Our earlier writings give a more intensive analysis for interested readers.[27,28]) From the standpoint of general theory in sociology, research on information transmittal employs principles from information theory, sociolinguistics, ethnomethodology, and various approaches to the problems of uncertainty and power. Four issues are examined: the problems of uncertainty and power, the definition of information, sociolinguistics and the diffidence of the sick poor, and ethnomethodology and common-sense constructs.

The Problem of Uncertainty and the Problem of Power

Sociologists and economists have discussed the uncertainty inherent in medical practice.[54–58] Although uncertainty affects both patient and doctor, the competence gap between them means that uncertainty generally is greater for the patient.[59] Previous research has shown that doctors tend to prolong patients' uncertainty, even when doctors' uncertainty about the course of disease or the efficacy of therapy is reduced.[60–65] One theoretical explanation of this observation is based on Crozier's[66] analysis of bureaucratic behavior: A physician's ability to preserve his or her own power over the doctor-patient relationship depends largely on the ability to control the patient's uncertainty. The postulated association between uncertainty and power may partially explain doctors' reluctance to provide information to dying patients and their use of a variety of tactics to avoid direct communication.[67,68] Under these circumstances, the communication of diagnosis would reveal the doctors' technical inability to cure the patient. On the other hand, it is expected that certain types of information transmittal increase patients' subsequent *autonomy* to deal with health issues. Autonomy-enhancing communications should be distinguishable from power-enhancing communications.

The Definition of Information

According to information theory, information may be defined as that which removes or reduces uncertainty.[69,70] Operationally, several investigators have treated the definition as a probabilistic one. A unit of language that has a high "transition probability" can be predicted easily from the units that precede or follow it: A high transition probability implies minimal uncertainty and minimal information transmitted. The "Cloze" technique, adapted from the experiments of Shannon[71] and Goldman-Eisler[72] may be used to estimate directly the information conveyed from doctor to patient.[73] In addition, the function of silences preceding or following information transmittal may be assessed.[72,74]

Sociolinguistics and the Diffidence of the Sick Poor

Many studies have documented the communication barrier related to class differences between doctors and patients.[75,76] In particular, working-class patients tend to be diffident in questioning their doctors about illness. However, despite their diffidence, working-class patients differ little from middle-class patients in their desire for information[1] or in their knowledge of medical terms.[77] The commonly expressed assumption that working-class patients do not wish a full explanation of illness seems to derive from the use of different sociolinguistic "codes" by doctors and patients[78] and particularly from working-class patients' hesitation in asking questions. Sociolinguistic observations by Bernstein[79-85] and Lawton,[86] as well as related studies in the rapidly growing field of sociolinguistics,[87-93] indicate that the communication gap between middle-class doctors and working-class patients may result from their customary use of different linguistic codes.

Ethnomethodology and Common-Sense Constructs

From the perspective of ethnomethodological theory and research,[94-97] doctors appear to develop "common-sense" decisional rules by which they "label" patients according to the desirability of information transmittal. If doctors adhere to the norms governing information that are stated in medical textbooks, they base decisions on patient characteristics such as education and prognosis. The actual nature of these common-sense decisional rules (which doctors apply to patients in general) and the "accounts" by which doctors might explain their informative behavior with specific patients have not been studied empirically.

Methods

General Goals

The overall methodological objective of the research project is to develop a research design that is based on these sociological perspectives and that permits reproducible and generalizable conclusions about the informative process in a variety of clinical settings. In prior

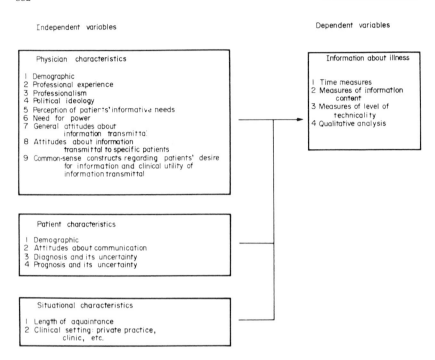

Independent variables   Dependent variables

Physician characteristics

1 Demographic
2 Professional experience
3 Professionalism
4 Political ideology
5 Perception of patients' informative needs
6 Need for power
7 General attitudes about
   information transmittal
8 Attitudes about information
   transmittal to specific patients
9 Common-sense constructs regarding patients' desire
   for information and clinical utility of
   information transmittal

Information about illness

1 Time measures
2 Measures of information
   content
3 Measures of level of
   technicality
4 Qualitative analysis

Patient characteristics

1 Demographic
2 Attitudes about communication
3 Diagnosis and its uncertainty
4 Prognosis and its uncertainty

Situational characteristics

1 Length of aquaintance
2 Clinical setting: private practice,
   clinic, etc.

Figure 1
Multivariate research model of the information process in medical care.

research, several methodological approaches have been used: participant observation, experimental communication, questionnaires and interviews, the case-study method, and the direct recording and analysis of doctor-patient interaction. In previous work that reviewed the strengths and weaknesses of each method in detail,[27] we concluded that the direct recording and analysis of interaction offered the greatest potential for valid and reproducible research on the informative process. The present research adopted this method of data collection by using audio and video taping of doctor-patient interaction.

One significant problem with previous studies was the research setting. Outpatient departments of university-affiliated teaching hospitals, for the most part, have been used. For this reason, the findings may not be generalizable to a broader population of physicians and patients. To increase the generalizability of the results, a stratified random sample of doctors and patients interacting in a variety of clinical settings was designed.

Figure 1 shows the multivariate research model of the informative process. The dependent variable, information transmittal, is measured from audio tape recordings and transcripts of doctor-patient interaction in four ways: time duration, information content, level of technicality, and qualitative analysis. In addition, several exploratory methods are being developed to analyze nonverbal and affective aspects of transmitted information from video tape recordings. Independent variables—doctor, patient, and situational characteristics—are measured by questionnaires and interviews administered to physicians and patients; these variables are also assessed by sampling techniques. Relationships are hypothesized between transmitted information and several independent variables (grouped under the headings of physician characteristics, patient characteristics, and situational characteristics).

Most of the methods have been subjected to a pretest with two physicians and ten patients. Techniques that proved unworkable, especially through problems of validity or reliability, were eliminated, and new questionnaire items were added. Results and hypotheses suggested by the pretest have been presented in an unpublished report.[98]

The Dependent Variable: Information about Illness
To measure this variable, doctor-patient interaction is directly recorded and analyzed. Physicians and their patients in the sample are asked to tape-record their entire interaction (see"Sample," below). Informed consent is obtained from patients and doctors by standardized permission forms. Transcripts are prepared of those parts of recorded interaction in which information is requested by patients and/or conveyed by doctors. From the tape recordings and transcripts of doctor-patient interaction, the dependent variable is measured in four ways:

(1) Time measures
Previous investigators have demonstrated the importance of simple temporal relationships in interaction and have developed automated methods for measuring these.[72, 99–101] In the present study, total interaction time is divided into several nominal categories: history taking; comments about the physical examination; further diagnostic tests; future visits, drugs or other treatment; general reassurance; silence; miscellaneous; and information about illness. The amount of time in the last category then is expressed both in absolute terms and as a proportion of total interaction time. This approach provides a quantitative measurement of the informative process and permits analysis of variability along this dimension. These measures focus on

verbal exchanges only. Nonverbal and affective aspects of communication are assessed in a phase of the project using video recordings.

Coding procedures developed for analysis of tape-recorded interaction are taught to five coders. Intercoder reliability is assessed
through a modification of the Spearman ρ nonparametric statistic of
association. A series of doctor-patient encounters are coded independently by all coders. Discrepancies in coding are discussed, and
procedures are standardized until intercoder reliability reaches an
acceptable level—arbitrarily defined as a modified Spearman ρ
greater than 0.8. Tapes are randomly and blindly divided among the
five coders. It is assumed that this random and blind assignment of the
tapes will minimize the possibility of "experimenter bias." [105]

(2) Measure of information content
According to information theory, information is that which removes
or reduces uncertainty.[69,70] The definition has been treated operationally as a probabilistic one. If a unit of language has a high
"transition probability," it can be predicted easily from those units
that precede or follow it. High transition probability implies that
little information is conveyed by that unit of language.

In the present research, the measure of information content derives
from information theory and utilizes the Cloze technique[73] modified
from the work of Shannon[71] and Goldman-Eisler.[72] Briefly, this
method is as follows: Transcripts are prepared for all portions of the
doctor-patient encounters in which information transmittal occurs.
Words are then randomly deleted from these transcripts (by a table of
random numbers) and are replaced by blanks. These modified transcripts are presented to a panel of naive judges, together with excerpts
from communication "controls" such as newspaper articles. The
judges' average ability to supply the missing words, as compared to
the controls, provides a measure of the transition probability (in-
versely correlated with information content, according to information theory) of the particular passage. Transition probabilities computed by this technique are used as a measure of information about
illness. This technique is an exploratory measure of the dependent
variable; its validity will need further assessment.

(3) Measures of level of technicality
The purpose of these measures is to assess the level of technicality in
physicians' explanations and the degree to which this level is congruent with the technical level of patients' requests for information. Of
particular interest are the extent to which physicians volunteer ex-

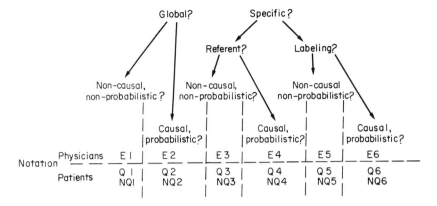

Figure 2
Measures of level of technicality.

planations that patients do not ask for, compared to their responses to patients' questions, and the discrepancies in the technical level between physicians' explanations and patients' questions.

The technical level of information transmitted and of questions asked is rated from transcripts by judges using a standard scale. The scale ranges from 1 to 6, where 1 is least and 6 most technical. Assignment of any given remark to one of the six ranks is determined by three criteria, applied successively (figure 2): globality vs. specificity of the remark; referent (body part, blood pressure, etc.) vs. labeling (disease name, numerical level of blood test, etc.): and noncausal, nonprobabilistic vs. causal, probabilistic nature of the explanation.

Illustrations of the scoring scheme, as applied to transcripts of doctor-patient communication, are as follows:

1. Physicians' explanations (E):
El You're fine. Everything's going to be all right.
E2 Your chances are good. Can't predict—everyone's different.
E3 There's something the matter with your arm. Your vessels to the brain are clear as a whistle. Blood pressure is OK.
E4 Often the swelling of the vein leaves a tag that protrudes. It's like scar tissue, nothing to worry about. Yes, blood pressure like that may just be a sign of age, but since the change was sudden, we're gonna check out the other possibilities.
E5 You've got diabetes. Your blood pressure is 120/80.
E6 Chances are 20 percent of your having diabetes with one parent having diabetes. Well, there's no significant difference between 170 and 180, especially when there's an error with measure-

ments. It's only about 5 percent. It's unlikely the Darvon caused the pancreatitis even though it may irritate the condition because you had been taking it regularly with no symptoms for two years.

2. Patients' questions (Q):
   Q1 How am I, doc?
   Q2 What are my chances?
   Q3 Is my heart OK? How's my blood pressure?
   Q4 But before you said the pain was nothing. Why are you going to do tests? Can I do anything to make my blood pressure go down?
   Q5 What's my blood pressure? What do I have?
   Q6 What are the complications which diabetes might lead to? Then about six months later, these pills and taking it easy, I suppose, brought it down to 165, which was just great. But now, you say it's 200, and I say, well, why?

3. Patients' nonquestions (NQ):
   NQ1 Oh; Yeah; Mm-hmm.
   The remaining NQ's tend to collapse to NQ1 or to repeat or to extend a doctor's remark.

The explanations offered in response to patients' questions, compared to spontaneous explanations, are calculated for each level of technicality. The degree of discrepancy in level of technicality between explanations and questions is determined for each recorded interaction. The reliability of scoring again is estimated by an adaptation of the Spearman ρ measure of association.

(4) Qualitative analysis of the informative process
From the pretest it became clear that the above quantitative measures of the dependent variable would not convey adequately many of the nuances of the interaction between doctors and patients. Therefore, a qualitative analysis of the informative process has been developed, based on transcripts of tape-recorded interaction. The qualitative analysis has two phases. First, transcripts are presented to a panel of judges, who are asked to rate the transcripts on dichotomous scales adapted from the semantic differential technique.[106] By this measure, transcripts are ranked along the dimension of autonomy-enhancing vs. power-enhancing communications. Second, the investigators perform a separate qualitative analysis of the transcripts. Gaps in communication are studied with reference to recorded materials. Of special interest are the discrepancies between patients' "ethnoscientific" understandings of illness and physicians' own explanatory re-

marks.[107] In addition, the process by which physicians translate scientific terms into the everyday language of patients is examined.

The above measurement techniques permit an assessment of the dependent variable, information transmittal. The measurement of the three sets of independent variables—physician, patient, and situational characteristics—is now described.

Independent Variables

Physician characteristics

Several investigators have hypothesized that a doctor's personal characteristics form the most important predictor of the tendency to convey information to patients.[108–110] In the present research, physician characteristics are assessed by a questionnaire which the physicians complete after their sessions with a sample of patients. The following physician characteristics are measured by the questionnaire:

- Demographic: sex, age, religion, income, occupational mobility, and race.

- Professional experience and practice: years since completion of medical school, years of specialty training after internship, type of specialty training, consultations used, consultations received, type of practice, patient visits per day, percent patients over 65, percent patients who are chronically ill, emergencies per week, participation on scientific advisory boards, malpractice insurance, and hospital affiliations. Many of these questions were adapted from Ford et al.[111]

- Professionalism (attitudes about professional life): satisfaction in professional accomplishments, colleagues' assessment of performance, attitudes toward chronically ill patients, attitudes toward elderly patients, self-rating of effectiveness, journals subscribed, journals read, thoroughness of reading, consideration of psychological factors in patients, distribution of time in professional activities, papers read at meetings, satisfaction from caring for patients and participation in refresher courses or seminars. Many of these questions were adapted from Ford et al.[111] and Wilensky.[112] A scale of professionalism has been constructed, based on physicians' responses to individual items. (The validity of this and other scales is discussed in a separate paper.[113])

- Political ideology: Attitudes are assessed by several questions adapted from Colombotos.[114] A scale of political ideology has been constructed.[113]

• Perception of patients' informative needs: This variable is measured by the degree to which the physician accurately perceives the patient's felt need for information. In a questionnaire which he or she fills out after all interaction sessions are completed, the physician is asked how much detailed information each patient desires and how helpful the communication of information would be for the patient's progress. The physician's responses are compared to the patient's actual attitudes, as assessed by a questionnaire administered to each patient after the recorded interaction. Perception of patients' informative needs is estimated as the correspondence between the physician's perceptions and the patient's actual attitudes.

• Need for power: The investigators considered this characteristic to be an important explanatory variable, given the sociological considerations guiding the study. Projective measures would be too cumbersome for a study of this type. In the pretest, an adaptation of the Machiavellianism scale, developed by Christie and Geis,[115] was used as a measure of the need for power. The pretest results, however, showed that the validity of these items was questionable. Subsequently, we have developed and used a series of questions designed to assess need for power within the doctor-patient relationship. These items appear to form a valid scale, based on sampled physicians' responses.[113]

• General attitudes about information transmittal: It is assumed that physicians' general attitudes about information transmittal are correlated with their actual behavior. However, the empirical relationship between attitudes and behavior along this dimension has not been studied in depth. The questionnaire in this study asks for physicians' attitudes about the danger in telling patients details about illness, the importance of keeping patients fully informed, the information that patients desire generally, the helpfulness of informing patients about illness, and the advantage of patients' not knowing all the facts. In addition, physicians' estimates of the time spent in communicating information about illness in a typical visit are assessed.

• Attitudes about information transmittal to specific patients: General attitudes about the informative process can be distinguished from attitudes relating to the transmittal of information to specific patients. It is of interest to observe how physicians' general attitudes differ from their attitudes about specific patients, and also to determine the association between general or specific attitudes and actual recorded communication. Physicians' specific attitudes about patients' desire for information and the helpfulness of informing the patient are measured by two items in the questionnaire which physicians complete for each patient whose interaction with the physician is recorded. Physicians' estimate of the time spent in communicating information to specific patients also is elicited so that it may be compared to the actual time as measured by the tape recordings.

• Common-sense decisional rules regarding patients' desire for information and the clinical utility of information transmittal: It is expected that the decisional rules by which physicians decide what information to communicate to patients contain subtleties of which physicians themselves are not fully aware. Several open-ended items are contained in the questionnaire, so that physicians' own verbalization of these decisional rules may be assessed. In addition, a smaller physician sample are asked to comment on transcripts of their own informational remarks. These retrospective "accounts" should provide the "background understandings" that guide decisions about information transmittal.[96]

Patient characteristics

Many writers have pointed out that a patient's characteristics, especially social class and educational background, influence the physician's communication.[14,116–119] We have theorized that these relationships may derive from sociolinguistic differences between practitioner and patient, because of which the patient is diffident about expressing a desire for information. The present research focuses on the association between information transmittal and the following patient characteristics:

• Demographic: sex, age, race, occupation, religion, education, marital status, children. These characteristics are ascertained by a questionnaire administered after the patient's interaction with the doctor has been recorded.

• Attitudes about communication: A questionnaire assesses attitudes about the informative process, especially the extent that these influence the patient's questioning the doctor. Also examined is the expressed need for information and judgments about its clinical helpfulness.

• Patients' diagnosis and its uncertainty: It is hypothesized that patients' medical diagnoses, and especially physicians' varying uncertainty about them, may influence the transmittal of information about illness. After doctor-patient interaction, questionnaires record patients' diagnoses and physicians' uncertainty about them.

• Patients' prognosis and its uncertainty: Similarly, it is reasonable to hypothesize that the patient's prognosis, as well as the physician's uncertainty about prognosis, may influence the informative process. Data regarding prognosis and uncertainty are elicited by the postvisit physician questionnaire.

Situational characteristics

Finally, the unique situation in which physician and patient interact may affect the transfer of information between them.

• Length of acquaintance: It is expected that the length of acquaintance between physician and patient may predispose to a certain communicative pattern. A natural history of the informative process may show, for example, relatively little information transmitted in early encounters between a physician and a new patient, followed by the revelation of more information in later sessions. The questionnaire which physicians complete for each patient asks how long the physician has known the patient. In addition, the sample includes one cohort of patients who are followed longitudinally over time, from their initial visit through several later visits, with all sessions recorded (see "Sample," below). This technique permits conclusions about the relationship between length of acquaintance and the informative process.

• Clinical setting: The clinical setting in which physician and patient interact—for example, private practice vs. hospital clinic—may be associated with different types of information transmittal. It might be expected that physicians in private practice would devote more effort to informing patients than physicians working in hospital clinics. The effect of clinical setting is assessed by selecting a sample of physicians who see patients in both hospital clinics and private practice (see "Sample," below). Since physicians record interaction in both settings, it is possible to determine whether the setting is associated with a characteristic informative pattern.

Sample

Nearly all previous studies employing direct recording and analysis of doctor-patient interaction have used samples derived from clinics associated with university teaching centers. The generalizability of findings to the population of physicians and patients outside university-hospital clinics has been greatly limited. In addition, there have been very few attempts to trace changes in the informative process longitudinally over the course of several meetings between physician and patients, although it might be expected that the physician's ability or inclination to convey information would differ between the initial and later visits by a given patient. The present research project attempted to overcome these problems of sample bias by constructing a sample which was representative of a broader population of physicians and patients and which also employed randomization in the sample selection. The total sample was stratified into the following three subsamples:

• The first subsample consisted of ten physicians randomly sampled from a list of licensed internists practicing in Middlesex County, Massachusetts. This phase of the study was conducted under the auspices of the Massachusetts Society of Internal Medicine, which agreed to support the study and to solicit the participation of sampled members. Cooperation was requested by letter, and noncooperating physicians were replaced by randomly selected substitutes. The initial cooperation rate was 72 percent. Noncooperators were asked to complete a questionnaire, to assess whether they differed in any systematic way from cooperators. The physicians who were chosen recorded interaction with 10 consecutive patients seen on a typical day in the physician's professional life. If the sampled physicians worked in different clinical settings, they were asked to record in whatever setting they spent most of their time. The total subsample of physicians was 10, and that of patients was 100.

• A second subsample comprised physicians who work in both outpatient clinics and private practice, to determine the effects of various situations in which physicians and patients interact. The technique of cluster sampling was used to construct this subsample. Three hospital outpatient departments were selected randomly (by a table of random numbers) from a list of all such departments in San Mateo and Santa Clara Counties, California. A list of physicians working both in the outpatient clinics and in private practice was obtained from hospital officials after approval of the study by the respective hospitals' staffs. Ten physicians from each hospital were randomly selected from this list. The initial cooperation rate for this subsample was 82 percent; noncooperation was treated as in the first subsample. Physicians were asked to record interaction with five consecutive patients seen on a typical day in the outpatient clinic and five consecutive patients in private practice. Differences in the information transmitted by the same physician may be inferred as reflecting the effect of clinical setting. The total subsample of physicians was 30, and that of patients was 300.

• The third subsample was constructed in a manner which permitted longitudinal observations of doctor-patient interaction over the course of multiple visits. Thirty-six patients, selected randomly, who were seen by six internists for the first time in the outpatient clinics at the Massachusetts General Hospital made up this subsample. The initial cooperation rate was 86 percent: noncooperation was treated as in the other subsamples. The first and all subsequent meetings between these patients and their physicians during a nine-month period were recorded. Changes in both quantitative and qualitative measures of information transmittal can be traced over time.

The total stratified sample includes 436 patients, 46 physicians, and 481 doctor-patient encounters.

Analysis

The initial analysis of the data consists of simple cross-tabulations and comparisons of means. Of interest are associations between the measures of information transmittal and each of the independent variables—physician, patient, and situational characteristics. Such preliminary exploration indicates which variables are worthy of further statistical analysis and controls. It then is possible to perform multivariate analyses, including analysis of variance and path analysis, to determine the explanatory power of the major independent variables and to assess possible causal relationships. Our working hypotheses are that physician characteristics (especially need for power, professionalism, and common-sense constructs), as well as organizational variables (especially clinical setting), will have the greatest explanatory power. In addition, as mentioned previously, the investigation includes a qualitative analysis of observed information transmittal and its variability.

One technical challenge faced in such research is the conversion of data on the dependent variable (time measures, measures of information, and measures of level of technicality) from the format of code sheets to a format appropriate for multivariate analysis with data on the independent variables. For example, the sequential listing of time spent in each category of interaction as it occurs on the code sheet must be converted to absolute and relative distribution of time in each category for each doctor-patient encounter. A time-sharing computer program has been developed which permits the conversion of raw data on the code sheets to overall data for each encounter. The general features of this program are summarized in figure 3. With this program, data from the code sheets can be converted to the desired format of the dependent variables and stored for later multivariate

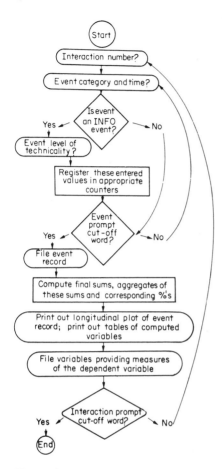

Figure 3
Simplified flow chart of computer programs for deriving dependent variables.

analysis. It is our belief that this program can be applied to the analysis of essentially any dyadic interaction that is coded according to nominal categories.

Conclusion

The informative process is a key element in health delivery systems. We have selected methods to examine the micro level in the hope that our observations will illumine the structural bases in everyday life of macro patterns of dominance and subordination in our society. We believe that the clinical importance of the informative process for health outcomes already has been demonstrated, and that further systematic study of the informative process itself is needed. Although we hope that our work may lead to improved clinical outcomes, our main goal is to heighten consciousness of the ways that stratified patterns emerge in the doctor-patient relationship, and in other "helping" relationships.

Acknowledgments

W. Richard Scott has participated as Co-Principal Investigator of the research project. Elliot G. Mishler has given valuable critical advice. Eric Beller, Sandra Chapek, June Fisher, Terence Fried, Alison Harlow, Carl Mons, Viviane Nathan, Bonnie Obrig, and Beverly Russell have made important contributions to this work.

This report is based on Working Paper No. 9, which was prepared as part of a research project, "The Informative Process in Medical Care," sponsored by grants HS 01565 and 5F01HS54,957 from the National Center for Health Services Research, and by the Robert Wood Johnson Foundation Clinical Scholars Program at Stanford University. Portions of the report were presented at the Annual Meeting of the Clinical Scholars Program, Rye, New York, April, 1975.

References

1. Cartwright, A. *Human Relations and Hospital Care*. Routledge & Kegan Paul. London, 1964.

2. McGhee, A. *The Patient's Attitude to Nursing Care*. Livingstone, Edinburgh, 1961.

3. Duff, R. S., and Hollingshead, A. B. *Sickness and Society*, Harper & Row, New York, 1968.

4. Skipper, J. K., and Leonard, R. C. (editors). *Social Interaction and Patient Care*. Lippincott, Philadelphia, 1965.

5. Titmuss, R. M. *Essays on The Welfare State*. Unwin, London, 1963.

6. Frank, D. A. Hospitals and Me don't Take: A Participant Observation Study of Physically Ill Adolescents. Honors thesis, Harvard University, 1970.

7. Waitzkin, H. Truth's search for power: The dilemmas of the social sciences. *Soc. Probl.* 15, 408, 1968.

8. Wintrobe, M. M., Thorn, G. W., Adams, R. D., et al. (editors). *Harrison's Principles of Internal Medicine*. McGraw-Hill, New York, 1974.

9. Blumgart, H. L. Caring for the patient. *New Engl. J. Med.* 270, 449, 1964.

10. Brauer, P. H. Should the patient be told the truth? In *Social Interaction and Patient Care* (edited by Skipper, J. K., and Leonard, R. C.). Lippincott, Philadelphia, 1965.

11. Standard, S., and Nathan, H. (editors). *Should the Patient Know the Truth?* Springer, New York, 1955.

12. Verwoerdt, A. *Communication with the Fatally Ill*. Thomas, Springfield, 1966.

13. Kant, I. *Critique of Practical Reason*. Bobbs-Merrill, Indianapolis, 1956.

14. Cabot, R. C. The use of truth and falsehood in medicine: An experimental study. *Am. Med.* 5, 344, 1903.

15. Cabot, R. C. Ethical Forces in the Practice of Medicine. Address before students of Harvard College, Harvard Union, 1905 (private printing).

16. Cabot, R. C. *Social Service and the Art of Healing*, Moffat, Yard. New York, 1909.

17. Cabot, R. C. *The Meaning of Right and Wrong*. Macmillan, New York, 1936.

18. Eustene, A. C. Explaining to the patient: A therapeutic tool and a professional obligation. *JAMA* 165, 1110, 1957.

19. Fletcher, J. *Morals and Medicine*. Beacon, Boston, 1954.

20. Katz, J. The education of the physician-investigator. *Daedalus* 98, 480, 1969.

21. White, L. P. The self-image of the physician and the care of dying patients. *Ann. N.Y. Acad. Sci.* 164, 822, 1969.

22. Collins, J. Should doctors tell the truth? *Harper's Mag.* 155, 320, 1927.

23. Henderson, L. J. Physician and patient as a social system. *New Engl. J. Med.* 212, 819, 1935.

24. Leake, C. D. (editor). *Percival's Medical Ethics*. Williams, Baltimore, 1927.

25. Sachs, B. Be an optimist. *J. Mt. Sinai Hosp.* 8, 323, 1942.

26. Treves, F. A modern religio medici: Sir Thomas Browne, *Br. Med. J.*, pp. 1197–1199, 1902.

27. Waitzkin, H., and Stoeckle, J. D. The communication of information about illness: Clinical, sociological and methodological considerations. *Adv. Psychosom. Med.* 8, 180, 1972.

28. Waitzkin, H., and Waterman, B. *The Exploitation of Illness in Capitalist Society*, Bobbs-Merrill, Indianapolis, 1974.

29. Weed, L. L. *Medical Records, Medical Education, and Patient Care*. Case Western Reserve Press, Cleveland, 1969.

30. Davis, M. S. Variations in patients' compliance with doctors' advice: An empirical analysis of patterns of communication. *Am. J. Publ. Hlth* 58, 274, 1968.

31. Francis, V., Korsch, B. M., and Morris, M. J. Gaps in doctor patient communication: Patients' response to medical advice. *New Engl. J. Med.* 280, 535, 1969.

32. Davis, M. S. Variation in patients' compliance with doctors' orders: Medical practice and doctor-patient interaction. *Psychiat. Med.* 2, 31, 1971.

33. Williams, T. F., Martin, D. A., Hogan, M. D., et al. The clinical picture of diabetes control, studied in four settings. *Am. J. Publ. Hlth* 57, 441, 1967.

34. Haggerty, R., and Roghmann, K. Noncompliance and self-medication. *Ped. Cl. N. Am.* 19, 101, 1972.

35. Blackwell, B. Patient compliance. *New Engl. J. Med.* 289, 249, 1973.

36. Inui, T. S. Effects of Post-Graduate Physician Education on the Management and Outcomes of Patients with Hypertension. School of Hygiene and Public Health, Johns Hopkins University, M.A. thesis, 1973.

37. Korsch, B. M., Gozzi, E. K. and Francis, V. Gaps in doctor-patient communication: Doctor-patient interaction and patient satisfaction. *Pediat.* 42, 855, 1968.

38. Korsch, B. M., and Negrete, V. F. Doctor-patient communication. *Sci. Am.* 227, 66, 1972.

39. Janis, I. L. *Psychological Stress: Psychoanalytic and Behavioral Studies of Surgical Patients.* Wiley, New York, 1958.

40. Egbert, L. D., Battit, G. E., Welch, C. E., and Bartlett, M. K. Reduction of post-operative pain by encouragement and instruction of patients. *New Engl. J. Med.* 270, 825, 1964.

41. Skipper, J. K., and Leonard, R. C. Children, stress, and hospitalization: A field experiment. *J. Hlth Soc. Behav.* 9, 275, 1968.

42. Hackett, T. P., Cassem, N. H., and Raker, J. W. Patient delay in cancer. *New Engl. J. Med.* 289, 14, 1973.

43. Bartlett, M. H., Johnston, A., and Meyer, T. C. Dial access library—Patient information service: An experiment in health education. *New Engl. J. Med.* 288, 994, 1973.

44. Leonard, C. O., Chase, G. A., and Childs, B. Genetic counseling: A consumers' view. *New Engl. J. Med.* 287, 433, 1972.

45. Glogow, E. The "bad" patient gets better quicker. *Soc. Policy,* 4, 72, 1973.

46. Schwartz, C. G. Strategies and tactics of mothers of mentally retarded children for dealing with the medical care system. In *Diminished People* (edited by Bernstein, N.). Little-Brown. Boston, 1970.

47. Shenkin, B. N. Giving the patient his medical record: A proposal to improve the system, *New Engl. J. Med.* 289, 688, 1973.

48. Horty, J. F. Informed consent: New rule puts burden of proof on patients, *Mod. Hosp.* 116, 74, 1971.

49. Ingelfinger, F. J. Informed (but uneducated) consent. *New Engl. J. Med.* 287, 465, 1972.

50. Alfidi, R. J. Informed consent: A study of patient reaction. *JAMA* 216, 1325, 1971.

51. Shaw, A. Dilemmas of informed consent in children. *New Engl. J. Med.* 289, 885, 1973.

52. Duff, R. S., and Campbell, A. G. M. Moral and ethical dilemmas in the special-care nursery. *New Engl. J. Med.* 289, 890, 1973.

53. Ingelfinger, F. J. Bedside ethics for the hopeless case. *New Engl. J. Med.* 289, 914, 1973.

54. Fox, R. C. Training for uncertainty. In *The Student-Physician* (edited by Merton, R. K., et al.). Harvard University Press, Cambridge, 1957.

55. Fox, R. C. *Experiment Perilous.* Free Press, Glencoe, 1959.

56. Fox, R. C. A sociological perspective on organ transplantation and hemodialysis. *Ann. N.Y. Acad. Sci.* 169, 406, 1970.

57. Arrow, K. J. Uncertainty and the welfare economics of medical care. *Am. Econ. Rev.* 53, 941, 1963.

58. Fuchs, V. R. The contribution of health services to the American economy. *Milbank Mem. F. Q* 44, 65, 1966.

59. Parsons, T. Research with human subjects and the professional complex. *Daedalus* 98, 325, 1969.

60. Davis, F. Uncertainty in medical prognosis: Clinical and functional. *Am. J. Sociol.* 66, 41, 1960.

61. Davis, F. *Passage through Crisis*. Bobbs-Merrill, Indianapolis, 1963.

62. Roth, J. A. Information and the control of treatment in tuberculosis hospitals. In *The Hospital in Modern Society* (edited by Freidson, E.). Free Press, Glencoe, 1963.

63. Roth, J. A. *Timetables*. Bobbs-Merrill, Indianapolis, 1963.

64. Freidson, E. *Profession of Medicine*. Dodd, Mead, New York, 1970.

65. Freidson, E. *Professional Dominance*. Atherton, New York, 1970.

66. Crozier, M. *The Bureaucratic Phenomenon*. University of Chicago Press, 1964.

67. Artiss, K., and Levine, A. Doctor-patient relation in severe illness. *New Engl. J. Med.* 288, 1210, 1973.

68. McIntosh, J. Processes of communication, information seeking and control associated with cancer: A selected review of the literature. *Soc. Sci. & Med.* 8, 167, 1974.

69. Cherry, C. *On Human Communication*. MIT Press, Cambridge, 1966.

70. Attneave, F. *Applications of Information Theory to Psychology*. Holt, New York, 1959.

71. Shannon, C. E. Prediction and entropy of printed English. *Bell Syst. Tech. J.* 30, 50, 1951.

72. Goldman-Eisler, F. *Psycholinguistics: Experiments in Spontaneous Speech*. Academic Press, London, 1968.

73. Robinson, W. P. *Language and Social Behavior*. Penguin, Baltimore, 1972.

74. Blos, P. Silence: A clinical exploration. *Psychoanalyt. Q* 11, 348, 1972.

75. Heagarty, M., and Robertson, L. Slave doctors and free doctors. *New Engl. J. Med.* 284, 636, 1971.

76. Shuy, R. W. Problems of Communication in the Cross-Cultural Medical Interview. Presented at meeting of American Sociological Association. New York, 1973.

77. McKinlay, J. B. Who is really ignorant—physician or patient? *J. Hlth Soc. Behav.* 16, 3, 1975.

78. Fletcher, C. M. *Communication in Medicine*. Oxford University Press, London, 1973.

79. Bernstein, B. Language and social class. *Br. J. Sociol.* 11, 271, 1961.

80. Bernstein, B. Linguistic codes, hesitation phenomena and intelligence. *Lang. & Speech* 5, 221, 1962.

81. Bernstein, B. Social class, linguistic codes and grammatical elements. *Lang. & Speech* 5, 31, 1962.

82. Bernstein, B. Elaborated and restricted codes: Their social origins and some consequences. *Am Anthropol.* 66, 55, 1964.

83. Bernstein, B. Social class, speech systems and psychotherapy. *Br. J. Sociol.* 15, 54, 1964.

84. Bernstein, B. *Class, Codes and Control—I: Theoretical Studies towards a Sociology of Language*. Routledge & Kegan Paul. London, 1971.

85. Bernstein, B. *Class. Codes and Control—II: Applied Studies towards a Sociology of Language*. Routledge & Kegan Paul, London, 1973.

86. Lawton, D. *Social Class, Language and Education*. Routledge & Kegan Paul, London, 1968.

87. Cook-Gumperz, J. *Social Control and Socialization: A Study of Class Differences in the Language of Maternal Control*. Routledge & Kegan Paul, London, 1973.

88. Labov, W. *Language in the Inner City: Studies in the Black English Vernacular*. University of Pennsylvania Press, Philadelphia, 1972.

89. Labov, W. *Sociolinguistic Patterns*. University of Pennsylvania Press, Philadelphia, 1972.

90. Grimshaw, A. D. On language in society—I. *Contemp. Sociol.* 2, 575, 1973.

91. Grimshaw, A. D. On language in society—II. *Contemp. Sociol.* 3, 3, 1974.

92. Fishman, J. A. *Advances in the Sociology of Language—I: Basic Concepts, Theories and Problems, Alternative Approaches*. Mouton. The Hague, 1971.

93. Gumperz, J. J., and Hymes, D. *Directions in Sociolinguistics: The Ethnography of Communication*. Holt, Rinehart & Winston, New York, 1972.

94. Schutz, A. *The Phenomenology of the Social World*. Northwestern University Press, Evanston, 1967.

95. Schutz, A. Concept and theory formation in the social sciences: Common-sense and scientific interpretation of human action. In *Philosophy of the Social Sciences* (edited by Nathanson, M.). Random House, New York, 1963.

96. Garfinkel, H. *Studies in Ethnomethodology*, Prentice-Hall, Englewood Cliffs, 1967.

97. Scheff, T. *Being Mentally Ill*. Aldine, Chicago, 1966.

98. Waitzkin, H. The Communication of Information about Illness: A Research Proposal and Results of a Pre-Test. Unpublished paper, Department of Sociology, Harvard University, 1971.

99. Goldman-Eisler, F. The measurement of time sequences in conversational behavior. *Br. J. Psychol.* 42, 355, 1951.

100. Goldman-Eisler, F. Individual differences between interviewers and their effect on interviewees' conversational behavior. *J. Ment. Sci.* 98, 660, 1962.

101. Chapple, E. D. Measuring human relations: An introduction to the study of the interaction of individuals. *Genet. Psychol. Monog.* 22, 3, 1940.

102. Chapple, E. D. The measurement of interpersonal behavior. *Trans. N.Y. Acad. Sci.* 4, 222, 1942.

103. Bales, R. F. *Interaction Process Analysis*. Addison-Wesley, Cambridge, 1950.

104. Jaffe, F., and Feldstein, S. *Rhythms of Dialogue*. Academic Press, New York, 1970.

105. Rosenthal, R. *Experimenter Effects in Behavioral Research*. Appleton-Century-Crofts, New York, 1966.

106. Snyder, J. G., and Osgood, C. E. *Semantic Differential Technique*. Aldine, Chicago, 1969.

107. Plaja, A. O., Cohen, L. M., and Samora, J. Communication between physicians and patients in outpatient clinics: Social and cultural factors. *Milbank Mem. F. Q* 46, 161, 1968.

108. Oken, D. What to tell cancer patients: A study of medical attitudes. *JAMA* 175, 1120, 1961.

109. Kübler-Ross, E. *On Death and Dying*. Macmillan, New York, 1969.

110. Dodge, J. S. Nurses' sense of adequacy and attitudes toward keeping patients informed. *J. Hlth Hum. Behav.* 2, 213, 1961.

111. Ford, A. B. et al. *The Doctor's Perspective*. Case Western Reserve Press, Cleveland, 1967.

112. Wilensky, H. L. The professionalization of everyone? *Am. J. Sociol.* 70, 137, 1964.

113. Waitzkin, H., Beller, E. and Mons, C. The Informative Process in Medical Care: Preliminary Statistical Results. Unpublished paper, Department of Sociology, University of Vermont, 1975.

114. Colombotos, J. Physicians and Medicare: A before-after study of the effects of legislation on attitudes. *Am. Sociol. Rev.* 34, 318, 1969.

115. Christie, R., and Geis, F. Some consequences of taking Machiavelli seriously. In *Handbook of Personality Theory and Research* (edited by Borgatta, E. F., and Lambert, W. W.). Rand McNally, Chicago, 1968.

116. Reader, G., Pratt, L., and Mudd, M. C. What patients expect from their doctors. *Mod. Hosp.* 89, 88, 1957.

117. Seligmann, A. W., McGrath, N. E., and Pratt, L. Level of medical information among clinic patients. *J. Chron. Dis.* 6, 497, 1957.

118. Samora, J., Saunders, L. and Larson, R. F. Knowledge about specific diseases in four selected samples. *J. Hlth Hum. Behav.* 3, 176, 1962.

119. Cartwright, A. Pilot Study of Communication between Doctors and Patients. Unpublished paper, Institute for Social Studies in Medical Care. London, 1973.

14

Chinese-Style and Western-Style Doctors in Northern Taiwan
Emily M. Ahern

In Sanhsia, a township on the southern edge of the Taipei basin, there are two distinct kinds of doctors: Chinese-style doctors (*Tiong-i-siêng*) and Western-style doctors (*Se-i-siêng*).[1] Although both kinds of doctors are Taiwanese who have been educated in Taiwan or Japan, their methods of diagnosis and treatment are very different. Chinese-style doctors diagnose by feeling the pulse or studying the complexion and dispense herbs or other substances from an extensive pharmacopoeia called *tiong-iôuq* (literally, Chinese medicine). Western-Style doctors diagnose with the help of instruments such as stethoscopes, thermometers, and sphygmomanometers and dispense powders, pills, or injections known collectively as *se-iôuq* (literally, Western medicine). Beyond these differences, the two kinds of doctors ordinarily practice in separate settings: Chinese-style doctors in small shops that open directly onto the street and Western-style doctors in offices or hospitals with examining rooms that open onto an inside corridor to afford a greater degree of privacy.[2] (See figure 1.)

Despite these distinctions, the separation between the two styles of medicine is not absolute; both Western medicine and Chinese medicine are often sold over the same counter in drug stores staffed by men or women knowledgeable about the uses of drugs. Neither can the two kinds of doctors always be rigidly distinguished. In my other chapter (2) in [*Medicine in Chinese Culture*] it is shown that in comparison with the gods neither Chinese-style nor Western-style doctors make much effort to provide patients with explanations for the cause of their illnesses. In what follows I explore further the texture of the relationship between doctors and their patients in order to refine the conclusions reached earlier. Although in some ways the relationship be-

Reprinted, with permission of the author, from *Medicine in Chinese Culture*, edited by A. Kleinman et al. (publication NIH75–653, Public Health Service, National Institutes of Health).

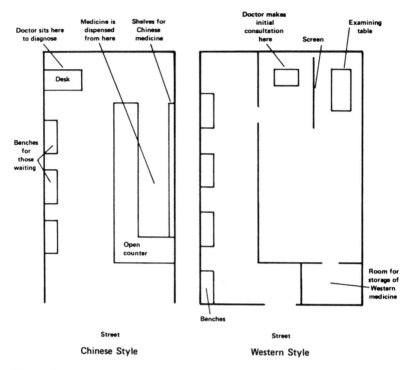

Figure 1
Floor plans of a Chinese-style doctor's shop (left) and a Western-style doctor's office (right).

tween both kinds of doctors and their patients is similar, in other ways there are striking differences in the way the two kinds of doctors communicate with their patients. Some of these differences can be shown to have important implications for the system of health care as a whole.

I

The following suggestions are based on transcripts of doctor-patient interactions that took place during at least one working day in the offices of seven Western-style and two Chinese-style doctors in Sanhsia. Each of the doctors kindly gave permission for my assistants to record these interactions, the Chinese-style doctors allowing an assistant to sit on one of the benches facing the open counter and the Western-style doctors allowing one of them to sit in an inconspicuous corner of the examination room.[3] (See figure 1.) Thus they were able to transcribe conversations between doctors and patients verbatim. The sample of doctors is by no means adequate to provide a definitive analysis of the population of doctors as a whole. I present this material merely to formulate initial hypotheses that might be tested more rigorously at another time.

Even without considering the evidence from the transcriptions of doctor-patient interactions, one might guess that Chinese-style doctors would be able to communicate about medical problems with their patients more easily than would Western-style doctors. Although in contrast to ordinary people Chinese-style doctors possess highly systematic, esoteric knowledge obtained through long training as apprentices to practicing doctors, it is evident even from casual conversations that both Chinese-style doctors and ordinary people use much the same vocabulary in discussing disease. This affinity between the medical notions used by Chinese-style doctors and their patients is revealed clearly in the following excerpts from interactions in the doctors' shops.

(1) [The doctor gives an adult woman an herb.]
Doctor: Stew this herb in water for several hours. This kind of herb is good for your health. It is used to clean your uterus.

(2) [The doctor gives an adult woman an herb.]
Doctor: Now don't take any other drugs to make you stronger because they would be bad for your health. And also don't eat duck. I'll treat your liver ailment first, then your leg pain later because the drugs for the liver and those for the legs are incompatible. Both your liver and kidneys are bad and so you can't eat duck or salt.
Patient: It is said that a shot works rapidly.
Doctor: Yes, it does. But shots only relieve symptoms, and after the medicine wears off they return again. Herbs not only eradicate the symptoms, they also cure completely.

(3) [The patient, an elderly woman, and the doctor face each other across the desk.]
Doctor: What's the matter?
Patient: [She describes her symptoms in detail for about 5 minutes, saying that one-half of her body feels numb, and that she often feels dizzy.]
Doctor: How do your *kûn* [nerves] feel? [He points to the back of his neck.]
Patient: They feel very uncomfortable. I never know which one will break next.
Doctor: You know that a person usually has an equal amount of *ch'i* [vital force] on each side of her body—half on each side. Your problem is that you have lost some *ch'i* from one side of your body. That side is different and so it feels numb. [The doctor then feels her pulse and writes out a prescription for herbs.]

In these examples the Chinese-style doctors utilize concepts and employ terms that are familiar to their patients. In example 1 certain substances clean dirty parts of the body; in example 2 some medicines are incompatible with each other and some diseases are incompatible with particular foods; in example 3 the doctor mentions *ch'i* and *kûn*, two entities commonly mentioned in every day conversations about illness. *Kun* are small nerve-like strands that run along the back of the neck. Old people, especially those suffering from a series of strokes, mention them frequently, saying their kûn feel uncomfortable and are liable to break.

A detailed study of the way these notions—such as incompatibility of foods—fit into the systematic knowledge of doctors as compared to the way they fit together with other beliefs of laymen has yet to be done. The outcome of such a study might be that, although doctors and patients use the same vocabulary, the underlying premises they accept are often different. In a study of the relationship between other experts and laymen—geomancers and their clients—I found that this was so, and it is possible that the same pattern exists in the case of doctors and their patients (Ahern 1973, pp. 175–190). Whether or not Chinese-style doctors and their patients share the same premises, it is clear that they use similar medical vocabularies in speaking to each other.

Western-style doctors, on the other hand, not only seldom offer explanations of the sort given in example 3 above but also seem to have far more difficulty dealing with the notions their patients have about disease. The two conversations below between Western-style doctors and their patients illustrate this.

(4) [The doctor examines a 1-year-old boy and gives him a shot.]
Doctor: Don't keep him too warm.
Patients mother: Will wind (*hông*) hurt him?
Doctor: That's not important. His temperature is nearly 40°C, so you must keep him cool.
Patient's mother: Does he have to take medicine?
Doctor: Yes, he does.
Patient's mother: Can he drink juices?
Doctor: Why don't you give him milk?
Patient's mother: He doesn't want to drink milk.
Doctor: If he's been used to drinking it, it will be all right. Be sure not to add too much sugar.

(5) [The doctor tells his patient, a young adult woman, that she has arthritis.]
Patient: It's said that arthritis is caused by wind (*hông*).
Doctor: It's literally called "wind-wet" but it's not caused by wind.
[The patient takes the medicine and leaves.]

In these examples, doctor and patient share a common vocabulary, but the patient's ideas about disease are either contradicted or ignored by the doctor. In both examples the patient brings up the notion of wind (*hông*). *Hông*, as used by laymen, sometimes refers to moving air—air that can make a baby that is inadequately covered fall sick. At other times *hông* refers to a substance that can get trapped inside the body when a bone is broken or when arthritis is contracted. The term *hông* is also frequently used by Chinese-style doctors, and they would probably have responded positively to the patients' use of it in the examples above. The Western-style doctors, however, say that *hông* is "not important" or that it does not cause arthritis. Similarly, the woman in example 4 asks whether her son can drink juice, probably out of concern that the juice will be incompatible with either the medicine or the illness. But the doctor evades her question in order to encourage her to feed the child normally. Patient and doctor talk past each other, the one bringing ideas unacceptable to the other, neither able to establish a common conceptual ground.

II

Perhaps in part because of the difficulty Western-style practitioners have in dealing with popular conceptions of diseases, there is no indication that Western medicine will supplant Chinese medicine on Taiwan. Chinese-style doctors flourish alongside Western-style doctors and are sought out by the same population. In a preliminary effort to discover whether there are different attitudes toward Western- or Chinese-style medicine among different segments of the population, I administered a questionnaire to 68 people in a village near Sanhsia.[4] Respondents represented segments of the population differentiated by sex, education, and stage of life cycle, as indicated in table 1.

The questionnaire was composed of twelve statements with which respondents were asked to agree or disagree, six indicating inclination toward Western-style medicine and doctors and six indicating inclination toward Chinese-style medicine and doctors. Examples of the former are "Western medicine can completely cure almost all common illnesses such as colds, coughs, diarrhea" and "The Western-style doctor's stethoscope and examination are more accurate means of determining what is wrong than the Chinese doctor feeling the pulse." Examples of the latter are "Western medicines are chemicals and hence harmful to the body" and "Shots make you feel better for only a little while."[5]

Table 1

Inclination toward Chinese or Western medicine according to sex, education, and stage of life cycle.**

Approximate ages	Stage of life cycle	Education	Female	N	Male	N
<20	not yet married	≦ middle school *	0	5	−0.2	5
		> middle school	−2	6	−1	5
20–40	married; living with parents or parents-in-law	≦ elementary school	+0.8	6	+0.7	3
		> elementary school	+2	7	−0.75	4
40–60	married; living in independent household or parents deceased	≦ elementary school	+1.8	11	+2	10
		> elementary school	−0.3	3	0	3

* Middle school (grades 7-9) has been mandatory since 1969.
**Positive scores indicate inclination toward Chinese-style medicine; negative scores indicate inclination toward Western-style medicine.

The questionnaire was then scored to give an estimate of each individual's adherence to one medical system or the other. Someone who agreed with all six statements favoring Chinese-style medicine and disagreed with all six statements favoring Western-style medicine would have a score of +6, indicating the strongest inclination to Chinese-style medicine; someone who agreed with all statements favoring Western-style medicine and disagreed with the rest would have a score of −6, indicating the strongest inclination to Western-style medicine. A score of 0 meant the person agreed with an equal number of pro-Chinese-style and pro-Western-style statements; a score of +2 or −2 meant the person agreed with two more pro-Chinese-style (+2) or pro-Western-style (−2) statements than statements favoring the other form of medicine. Averages of these scores for the twelve population segments are set out in table 1.

Although this kind of measure (used of necessity during this short-term pilot project) is an extremely imperfect instrument with which to summarize people's attitudes about illness and curing, it does divulge several clear trends:

• There is considerable variation among the population, with some segments inclined toward Chinese-style medicine and others toward Western-style medicine.

• On the whole, women, older people, and less-educated people tend to be more inclined toward Chinese-style medicine.[6]

The question that arises at this point is this: Given that both Chinese-style and Western-style doctors are readily available, could it be that those segments of the population who indicate on this questionnaire that they are inclined toward one style of medicine actually make more use of doctors practicing that style of medicine? This question is particularly crucial because those people most responsible for the health of their families—married women—are also those most inclined toward Chinese-style medicine. Unfortunately, no study of differences in the use of different kinds of doctors is yet available. I can only offer evidence of another kind from a question asked of the same people represented in table 1. They were asked what kind of professional help they thought they would seek for a variety of different kinds of ailments, from a skin rash to severe stomach pain. Despite the variation in attitudes disclosed in table 1, practically the entire sample indicated they would make greater use of Western-style practitioners. Of course, this fact cannot be taken as evidence that most everyone actually makes more use of Western-style doctors; it is only an indication that the use of Western-style doctors is not insignificant even among those whose attitudes as described in table 1 incline them toward Chinese-style medicine.

We have then a situation in which three conditions uneasily coexist:

• Many people, especially women and those in older age groups, say in one context that they find Chinese-style doctors and medicine more satisfactory than western-style doctors and medicine (table 1).

• Chinese-style doctors provide more support for laymen's notions about disease than Western-style doctors.

• People generally, including those strongly pro-Chinese medicine in table 1, at least sometimes make use of Western-style doctors.

The uneasiness in this is that those who are avowedly more sympathetic to Chinese-style doctors and medicine in table 1 (perhaps partly because they provide support for laymen's ideas about disease) are willing to confront Western-style doctors despite the difficulty in communication that we have seen exists. Similar problems in communication probably also exist—though perhaps to a lesser extent—for those in table 1 whose inclinations are more toward Western-style medicine. Even though people may say Western-style medicine *works* better, when they talk about disease they still utilize the traditional notions so much a part of Chinese medicine.

There is little evidence that ideas about germs' causing disease or antiseptics' killing germs have gained general acceptance among any portion of the population—ideas that might make it easier for Western-style doctors to communicate with their patients.[7]

In this part of Taiwan, for the moment at least, a population of laymen with certain ideas about what disease is confront one set of experts (Chinese-style doctors) with roughly similar ideas and another set of experts (Western-style doctors) with substantially different ideas.

III

One need not assume, of course, that anything will happen to bring the elements of this situation into closer fit. It may be that ideas compatible with Western-style doctors' understanding of illness will become part of ordinary people's understanding of illness, or it may not. I know of no way to make a prediction. It is interesting nonetheless to consider the opinions of the people in this situation about whether or not things are likely to change. All nine doctors (seven Western-style, two Chinese-style) interviewed thought that no change was likely in the next decade. They predicted that an uneven balance between the two forms of medicine would persist, with virtually all state funding for schools and research going toward Western-style medicine while Chinese-style doctors depend on private training. Asked what changes they thought would be desirable, all but two of the doctors said that more Chinese-style doctors were urgently needed, provided they were adequately trained. On the other hand, most villagers I asked about future trends said that Chinese-style medicine would surely die out in the next generation because its doctors will only pass on their knowledge to young apprentices, and young people are no longer interested in this profession.

Taken together, these responses seem to indicate that there are two possible directions for future development. Chinese-style medicine can be kept as a second-class partner to Western-style medicine, in which case educated youth may be attracted to Western-style medicine. If the villagers are right, one consequence may be that Chinese-style medicine will "die," if not completely, then insofar as its development will be far inferior to that of Western-style medicine. Or, as the doctors recommend, a way could be found to increase the numbers of Chinese-style doctors and train them systematically, thus guaranteeing preservation of at least one set of medical experts who speak the same language as their patients.

The subject is too large to be pursued here, but it is interesting that the second alternative is precisely the route taken by the government of the People's Republic of China as of the mid-1950s, by providing state support for both forms of medicine (Croizier 1968, pp. 157–209). One reason for this, in addition to the many practical and political ones, may have been that this was one more way of ensuring a link between those who are trained to administer medical services and those whom they serve. One need only assume that the pattern described here for Taiwan existed on the mainland before 1949, such that patients' understanding of disease was closer to that of Chinese-style doctors than to that of Western-style doctors; the link in question would be a closer conceptual fit between popular and expert ideas about the causes and mechanisms of disease.

Notes

1. Taiwanese words are spelled according to the system outlined in Nicholas C. Bodman's *Spoken Amoy Hokkien* (1955). They are italicized, and marked for tone on first occurrence only. Mandarin is used for place names and for words that commonly appear in their Mandarin forms.

2. See Katherine Martin's chapter in [*Medicine in Chinese Culture*] for a discussion of some of the social differences between the two kinds of doctors.

3. I would like to express my deep appreciation for the cooperation of the nine doctors, who shall remain anonymous, and the labors of my two assistants, Liu Hsiou-yüan and Chou Pi-se.

4. There was no attempt made to choose a random sample of respondents. The questionnaire was simply administered during the course of other interviewing as people were willing to fill it out. Consequently these results cannot be taken as representative of the population.

5. An English version of the complete questionnaire is as follows. Agreement with statements 1, 2, 7, 8, 10, and 11 indicates inclination toward Chinese-style medicine; agreement with statements 3, 4, 5, 6, 9, and 12 indicates inclination toward Western-style medicine.

(1) If a young person doesn't take tonic medicine [a "hot," strengthening potion] at puberty, he won't grow up properly.
(2) Only Chinese-style medicine can really cure the root cause of illness.
(3) The substances used in Western-style medicines are the same as those found in herbal medicine, only more refined. One might as well take Western-style medicine.
(4) Western-style medicine can completely cure almost all common illnesses, such as colds, coughs, diarrhea.
(5) Nowadays we don't need Chinese-style medicine anymore.
(6) The Western-style doctor says we must operate for appendicitis to save a boy's life but the Chinese-style doctor says it's not necessary to operate because herbal medicine will heal him slowly but surely. In this situation we should definitely operate.
(7) There are some illnesses such as *phà:kia:tiôuq* [literally "fright"; a childhood malady] that no Western-medicine can cure.

(8) The best cure for *tiôuq-káu* [literally "hit by a monkey"; a childhood malady] is to banish the monkey by burning chicken feathers and feces.

(9) Measles vaccine is effective and good for children. Therefore, every child should have it.

(10) Shots make you feel better for only a little while.

(11) Western-style medicines are chemicals and hence harmful to the body.

(12) The Western-style doctor's stethoscope and examination are more accurate means of determining what is wrong than the Chinese-style doctor feeling the pulse.

6. The one figure that contradicts the statement that more-educated people are more inclined to Western medicine is the score of +2 for married women living with their parents or parents-in-law who have more than an elementary-school education. This may be a result of influence from the mothers-in-law, who are living under the same roof. For one thing, much readily available advice about illness comes from a woman's mother-in-law. For another, the more a young woman cooperates with her mother-in-law the smoother her relationship with the rest of the family will be.

7. This is a subject that needs further study, especially because elementary and middle-school texts on health and hygiene make use of ideas about germs in their discussions of disease.

References

Ahern, E. M. 1973. *The Cult of the Dead in a Chinese Village*. Stanford University Press.

Bodman, N. C. 1955. *Spoken Amoy Hokkien*. Kuala Lumpur: Charles Grenier and Son, Ltd.

Croizier, R. C. 1968. *Traditional Medicine in Modern China*. Harvard University Press.

VI

The Good Relation

The ideal of the good doctor-patient relation—one that might withstand the criticism of the participants, of students of the relation, and of the public—has received attention not only from clinicians (T. Szasz, W. Knoff, and M. H. Hollender, "The Doctor-Patient Relationship and Its Historical Context," *Am. J. Psych.* 115 [1958]: 522), sociologists, and psychologists, but from philosophers as well (M. Mayerhoff, *On Caring* [Harper and Row, 1971]).

Francis Peabody is probably the most frequently quoted clinician. His 1927 paper "The Care of the Patient," reproduced in part here, contains the admonition that "the secret of caring for the patient is to care for him," which serves also as a reminder not to reject him. When Peabody wrote this essay he was seriously ill with liposarcoma of the stomach (T. F. Williams, "Cabot, Peabody, and the Care of the Patient," *Bull. Hist. Med.* 214 [1950]: 462) and may well have been aware of how the dying feel rejected. His words, written while he was working part-time in Boston City Hospital (a municipal hospital for the "sick poor") are also a powerful appeal for the maintenance of the tradition of not abandoning indigent patients. (No appeal was needed, apparently, for the care of others.) Peabody noted with regret that students were not exposed to private office practice, where personal care and intimacy—the real care of the patient—actually did take place and could be more easily learned. Hospital-based and outside the organization of private practice, medical education then did not provide students with office learning experience such as is provided by educational programs for primary care today. A recent version of this caring theme is Eric Cassell's *The Healer's Art* (Lippincott, 1976). More than an appeal, it also contains the details of negotiating the elements of care with the patient—particularly the dying patient.

While speaking more about a psychotherapeutic relation, Carl Rogers ("Characteristics of a Helping Relation," in *On Becoming a*

Person [Houghton Mifflin, 1961]) defined the features that may benefit both doctors and patients in many of their encounters. Rogers stressed a more open, egalitarian relation, which is most important for the modern task of caring for the chronically ill and dealing with the psychological distress that accompanies their illness. Such a relation can also enhance the patient's self-care and treatment, which are vital for facilitating and sharing the long-term task of optimal maintenance. Acceptance, respect, and empathy for the patient are at the core of Rogers's therapeutic relation, a psychological appeal that has philosophical and religious roots.

As a relationship develops, the doctor has important affective responses to the patient. Harry Wilmer's 1968 essay "The Doctor-Patient Relationship and the Issues of Pity, Sympathy, and Empathy" (included here) distinguishes among these three human responses. The doctor is privy to numerous accounts of existential despair in his encounters with patients—despair that may have its origins in illness or, quite apart from it, in the "everydayness" of a patient's life, in the dissatisfactions from lost chances, or in the disappointments of family attachments, failed achievements, or injured relationships. The nature and the dynamics of the doctor's empathetic response are, as Wilmer and others (e.g., A. Margulies ["Toward Empathy: The Uses of Wonder," *Am. J. Psych.* 141 (1984): 1025]) note, are important for the maintenance of the patient's autonomy.

To date, the measurement of the caring qualities of medical practice has not been regularly undertaken. Attention has been devoted to other topics, to the use of objective tests, procedures, and examinations in medical diagnosis, or to the use of the relation for such outcomes as compliance. However, beginnings have been made that go beyond the traditional interpersonal themes of care that rate intimacy vs. distance, dominance vs. submissiveness, or satisfactions vs. dissatisfactions in relations. From the social-psychology literature, W. Bemmis, D. Berlow, E. Sihen, and F. Steele ("Toward Better Interpersonal Relationships," part 5, in *Interpersonal Dynamics* [Dorsey, 1973]) have described criteria for judging the quality of relations by three dimensions: goals, content, and outcomes. For outcomes they would include solidarity, reality confirmation, growth, and competence. In the final reprinted paper, "Studies on a Negotiated Approach to Patienthood," Aaron Lazare, Sherman Eisenthal, Arlene Frank, and John D. Stoeckle summarize their research on the relation. Typifying it as a negotiated exchange, and again borrowing concepts from social psychology, they argue that the situation of modern medical practice calls for the recognition of an innately conflicted relation and that the goals of the doctor and the requests of the patient must be continuously negotiated throughout the encounter. Both the patient and the doctor are more satisfied if negotiation is part of all the clinical tasks of care: making the diagnosis, obtaining tests, undertaking treatment, and even establishing a particular relation with the patient. Perhaps of greater importance, the patient is, as a result, more informed, and his rational autonomy is enhanced, improving the patient's control of his own illness. This releases the doctor from the burden of "omnipotence," and medicine from the burden of "magic" and "cure." Doctor and patient can finally become partners or collaborators in a mutual consultation for rehabilitation, relief, and maintenance. And yet, in our society, with its diversity of cultures, class, ethnicities, and life styles, every patient may not want precisely this relationship, which has become the modern ideal in lay and professional writing on the subject.

Indeed, the writings on the relation and on the teaching of the medical interview contain the modern ideology and directions of the good relation (J. D. Stoeckle and J. A. Billings, "On Questioning, Listening and Talking, A History of the Interview and Its Instructions" [*J. Gen. Med.*, to appear]). The up-to-date instructions on how doctors should behave with patients may be summarized as follows:

1. Make the relation more democratic by giving the patient choices in decisions about the scope of diagnosis and alternatives in treatment.

2. Develop this patient participation by transmitting the necessary information about diagnosis and treatment so that the patient can make those choices.

3. Attend to the patient's feelings about illness and treatment by respect, genuine concern, and empathy.

4. Provide helping actions that are person-centered by eliciting, acknowledging, and responding to the patient's perspectives on their illness and care.

5. Negotiate with the patient about choices, decisions, and requests, similarly acknowledging and negotiating conflict in the relationship itself.

6. Promote health education and self-help by communicating information about diagnosis, treatment, health maintenance, and prevention.

7. Convey respect to the person of the patient without regard to the patient's gender, race, ethnicity, or age.

Some would say that these explicit directions for the modern conduct of the relation are not therapeutic imperatives themselves, only an adaptation of the relation to larger changes in a culture where authority and expertise are being questioned and where individuals must now reestablish their mutual ground rules for obtaining and using help. The good relation does not deny this influence; rather, it seeks only to separate true authority from authoritarianism and true expertise from mystification.

Could this modernization of the relationship and these new directions for it be dismissed as common knowledge? If only they were, and systematically acted on. That action requires leadership and education. In a relation that is so fundamentally asymmetrical in favor of the doctor, improvement rests largely with leadership. However, much of current thinking would argue only for the necessity of patient education to change the relation and to narrow the gap between the participants. While these readings may educate both doctors and patients, they are particularly for doctors, who, unlike patients, have the position, time, capacity, and responsibility to enhance their relationships. For this task, professional leadership and commitment are needed alongside a more educated patient in a more humane and equitable society,

15

The Care of the Patient
Francis W. Peabody

It is probably fortunate that systems of education are constantly under the fire of general criticism, for if education were left solely in the hands of teachers the chances are good that it would soon deteriorate. Medical education, however, is less likely to suffer from such stagnation, for whenever the lay public stops criticizing the type of modern doctor, the medical profession itself may be counted on to stir up the stagnant pool and cleanse it of its sedimentary deposit. The most common criticism made at present by older practitioners is that young graduates have been taught a great deal about the mechanism of disease, but very little about the practice of medicine—or, to put it more bluntly, they are too "scientific" and do not know how to take care of patients.

One is, of course, somewhat tempted to question how completely fitted for his life work the practitioner of the older generation was when he first entered on it, and how much the haze of time has led him to confuse what he learned in the school of medicine with what he acquired in the harder school of experience. But the indictment is a serious one, and it is concurred in by numerous recent graduates who find that in the actual practice of medicine they encounter many situations which they had not been led to anticipate and which they are not prepared to meet effectively. Where there is so much smoke, there is undoubtedly a good deal of fire, and the problem for teachers and for students is to consider what they can do to extinguish whatever is left of this smoldering distrust.

To begin with, the fact must be accepted that one cannot expect to become a skilful practitioner of medicine in the four or five years allotted to the medical curriculum. Medicine is not a trade to be learned but a profession to be entered. It is an ever widening field that

Reprinted, with permission, from *Journal of the American Medical Association* 88 (1927): 877–882. Copyright 1927 by American Medical Association.

requires continued study and prolonged experience in close contact with the sick. All that the medical school can hope to do is to supply the foundations on which to build. When one considers the amazing progress of science in its relation to medicine during the last thirty years, and the enormous mass of scientific material which must be made available to the modern physician, it is not surprising that the schools have tended to concern themselves more and more with this phase of the educational problem. And while they have been absorbed in the difficult task of digesting and correlating new knowledge, it has been easy to overlook the fact that the application of the principles of science to the diagnosis and treatment of disease is only one limited aspect of medical practice. The practice of medicine in its broadest sense includes the whole relationship of the physician with his patient. It is an art, based to an increasing extent on the medical sciences, but comprising much that still remains outside the realm of any science. The art of medicine and the science of medicine are not antagonistic but supplementary to each other. There is no more contradiction between the science of the medicine and the art of medicine than between the science of aeronautics and the art of flying. Good practice presupposes an understanding of the sciences which contribute to the structure of modern medicine, but it is obvious that sound pro-fessional training should include a much broader equipment.

The problem that I wish to consider, therefore, is whether this larger view of the profession cannot be approached even under the conditions imposed by the present curriculum of the medical school. Can the practitioner's art be grafted on the main trunk of the funda-mental sciences in such a way that there shall arise a symmetrical growth, like an expanding tree, the leaves of which may be for the "healing of the nations"?

One who speaks of the care of patients is naturally thinking about circumstances as they exist in the practice of medicine; but the teacher who is attempting to train medical students is immediately confron-ted by the fact that, even if he would, he cannot make the conditions under which he has to teach clinical medicine exactly similar to those of actual practice.

The primary difficulty is that instruction has to be carried out largely in the wards and dispensaries of hospitals rather than in the patient's home and the physician's office. Now the essence of the practice of medicine is that it is an intensely personal matter, and one of the chief differences between private practice and hospital practice is that the latter always tends to become impersonal. At first sight this may not appear to be a very vital point, but it is, as a matter of fact, the crux of the whole situation. The treatment of a disease may be entirely impersonal; the care of a patient must be completely personal. The significance of the intimate personal relationship between physician and patient cannot be too strongly emphasized, for in an extraordinarily large number of cases both diagnosis and treatment are directly dependent on it, and the failure of the young physician to establish this relationship accounts for much of his ineffectiveness in the care of patients.

Instruction in Treatment of Disease

Hospitals, like other institutions founded with the highest human ideals, are apt to deteriorate into dehumanized machines, and even the physician who has the patient's welfare most at heart finds that pressure of work forces him to give most of his attention to the critically sick and to those whose diseases are a menace to the public health. In such cases he must first treat the specific disease, and there then remains little time in which to cultivate more than a superficial personal contact with the patients. Moreover, the circumstances under which the physician sees the patient are not wholly favorable to the establishment of the intimate personal relationship that exists in private practice, for one of the outstanding features of hospitalization is that it completely removes the patient from his accustomed environment. This may, of course, be entirely desirable, and one of the main reasons for sending a person into the hospital is to get him away from home surroundings, which, be he rich or poor, are often unfavorable to recovery; but at the same time it is equally important for the physician to know the exact character of those surroundings.

Everybody, sick or well, is affected in one way or another, consciously or subconsciously, by the material and spiritual forces that bear on his life, and especially to the sick such forces may act as powerful stimulants or depressants. When the general practitioner goes into the home of a patient, he may know the whole background of the family life from past experience; but even when he comes as a stranger he has every opportunity to find out what manner of man his patient is, and what kind of circumstances make his life. He gets a hint of financial anxiety or of domestic incompatibility; he may find himself confronted by a querulous, exacting, self-centered patient, or by a gentle invalid overawed by a dominating family; and as he appreciates how these circumstances are reacting on the patient he dispenses sympathy, encouragement, or discipline. What is spoken of as a "clinical picture" is not just a photograph of a man sick in bed; it is an impressionistic painting of the patient surrounded by his home, his work, his relations, his friends, his joys, sorrows, hopes, and fears. Now, all of this background of sickness which bears so strongly on the symptomatology is liable to be lost sight of in the hospital: I say "liable to" because it is not by any means always lost sight of, and because I believe that by making a constant and conscious effort one can almost always bring it out into its proper perspective. The difficulty is that in the hospital one gets into the habit of using the oil immersion lens instead of the low power, and focuses too intently on the center of the field.

When a patient enters a hospital, one of the first things that commonly happens to him is that he loses his personal identity. He is generally referred to, not as Henry Jones, but as "that case of mitral stenosis in the second bed on the left." There are plenty of reasons why this is so, and the point is, in itself, relatively unimportant; but the trouble is that it leads, more or less directly, to the patient being treated as a case of mitral stenosis, and not as a sick man. The disease is treated, but Henry Jones, lying awake nights while he worries about his wife and children, represents a problem that is much more complex than the pathologic physiology of mitral stenosis, and he is apt to improve very slowly unless a discerning intern happens to discover why it is that even large doses of digitalis fail to slow his heart rate. Henry happens to have heart disease, but he is not disturbed so much by dyspnea as he is by anxiety for the future, and a talk with an understanding physician who tries to make the situation clear to him, and then gets the social service worker to find a suitable occupation, does more to straighten him out than a book full of drugs and diets. Henry has an excellent example of a certain type of heart disease, and he is glad that all the staff find him interesting, for it makes him feel that they will do the best they can to cure him; but just because he is an interesting case he does not cease to be a human being with very human hopes and fears. Sickness produces an abnormally sensitive emotional state in almost every one, and in many cases the emotional state repercusses, as it were, on the organic disease. The pneumonia would probably run its course in a week, regardless of treatment, but the experienced physician knows that by quieting the cough, getting the patient to sleep, and giving a bit of encouragement, he can save his patient's strength and lift him through many distressing hours. The institutional eye tends to become focused on the lung, and it forgets that the lung is only one member of the body.

Patients Who Have "Nothing the Matter With Them"

But if teachers and students are liable to take a limited point of view even toward interesting cases of organic disease, they fall into much more serious error in their attitude toward a large group of patients who do not show objective, organic pathologic conditions, and who are generally spoken of as having "nothing the matter with them." Up to a certain point, as long as the are regarded as diagnostic problems, they command attention; but as soon as a physician has assured himself that they do not have organic disease, he passes them over lightly.

Take the case of a young woman, for instance, who entered the hospital with a history of nausea and discomfort in the upper part of the abdomen after eating, Mrs. Brown had "suffered many things of many physicians." Each of them gave her a tonic and limited her diet. She stopped eating everything that any of her physicians advised her to omit, and is now living on a little milk with a few crackers; but her symptoms persist. The history suggests a possible gastric ulcer or gallstones, and with a proper desire to study the case thoroughly, she is given a test meal, gastric analysis, and duodenal intubation, and roentgen-ray examinations are made of the gastro-intestinal tract and gallbladder. All of these diagnostic methods give negative results; that is, they do not show evidence of any structural change. The case is immediately much less interesting than if it had turned out to be a gastric ulcer with atypical symptoms. The visiting physician walks by and says: "Well, there's nothing the matter with her." The clinical clerk says: "I did an awful lot of work on that case and it turned out to be nothing at all." The intern, who wants to clear out the ward so as to make room for some interesting cases, says: "Mrs. Brown, you can send for your clothes and go home tomorrow. There really is nothing the matter with you, and fortunately you have not got any of the serious troubles we suspected. We have used all the most modern and scientific methods and we find that there is no reason why you should not eat anything you want to. I'll give you a tonic to take when you go home." Same story, same colored medicine! Mrs. Brown goes home, somewhat better for her rest in new surroundings, thinking that nurses are kind and physicians are pleasant, but that they do not seem to know much about the sort of medicine that will touch her trouble. She takes up her life and the symptoms return—and then she tries chiropractic, or perhaps it is Christian Science.

It is rather fashionable to say that the modern physician has become "too scientific." Now, was it too scientific, with all the stomach tubes and blood counts and roentgen-ray examinations? Not at all. Mrs. Brown's symptoms might have been due to a gastric ulcer or to gallstones, and after such a long course it was only proper to use every method that might help to clear the diagnosis. Was it, perhaps, not scientific enough? The popular conception of a scientist as a man who works in a laboratory and who uses instruments of precision is as inaccurate as it is superficial, for a scientist is known, not by his technical processes, but by his intellectual processes; and the essence of the scientific method of thought is that it proceeds in an orderly manner toward the establishment of a truth. Now the chief criticism to be made of the way Mrs. Brown's case was handled is that the staff was contented with a half truth. The investigation of the patient was decidedly unscientific in that it stopped short of even an attempt to determine the real cause of the symptoms. As soon as organic disease could be excluded the whole problem was given up, but the symptoms persisted. Speaking candidly, the case was a medical failure in spite of the fact that the patient went home with the assurance that there was "nothing the matter" with her.

A good many "Mrs. Browns," male and female, come to hospitals, and a great many more go to private physicians. They are all characterized by the presence of symptoms that cannot be accounted for by organic disease, and they are all liable to be told that they have "nothing the matter" with them. Now my own experience as a hospital physician has been rather long and varied, and I have always found that, from my point of view, hospitals are particularly interesting and cheerful places; but I am fairly certain that, except for a few low grade morons and some poor wretches who want to get in out of the cold, there are not many people who become hospital patients unless there is something the matter with them. And, by the same token, I doubt whether there are many people, except for those stupid creatures who would rather go to the physician than go to the theater, who spend their money on visiting private physicians unless there is something the matter with them. In hospital and in private practice, however, one finds this same type of patient, and many physicians whom I have questioned agree in saying that, excluding cases of acute infection, approximately half of their patients complained of symptoms for which an adequate organic cause could not be discovered. Numerically, then, these patients constitute a large group, and their fees go a long way toward spreading butter on the physician's bread. Medically speaking, they are not serious cases as regards prospective death, but they are often extremely serious as regards prospective life. Their symptoms will rarely prove fatal, but their lives will be long and miserable, and they may end by nearly exhausting their families and friends. Death is not the worst thing in the world, and to help a man to a happy and useful career may be more of a service than the saving of life.

Physiologic Disturbances From Emotional Reactions

What is the matter with all these patients? Technically, most of them come under the broad heading of the "psychoneuroses"; but for practical purposes many of them may be regarded as patients whose subjective symptoms are due to disturbances of the physiologic activity of one or more organs or systems. These symptoms may depend on an increase or a decrease of a normal function, on an abnormality of function, or merely on the subject's becoming conscious of a wholly normal function that normally goes on unnoticed; and this last conception indicates that there is a close relation between the appearance of the symptoms and the threshold of the patient's nervous reactions. The ultimate causes of these disturbances are to be found, not in any gross structural changes in the organs involved, but rather in nervous influences emanating from the emotional or intellectual life, which, directly or indirectly, affect in one way or another organs that are under either voluntary or involuntary control.

Every one has had experiences that have brought home the way in which emotional reactions affect organic functions. Some have been nauseated while anxiously waiting for an important examination to begin, and a few may even have vomited; others have been seized by an attack of diarrhea under the same circumstances. Some have had polyuria before making a speech, and others have felt thumping extrasystoles or a pounding tachycardia before a football game. Some have noticed rapid shallow breathing when listening to a piece of bad news, and others know the type of occipital headache, with pain down the muscles of the back of the neck, that comes from nervous anxiety and fatigue.

These are all simple examples of the way that emotional reactions may upset the normal functioning of an organ. Vomiting and diarrhea are due to abnormalities of the motor function of the gastro-intestinal tract—one to the production of an active reversed peristalsis of the stomach and a relaxation of the cardiac sphincter, the other to hyperperistalsis of the large intestine. The polyuria is caused by vasomotor changes in renal circulation, similar in character to the vasomotor changes that take place in the peripheral vessels in blushing and blanching of the skin, and in addition there are quite possibly associated changes in the rate of blood flow and in blood pressure. Tachycardia and extrasystoles indicate that not only the rate but also the rhythm of the heart is under a nervous control that can be demonstrated in the intact human being as well as in the experimental animal. The ventilatory function of the respiration is extraordinarily subject to nervous influences; so much so, in fact, that the study of the respiration in man is associated with peculiar difficulties. Rate, depth, and rhythm of breathing are easily upset by even minor stimuli, and in extreme cases the disturbance in total ventilation is sometimes so great that gaseous exchange becomes affected. Thus, I remember an emotional young woman who developed a respiratory neurosis with deep and rapid breathing, and expired so much carbon dioxide that the symptoms of tetany ensued. The explanation of the occipital headaches and of so many pains in the muscles of the back is not entirely clear, but they appear to be associated with changes in muscular tone or with prolonged states of contraction. There is certainly a very intimate correlation between mental tenseness and muscular tenseness, and whatever methods are used to produce mental relaxation will usually cause muscular relaxation, together with relief of this type of pain. A similar condition is found in the so-called writers' cramp, in which the painful muscles of the hand result, not from manual work, but from mental work.

One might go on much further, but these few illustrations will suffice to recall the infinite number of ways in which physiologic functions may be upset by emotional stimuli, and the manner in which the resulting disturbances of function manifest themselves as symptoms. These symptoms, although obviously not due to anatomic changes, may, nevertheless, be very disturbing and distressing, and there is nothing imaginary about them. Emotional vomiting is just as real as the vomiting due to pyloric obstruction, and so-called "nervous headaches" may be as painful as if they were due to a brain tumor. Moreover, it must be remembered that symptoms based on functional disturbances may be present in a patient who has, at the same time, organic disease, and in such cases the determination of the causes of the different symptoms may be an extremely difficult matter. Every one accepts the relationship between the common functional symptoms and nervous reactions, for convincing evidence is to be found in the fact that under ordinary circumstances the symptoms disappear just as soon as the emotional cause has passed. But what happens if the cause does not pass away? What if, instead of having to face a single three-hour examination, one has to face a life of being constantly on the rack? The emotional stimulus persists, and continues to produce the disturbances of function. As with all nervous reactions, the longer the process goes on, or the more frequently it goes on, the easier it is for it to go on. The unusual nervous track becomes an established path. After a time, the symptom and the subjective discomfort that it produces come to occupy the center of the picture, and the causative factors recede into a hazy background. The patient no longer thinks "I cannot stand this life," but he says out loud "I cannot stand this nausea and vomiting. I must go to see a stomach specialist."

Quite possibly the comment on this will be that the symptoms of such "neurotic" patients are well known, and they ought to go to a neurologist or a psychiatrist and not to an internist or a general practitioner. In an era of internal medicine, however, which takes pride in the fact that it concerns itself with the functional capacity of organs rather than with mere structural changes and which has developed so many "functional tests" of kidneys, heart, and liver, is it not rather narrow minded to limit one's interest to those disturbances of function which are based on anatomic abnormalities? There are other reasons, too, why most of these "functional" cases belong to the field of general medicine. In the first place, the differential diagnosis between organic disease and functional disturbance is often extremely difficult, and it needs the broad training in the use of general clinical and laboratory methods which forms the equipment of the internist. Diagnosis is the first step in treatment. In the second place, the patients themselves frequently prefer to go to a medical practitioner rather than to a psychiatrist, and in the long run it is probably better for them to get straightened out without having what they often consider the stigma of having been "nervous" cases. A limited number, it is true, are so refractory or so complex that the aid of the psychiatrist must be sought, but the majority can be helped by the internist without highly specialized psychologic technic, if he will appreciate the significance of functional disturbances and interest himself in their treatment. The physician who does take these cases seriously—one might say scientifically—has the great satisfaction of seeing some of his patients get well, not as the result of drugs or as the result of the disease having run its course, but as the result of his own individual efforts.

Here, then, is a great group of patients in which it is not the disease but the man or the woman who needs to be treated. In general hospital practice physicians are so busy with the critically sick, and in clinical teaching are so concerned with training students in physical diagnosis and attempting to show them all the types of organic disease, that they do not pay as much attention as they should to the functional disorders. Many a student enters practice having hardly heard of them except in his course in psychiatry, and without the faintest conception of how large a part they will play in his future practice. At best, his method of treatment is apt to be a cheerful reassurance combined with a placebo. The successful diagnosis and treatment of these patients, however, depends almost wholly on the establishment of that intimate personal contact between physician and patient which forms the basis of private practice. Without this, it is quite impossible for the physician to get an idea of the problems and troubles that lie behind so many functional disorders. If students are to obtain any insight into this field of medicine, they must also be given opportunities to build up the same type of personal relationship with their patients.

Student's Opportunity in the Hospital

Is there, then, anything inherent in the conditions of clinical teaching in a general hospital that makes this impossible? Can you form a personal relationship in an impersonal institution? Can you accept the fact that your patient is entirely removed from his natural environment and then reconstruct the background of environment from the history, from the family, from a visit to the home or workshop, and from the information obtained by the social service worker? And while you are building up this environmental background, can you enter into the same personal relationship that you ought to have in private practice? If you can do all this, and I know from experience that you can, then the study of medicine in the hospital actually becomes the practice of medicine, and the treatment of disease immediately takes its proper place in the larger problem of the care of the patient.

When a patient goes to a physician he usually has confidence that the physician is the best, or at least the best available, person to help him in what is, for the time being, his most important trouble. He relies on him as on a sympathetic adviser and a wise professional counselor. When a patient goes to a hospital he has confidence in the reputation of the institution, but it is hardly necessary to add that he also hopes to come into contact with some individual who personifies the institution and will also take a human interest in him. It is obvious that the first physician to see the patient is in the strategic position— and in hospitals all students can have the satisfaction of being regarded as physicians.

Here, for instance, is a poor fellow who has just been jolted to the hospital in an ambulance. A string of questions about himself and his family have been fired at him, his valuables and even his clothes have been taken away from him, and he is wheeled into the ward on a truck, miserable, scared, defenseless, and, in his nakedness, unable to run away. He is lifted into a bed, becomes conscious of the fact that he is the center of interest in the ward, wishes that he had stayed at home among friends, and, just as he is beginning to take stock of his surroundings, finds that a thermometer is being stuck under his tongue. It is all strange and new, and he wonders what is going to happen next. The next thing that does happen is that a man in a long white coat sits down by his bedside, and starts to talk to him. Now it happens that according to our system of clinical instruction that man is usually a medical student. Do you see what an opportunity you have? The foundation of your whole relation with that patient is laid in those first few minutes of contact, just as happens in private practice. Here is a worried, lonely, suffering man, and if you begin by approaching him with sympathy, tact, and consideration, you get his confidence and he becomes your patient. Interns and visiting physicians may come and go, and the hierarchy gives them a precedence; but if you make the most of your opportunities he will regard you as his personal physician, and all the rest as mere consultants. Of course, you must not drop him after you have taken the history and made your physical examination. Once your relationship with him has been established, you must foster it by every means. Watch his condition closely and he will see that you are alert professionally. Make time to have little talks with him—and these talks need not always be about his symptoms. Remember that you want to know him as a man, and this means you must know about his family and friends, his work and his play. What kind of a person is he—cheerful, depressed, introspective, careless, conscientious, mentally keen or dull? Look out for all the little incidental things that you can do for his comfort. These, too, are a part of "the care of the patient." Some of them will fall technically in the field of "nursing," but you will always be profoundly grateful for any nursing technic that you have acquired. It is worth your while to get the nurse to teach you the right way to feed a patient, change the bed, or give a bed pan. Do you know the practical tricks that make a dyspneic patient comfortable? Assume some responsibility for these apparently minor points and you will find that it is when you are doing some such friendly service, rather than when you are a formal questioner, that the patient suddenly starts to unburden himself, and a flood of light is thrown on the situation.

Meantime, of course, you will have been active along strictly medical lines, and by the time your clinical and laboratory examinations are completed you will be surprised at how intimately you know your patient, not only as an interesting case but also as a sick human being. And everything you have picked up about him will be of value in the subsequent handling of the situation. Suppose, for instance, you find conclusive evidence that his symptoms are due to organic disease; say, to a gastric ulcer. As soon as you face the problem of laying out his regimen you find that it is one thing to write an examination paper on the treatment of gastric ulcer and quite another thing to treat John Smith who happens to have a gastric ulcer. You want to begin by giving him rest in bed and a special diet for eight weeks. Rest means both nervous and physical rest. Can he get it best at home or in the hosptial? What are the conditions at home? If you keep him in the hospital, it is probably good for him to see certain people, and bad for him to see others. He has business problems that must be considered. What kind of a compromise can you make on them? How about the financial implications of eight weeks in bed followed by a period of convalescence? Is it, on the whole, wiser to try a strict regimen for a shorter period, and, if he does not improve, take up the question of operation sooner than is in general advisable? These and many similar problems arise in the course of the treatment of almost every patient, and they have to be looked at, not from the abstract point of view of the treatment of the disease, but from the concrete point of view of the care of the individual.

Suppose, on the other hand, that all your clinical and laboratory examinations turn out entirely negative as far as revealing any evidence of organic disease is concerned. Then you are in the difficult position of not having discovered the explanation of the patient's symptoms. You have merely assured yourself that certain conditions are not present. Of course, the first thing you have to consider is whether these symptoms are the result of organic disease in such an early stage that you cannot definitely recognize it. This problem is often extremely perplexing, requiring great clinical experience for its solution, and often you will be forced to fall back on time in which to watch developments. If, however, you finally exclude recognizable organic disease, and the probability of early or very slight organic disease, it becomes necessary to consider whether the symptomatology may be due to a functional disorder which is caused by nervous or emotional influences. You know a good deal about the personal life of your patient by this time, but perhaps there is nothing that stands out as an obvious etiologic factor, and it becomes necessary to sit down for a long intimate talk with him to discover what has remained hidden.

Sometimes it is well to explain to the patient, by obvious examples, how it is that emotional states may bring about symptoms similar to his own, so that he will understand what you driving at and will cooperate with you. Often the best way is to go back to the very beginning and try to find out the circumstances of the patient's life at the time the symptoms first began. The association between symptoms and cause may have been simpler and more direct at the onset at least in the patient's mind, for as time goes on and the symptoms become more pronounced and distressing there is a natural tendency for the symptoms to occupy so much of the foreground of the picture that the background is completely obliterated. Sorrow, disappointment, anxiety, self-distrust, thwarted ideals or ambitions in social, business, or personal life, and particularly what are called maladaptations to these conditions—these are among the commonest and simplest factors that initiate and perpetuate the functional disturbances. Perhaps you will find that the digestive disturbances began at the time the patient was in serious financial difficulties, and they have recurred whenever he is worried about money matters. Or you may find that ten years ago a physician told the patient he had heart disease, cautioning him "not to worry about it." For ten years the patient has never mentioned the subject, but he has avoided every exertion, and has lived with the idea that sudden death was in store for him. You will find that physicians, by wrong diagnoses and ill-considered statements, are responsible for many a wrecked life, and you will discover that it is much easier to make a wrong diagnosis than it is to unmake it. Or, again, you may find that the pain in this woman's back made its appearance when she first felt her domestic unhappiness, and that this man's headaches have been associated, not with long hours of work, but with a constant depression due to unfulfilled ambitions. The causes are manifold and the manifestations protean. Sometimes the mechanism of cause and effect is obvious; sometimes it becomes apparent only after a very tangled skein has been unraveled.

If the establishment of an intimate personal relationship is necessary in the diagnosis of functional disturbances, it becomes doubly necessary in their treatment. Unless there is complete confidence in the sympathetic understanding of the physician as well as in his professional skill, very little can be accomplished; but granted that you have been able to get close enough to the patient to discover the cause of the trouble, you will find that a general hospital is not at all an impossible place for the treatment of functional disturbances. The hospital has, indeed, the advantage that the entire reputation of the institution, and all that it represents in the way of facilities for diagnosis and treatment, go to enhance the confidence which the patients has in the individual physician who represents it. This gives the very young physician a hold on his patients that he could scarcely hope to have without its support. Another advantage is that hospital patients are removed from their usual environment, for the treatment of functional disturbances is often easier when patients are away from friends, relatives, home, work, and, indeed, everything that is associated with their daily life. It is true that in a public ward one cannot obtain complete isolation in the sense that this is a part of the Weir Mitchell treatment, but the main object is accomplished if one has obtained the psychologic effect of isolation which comes with an entirely new and unaccustomed atmosphere. The conditions, therefore, under which you, as students, come into contact with patients with functional disturbances are not wholly unfavorable, and with very little effort they can be made to simulate closely the conditions in private practice.

Importance of Personal Relationship

It is not my purpose, however, to go into a discussion of the methods of treating functional disturbances, and I have dwelt on the subject only because these cases illustrate so clearly the vital importance of the personal relationship between physician and patient in the practice of medicine. In all your patients whose symptoms are of functional origin, the whole problem of diagnosis and treatment depends on your insight into the patient's character and personal life, and in every case of organic disease there are complex interactions between the pathologic processes and the intellectual processes which you must appreciate and consider if you would be a wise clinician. There are moments, of course, in cases of serious illness when you will think solely of the disease and its treatment; but when the corner is turned and the immediate crisis is passed, you must give your attention to the patient. Disease in man is never exactly the same as disease in an experimental animal, for in man the disease at once affects and is affected by what we call the emotional life. Thus, the physician who attempts to take care of a patient while he neglects this factor is as unscientific as the investigator who neglects to control all the conditions that may affect his experiment. The good physician knows his patients through and through, and his knowledge is bought dearly. Time, sympathy, and understanding must be lavishly dispensed, but the reward is to be found in the personal bond which forms the greatest satisfaction of the practice of medicine. One of the essential qualities of the clinician is interest in humanity, for the secret of the care of the patient is in caring for the patient.

16

The Doctor-Patient Relationship and the Issues of Pity, Sympathy, and Empathy
Harry A. Wilmer

A wise man has said that no matter what we teach our children they insist on behaving as we do. Our patients likewise tend to behave as we do. The more our anxiety and aggression are under control, the more theirs are likely to be. It is not enough to examine the psychology of the patient; the psychology of the professional staff must also be studied.

Physicians, by tradition and design, tend to consider their patients' behavior as if it had nothing to do with their own behavior (unless it be exemplary). However, destructive and agressive behavior can also have its genesis in the doctor-patient relationship. If we do not trust our patients, or if we expect bad behavior, defiance, and the like, if we hold that bad behavior calls for stringent punitive regimentation— we shall in all probability find what we expect.

"We may give advice, but we cannot give conduct," says *Poor Richard's Almanac*. We do not control our patients; they control them-selves. Doctors deal with the anti-social members of our society—the psychopaths, the character disorders—and sooner or later must face the frustration of disobedience and rebellion. The more you pursue such patients with punitive reactions, the more aggressive they become. The way lies not in more and more external control, but in the cultivation of understanding of his patients by the physician to facilitate the patient's internal control. Understanding involves the qualities of pity, sympathy, and empathy. It involves also firmness, confidence, honesty, and genuinely *caring* for patients as people. Sincerity, self-control, and understanding of *oneself* are essential. Understanding, like charity, begins at home.

Reprinted, with permission of the author, from *British Journal of Medical Psychology* 41 (1968): 243–248.

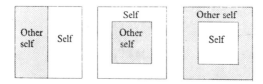

Figure 1
Model of concepts of pity, sympathy, and empathy. The block model is composed
of two elements: the self and the other self (the object of the relationship feeling).
The straight linear separation in pity is shown by a line drawn between the "two
halves." While this model is thought to be conceptually sound, in operation the
"self" progressively encroaches on the "other self," diminishing it in size and
importance. In the case of sympathy, the "self" surrounds the "other self,"
encompasses it, and is in contact with the outer boundaries of the "other self." In
the empathy model, the "self" is within the "other self," in contact with its inner
boundaries. However, only the outer boundaries of the "self" are in contact. To
be more precise, the boundaries are to be thought of not as one might think of
physical geographic borders, but as dynamic interfaces with the characteristics of
semi-permeable enclosure areas. (a) Pity: feeling—looks at and feels as if his
suffering were unbearable. (b) Sympathy: sharing—feels together with the
sufferer as if the pain were both of ours. (c) Empathy: understanding—enters into
sufferer, sees and feels from within as if pain were ours, but remains his.

Pity

Let us explore the three great qualities of human understanding so
important in the doctor-patient relationship: pity, sympathy, and
empathy. Understanding begins with consideration of the other
human being as a person and not an object or an *it*. In our scientific
laboratories we learn more and more about *its* and less and less about
him and her. If I say to someone "I pity you," he may not be pleased.
But if I am "moved to mercy and pity for a sufferer," this may suggest
a high quality of tenderness and feeling for suffering. Pity, unfortunately, has other connotations; "self-pity" is bad, and to be pitiful is
often to be contemptible. To feel pity for another may be a defense
against the unconscious feeling of cruelty toward him. Pity may also
be a defense against identification. Many people pity the poor and
downtrodden, but nevertheless tread on the downtrodden.

Of the three qualities under discussion, *pity* is historically the most
ancient word used to describe a feeling of tenderness aroused by
suffering or misfortune in others and prompting a desire for its relief.
It was first used in ths sense in 1290, in Middle English. In 1386,
Chaucer wrote: *"Pfor pitee renneth sonne in gentil herte."* The *Oxford
Dictionary* tells us that, in Middle English, both 'pite' and 'piete' are

used in the sense of 'piety' and were not completely differentiated before the 17th century. The Psalmist cried:

Turn me to have pity, for I am lonely and low;
Relieve the anguish of my heart, free me from all this pressure.

Three broadly different meanings attach to the words *piteous*, *pitiable*, and *pitiful*: to feel pity, to excite pity, to excite contempt. The person who feels pity in the first and second sense has compassion and a degree of emotional understanding. It is more likely to be felt by a physician for a poor patient than for a man of means. Pity, at best, is compassion; at worst, it is contempt.

Sympathy

Not so with sympathy. One may have pity 'for' another, but it is improper English to say 'sympathy for'. Our usage of the word *sympathy* is followed by 'with'. While pity may be a defense against identification, sympathy is identification—even sometimes to the point of loss of personal identity in fusion with another. Here is the distinction: Pity implies the strong and the weak, the rich and the poor, the big and the small. Pity may be commiseration, but sympathy is a sharing on an emotional level. But there cannot be complete equality or complete sharing, for, if this were reached, the sympathizer would be in the same plight as the other and therefore unable to help, for he himself would need help as much. Christopher Fry has remarked that "equality is a mortuary word." To help the sufferer, the helper must still remain somewhat unequal in being stronger. He must not merge his identity with that of the sufferer.

Sympathy has no "bad" connotations when concerned with human relationships. There are ancient uses of this word. At about the beginning of the 17th century it was used to describe the quality or state of being affected by the suffering or sorrow of another; a feeling of compassion. The qualities of accord and agreeableness, community of feeling, and harmony of disposition took on new meaning six decades later, when the word began to be used to describe the capacity for fellow-feeling, for sharing or entering into another's feeling. Milton, in *Paradise Lost*, wrote of "answering looks of sympathy and tone."

While the quality of sympathy is a positive attribute in human understanding, it may be contaminated with sentimentality, but then it is no longer sympathy.

Sympathy is also a quality of human communication we sometimes wish to shun. In 1872, Thomas Henry Huxley wrote a friend who had lost a son: "I hardly know whether I do well in writing to you. If such trouble befell me, there are very few people in the world from whom I could bear even sympathy."

One can feel sympathy with a person one has never known, and it can be coupled with advice. "Take the advice of a friend," wrote Abraham Lincoln in 1862 to a West Point cadet, "who though he never saw you, deeply sympathizes with you, and stick to your purpose." In the same letter, he adds, by way of establishing a relationship: "I am older than you, have felt badly myself, and know what I tell you is true. Adhere to your purpose and you will soon feel as well as you ever did. On the contrary, if you falter and give up, you will lose the power of keeping any resolution and will regret it all your life." Note that Lincoln looked within himself to find his understanding for the other. In modern times, all of physics and much in our world has been changed because Einstein put the observer into the equations, so relationships could be understood and hence biases and distortions removed; in interpersonal relationships we become participant observers.

If we think of sympathetic advice in terms of the doctor-patient relationship, it is the humanness of the doctor, his *being*, that permits the sympathetic reaction in a patient. When we attempt to understand someone by the process of sympathetic identification, we imagine how we would feel if we were in his place; that is, if we ourselves were in his circumstances. We share his suffering, imagining how we would feel if we were similarly afflicted. "If I were in his place" states the case for sympathy. In pity, on the other hand, there is a withdrawal from active identification, though there is a passive identification. In pity, the emotion we experience viewing the sufferer is a rebellion against identification. Pity arises from a more primitive imagining than does sympathy, for it is more completely within ourselves. The distinction between "self" and "other self" is much clearer in pity than in sympathy, where the "fellow-feeling" process begins. Sympathy remains a step toward empathy. Sympathy (*syn pathos*—together with suffering) is a process in which the feelings of the imitator remain essentially within himself. When both share similar feelings based on some unconscious quality, *identification* would be a more proper term, literally meaning "to make the same."

Empathy

Empathy is concerned with a much higher order of human relationship and understanding. If there is empathy there is real understanding of the other as another person. Here we understand his suffering in relationship to his personal and social world. We share, we feel for him and with him; psychologically, we get inside him for the purpose of understanding how he feels. In empathy it is as if: "If I were he."

To achieve an empathetic relationship, we use ourselves as the instrument for understanding, but by the same token we keep our own identity clearly separate. We understand the other as he feels by the process of being a participant observer. An empathetic observer enters into the equation and is then removed. In this situation the observer guards against his biases and misperceptions, and must therefore understand himself. Empathy involves two acts: identification with another person and awareness of one's own feelings after the identification (and thus awareness of the other's feelings). With empathy, true understanding is achieved by the power of entering into the experience or emotions of others.

The concept of empathy originated in 1912 when the German psychologist Theodor Lipps used the word *Einfühlung* (literally 'in-feeling') in an attempt to explain the emotional and kinaesthetic responses of the human observer to perceived objects. Its use was part of a theory which hypothesized that the understanding of another depends upon the capacity to imitate behavior. Empathic imitative behavioral responses are largely unconscious, and, while they may coexist with sympathy, they can be distinguished from sympathy as a sharing of activity or emotion rather than a sharing of attitude. A man will do unto others as he would have them do unto him so that he can diminish their suffering as he does his own.

Empathy signifies the imaginative projection of one's own consciousness into an object or person outside oneself. We sympathize with another human being when we share and suffer with him. An empathetic relationship is closer: We enter imaginatively into his life and feel as if it were our own. We cease being an outsider and become an insider. We borrow his feelings, look at them feel and understand them. We do not take them; we only enter into them to understand how he feels. One might say that pity rarely helps, sympathy commonly helps, empathy always helps.

Some people are reluctant to enter into the feeling world of another because it is too threatening. For example, if a patient comes with a long written list of complaints, the doctor may feel such disappointment and frustration that he begins at once to "write the patient off." He may order exhaustive laboratory tests to rule out the myriad of organic possibilities and may concentrate on these rather than on the patient's anxiety and emotional reasons for making a test which will reveal that "there is nothing wrong with the patient," when both doctor and patient know there is a lot wrong with him. This "wrong" is often his lot in life, as he sees it.

If the physician will really listen and try to understand by the process of imaginative projection into the other, he may find the clue to the patient's trouble. He must not be deceived by the cobweb of complaints spun like Mahomet's web. When Mahomet fled from Mecca, he hid in a cave and a spider wove its web over the entrance. The pursuing Koreishites passed by, convinced that no one had entered the cave because the cobweb was intact.

Let us consider empathy in action. Suppose a patient has lost a child and faces you in all the sadness of the moment. You may be moved by a great sense of pity, in which case you are overwhelmed by lack of power to bring back the dead child and by the tragedy of early death. If you say or wish to say "I know how you feel," you have committed an act of sympathy, but in truth you don't know how he feels. You only imagine how you would feel if you were in his position, if you shared common feelings. If you were to say this, the patient's inner voice might say: "How does he know how I feel? Did he lose his child? Can anyone ever know?" In his grief, the parent may hear only the warmth of your voice and sense the desire of one human being to comfort another. But these words have an omnipotent ring: If you really identified and projected yourself into the grieving one, you too would be struck by the overwhelming loss and would yourself need sympathy. You would be moved to tears and anguish and, like the sufferer, long for comfort.

A child's awareness of lack of empathy is vividly illustrated by a fragment from Pär Lagerkvist's story "Father and I":

We went on. Father was so calm as he walked there in the darkness with even strides, not speaking, thinking to himself. I couldn't understand how he could be so calm when it was so murky. I looked all around me in fear. Nothing but darkness everywhere.... Hugging closer to father, I whispered, "Father, why is it so horrible when it's dark?" "No, my boy, it's not horrible," he said, taking me by the hand. "Yes, father, it is." "No, my child, you mustn't think that, not when we know there is a God." I felt so lonely, forsaken. It was so strange that only I was afraid, not father, that we did not think the same. And strange that what he said didn't help me and stop me from being afraid. Not even what he said about God helped me....

In this fragment, the child sees his father as strong and unafraid and senses an incomprehensible fearlessness. Darkness itself is frightening, for he does not know what the unseen world is like. He reaches for his father, hugging for closeness, and asks why it is horrible when it is dark. what he is really saying is: "Why does it seem horrible to *me*?" But the father, in effect, says: "It is not horrible to *me*." Each is speaking for himself. Trying to reassure the child, the father reaches for his hand; but the child will not be put off and says that it is horrible to him. Again the father contradicts the child, denies that the child has any reason to be horrified. Defeated in his advice, the father tells the child what *not* to think, tells him he mustn't think as he does. Realizing he cannot have his own word accepted, father ends by appealing to the omnipotent Father of us all. Hence the child becomes silent, thinking inwardly, for there is no longer anything to say to father. The child now feels alone and forsaken, or rejected. And he tells us why: because he and his father do not think (that is, feel) the same. It is because his father was unable to put himself in the child's place, to understand that the child had his own childish, irrational or emotional reasons, more powerfully affecting him than the father's rational ones, for being afraid. The child felt it strange that his father was unable to stop him from being afraid. Not even the appeal to the presence of God could do it. Perhaps if that father could truly have empathized, the appeal to faith might have been successful. Faith can help people through trials, but it is understood by means of human relationships when we call upon it to explain and help us with human affairs.

The patient is the only person who has experienced precisely the problem he consults the doctor about. Once, in the Navy, I saw a sailor in a psychiatric consultation. He had jumped overboard to save a shipmate who had fallen into the sea. Though swimming desperately fast, he could not reach his friend and was horrified to see him sink beneath the waves. Back aboard ship, the sailor began to feel depressed. He was tormented by feelings of guilt—if only he hadn't hesitated those few seconds; if only he had swum harder; if only . . . if only. . . . Sleepless night followed sleepless night; nightmares and depression made him unfit for duty, and he was evacuated to a hospital, where the doctor, on admission, said, trying to help, "Other people have had similar things happen to them," to which the patient replied, "But it never happened to *me* before, sir." And this is really the point.

There is no short course to empathy. It is a lifetime pursuit. It is not TLC (tender loving care), so often prescribed. Can one really prescribe such things? Is it not a strange commentary that one writes an order for TLC? If special cases are singled out for special loving care, what about the others? Caring for every patient and striving always for empathy should be the everyday attitudes of staff members. The more natural and relaxed the caring, the better for everyone.

To paraphrase Saint Paul: "Then, there abide pity, sympathy, empathy, these three: but the greatest of these is empathy."

Identification for What?

How attentive is the listener to the problem placed before him? How sincere are his replies? Can he identify with the other person so as to know what he is really asking? What may occur if he does not possess those qualities is illustrated by a poignant episode of a young child who brought her crayon drawings home from school each evening for her father's inspection. Every night her father praised them. One day it occurred to her that father always used identical words of praise, so she decided to test him. She took a crayon and scribbled all over the paper. That night she waited anxiously for her father. He looked at the scribble and said, as he had every other time, "It's fine, daughter, it's very good," as he reached for the evening newspaper. He was astonished to see her burst into tears. He failed utterly to comprehend his daughter's discernment of his shallow pose of interest and the consequent undermining of her trust.

Many a doctor has conquered an illness he later seeks to treat and cure in others. When he remains silent about his own suffering, his strength is greater; when he is honest and matter-of-fact about his understanding by virtue of having been so afflicted, his therapeutic effectiveness is often enhanced. However, when he preaches or exhorts patients to endure and bases recovery on what he himself has overcome or learned to live with, he treads treacherous ground. By the belief "what I bore you can bear," generations of parents have sought revenge upon their children for the acts of their own parents, as teachers occasionally seek revenge for their parents and teachers before them.

Traditionally, the patient is expected to adapt himself to a more or less authoritarian medical social structure. He is expected to behave, to be good, to cause little trouble, to be cooperative and get well. If he misbehaves, becomes uncooperative, or fails to get well as expected, this awakens anxiety and occasionally depression in physicians. Since the vast majority of patients do behave, cooperate, and recover, the "logical" conclusion is that the one who does not is different in a disagreeable way. Further "logic" leads to the conclusion that it is all his fault and in no part ours, and this justifies our anger. He has brought it on himself, we think, and therefore we need not feel guilty for any part we might have had in his behavior. But often the doctor wishes that he would go away and not torment and upset composure and recovery rates. He is a nuisance, and we wish no more of him. We wish he were someone else's patient. In a word, we reject him, and he perceives this and thus loses trust and faith in us. And he begins to wish he were someone else's patient. He may remain to torment us or he may desert us, not because he is bad or recalcitrant but because, in effect, our wishes coincide with his destructive wishes.

We must learn how to become more understanding, tolerant, firm, and consistent. Increasing regimentation and rigidity will only foster more rebellion, and such rebellion is precisely "what the doctor ordered." We must search diligently for the way to empathy.

Ah, that I—you would have it so; George Dandin, you would have it so! This suits you nicely, and you are served right; you have precisely what you deserve.
Jean Molière, *George Dandin* (1668), Act 1, Scene 9.

References

Gould, J., and W. L. Kolb. *A Dictionary of the Social Sciences*. Free Press, 1965. See pp. 235–236.

Lagerkvist, P. "My father and I." In *The Eternal Smile and Other Stories*. Random House, 1954.

Wilmer, H. A. "Pity, sympathy and empathy." In *Personality, Stress and Tuberculosis*, ed. P. J. Sparer. International Universities Press.

Wilmer, H. A. "Rehabilitation: Being is belonging." *J. Chron. Dis.* 4 (1956): 212–215.

Wilmer, H. A. "Empathy and sensibility of heart." *N. Y. State J. Med.* 57 (1957): 2410–2413.

Studies on a Negotiated Approach to Patienthood
Aaron Lazare, Sherman Eisenthal, Arlene Frank, and John D. Stoeckle

In this paper we describe our clinical and research findings on a negotiated approach to the doctor-patient relationship. This work was stimulated by our clinical responsibility for a large number of patients seeking help at the psychiatric walk-in clinic of Massachusetts General Hospital and by our training responsibilities for first-year residents in psychiatry who staff the clinic. In this overview we shall show that the negotiation model can lead to a fruitful investigation of the doctor-patient relationship, that it can provide a conceptual framework that puts meaning and excitement in a clinical process that may otherwise be regarded as routine and tedious, and that it can serve as a prescription for physicians in relating to patients. This approach is based on the psychiatrist-patient relationship during the initial interview in a walk-in clinic. Our clinical work in other settings, however, leads us to believe that these concepts can be applied to other helping relationships in various settings at any stage of treatment.

Patient Requests

Our work began with a search for what patients wanted from the clinicians who were there to serve them. It was our initial belief that by learning what patients requested, we would have a better idea of how we might help. Our implicit assumption was that patients had requests in mind that they would share with the clinician under the proper conditions (Lazare et al. 1972).

It then became necessary to distinguish requests from other kinds of data which, together with requests, constitute what we term "the patient's perspective." This category of data includes the following:

Reprinted, with permission of the authors, from *The Doctor-Patient Relationship in International Perspective*, ed. E. Gallagher (Washington, D.C.: Fogarty Center, 1978).

(1) The *complaint*, or what the patient says is bothering him (" I am depressed and anxious"); (2) the *definition of the problem*, which may be an elaboration of the chief complaint; (3) the *goal*, or how the patient would ultimately like to feel, think, or act ("I would like to feel well enough so I can return to work"); (4) the *illness attribution*, or the patient's theory of the causes of what is wrong ("The reason I am so depressed is that my wife is threatening to leave me"); (5) the *expectation*, or what the patient anticipates will happen in and as a result of treatment ("I expect you will give me some pills to calm my nerves and make me feel less depressed"); and (6) the *request*, or what the patient wishes the clinician would do to achieve the desired goals ("I hope you can arrange to meet with my wife and me so we can figure out how to keep her from leaving me"). Each of these elements of the patient's perspective plays an important part in the negotiation *process* (Lazare et al. 1975a).

In the clinical literature, what patients want (requests) and what they anticipate will happen (expectations) have been regarded as the same. We have shown that expectations and requests are overlapping but not identical concepts (Eisenthal, Frank, and Lazare, unpublished). Each of the 14 request scales using our Patient Request Form (Lazare et al. 1975b, Lazare and Eisenthal, unpublished) was correlated to each of five expectations using the Williams (Williams et al. 1967) modifications of the Overall and Aronson (1963) Patient Expectations Questionnaire. From the resulting matrix of 70 correlations, we found 38 to be significant, with a median significant correlation of 0.27. A patient who expects that the clinic will provide medications or psychodynamic insight does not necessarily want these forms of treatment. Similarly, a patient who wants medication or psychodynamic insight does not necessarily expect that the clinic will provide these forms of treatment. This distinction, we believe, has been overlooked in some of the research on expectations.

To determine the range and definition of patient requests, we conducted brief interviews of several hundred patients who were waiting for initial evaluation in the walk-in clinic. Most patients who came of their own volition were willing to state a request when the investigators asked the questions with enough persistence and compassion. We were then able to compose definitions of what we believed to be 14 distinct requests in language that was respectful and understandable to the patient while meaningful to the clinician. The requests include *administrative request, advice, clarification, community triage, confession, control, medical, nothing, psychodynamic insight, psychological expertise, reality contact, social intervention, succorance,* and *ventilation*

(Lazare et al. 1972, Lazare et al. 1975b). These categories were settled upon only after numerous investigators on our research team attempted to elicit the full range of requests from different patients in the clinic. Simultaneously, we developed several versions of the Patient Request Form (PRF), a self-rating questionnaire easily completed by patients in the waiting room of the walk-in clinic. The third and most recent version of the PRF consists of 84 items which measure the 14 hypothesized requests (Lazare and Eisenthal, unpublished). We tested the hypothesis that 14 clinically derived categories of patient requests are relatively independent mathematically by factor-analyzing 84 PRF scores of 296 patients. Thirteen of the factors corresponded to 13 of the 14 hypothesized request categories. Only *nothing* did not receive clear confirmation as a request category. (The appendix describes each of the 14 requests and the sample items of PRF that measure it.)

These 14 request-category scores were then factor-analyzed to establish higher-level dimensions. Three distinct request dimensions were found. For the first dimension (*reality contact, control, succorance, medical,* and *ventilation*), the problem is seen as residing within the patient, is felt to be serious, has an affective-urgent quality, and stresses the passive desire for someone to take over in an active and giving manner. For the second dimension (*clarification, psychodynamic insight, psychological expertise,* and *community triage*), the problem is also seen as residing within the patient, but is not necessarily felt to be serious, and asks that the patient's role be active, collaborative, and more cognitive than emotional. For the third dimension (*administrative request, social intervention, nothing,* and *advice*), the problem is seen as residing outside the patient and stresses action by the clinician with minimal involvement on the part of the patient.

In order to study the degree of endorsement of the various requests, we devised an index of endorsement. It is based on the percentage of patients who say for each request "This is exactly what I want." The rank order was *clarification* (55 percent), *psychological expertise* (51 percent), *psychodynamic insight* (47 percent), *control* (44 percent), *ventilation* (41 percent), *medical* (36 percent), *succorance* (36 percent), *reality contact* (31 percent), *advice* (27 percent), *community triage* (26 percent), *confession* (20 percent), *administrative request* (10 percent), *social intervention* (9 percent), and *nothing* (9 percent).

To appreciate the depth of suffering of many patients as well as their willingness to acknowledge the importance of specific interventions which they feel will help, one must study the individual items of the PRF and their degree of endorsement. For instance, 31 percent of patients say what they "exactly want" is "I need to talk to someone so I will keep in touch with reality," 46 percent of patients say what they "exactly want" is "I want you to stop my feelings before they overpower me," and 24 percent of patients say what they "exactly want" is "If I can feel less guilty, I would be helped." Contrary to the widely held belief that our predominantly lower-class patient population wants "just support" or medication, we found that the most common requests were for some type of psychological understanding (*clarification, psychodynamic insight,* and *psychological expertise*).

A cross-validation of the PRF on a sample of college students at a university mental-health service yielded a factor structure nearly identical to that described above. Only *succorance* and *nothing* failed to receive clear confirmation as request categories. Thus, the PRF items and the request categories seem to be applicable to populations of different ages and in different clinical settings (Eisenthal, Lazare, and Solomon, unpublished).

The Expression of Patient Requests

Patient requests have, for the most part, been ignored in the psychiatric literature. Several investigators, however, have studied concepts related to patient requests. Hill (1969) identified and described seven clusters of patient purposes in therapy; Wilson (1973) and others have studied patients' goals, and several investigators have investigated patient expectations in an attempt to understand premature terminations from psychotherapy as a function of incongruent expectations between therapist and patient (Overall and Aronson 1963; Heine and Trosman 1960; Garfield and Wolper 1963; Goin et al. 1965; Borghi 1968).

Patient requests have also been ignored in the conduct of the interview. Clinicians describe several reasons why they do not elicit patient requests (Lazare et al. 1975a). Some believe that: (1) Patients do not know what they want. (2) The request is irrelevant because it is a distortion of an unconscious need. (3) The clinician's elicitation of the request would be tantamount to turning over authority to the patient and might even result in the patient's regarding the clinician as unprofessional. (4) Eliciting the request would open a Pandora's box of insatiable demands that would overwhelm the clinician.

While many clinicians fail to elicit requests, many patients will not spontaneously verbalize requests, thereby joining the clinician in an apparent conspiracy of not sharing and not exploring. Patients explain their behavior in several ways: (1) They may believe that it is not their role as patient to state a request. (2) They may view the clinician as an adversary who has the ultimate power to refuse the request, so that its expression must be carefully worded and timed. (3) They may fear that in expressing a request they may be exposing themselves to rejection and humiliation by the clinician.

For the clinician who is intent on eliciting patient requests, we have several suggestions based on our own experience. The request is best elicited after some meaningful interaction—such as a discussion of the nature of the problem—has occurred. This helps foster the necessary rapport. Eliciting the request at the very start of the interview may communicate to the patient that the clinician is more interested in a disposition than in knowing what is wrong. Eliciting the request at the end of the interview deprives both parties of time for the opportunity to enter into negotiations over the request. In eliciting the request, it is most useful to ask questions such as "What do you hope (or wish) I (the clinic) can do to help you with the problem?" This approach encourages the patient to ask for things he wants but may not even feel are possible to have. In contrast, a question such as "What do you want?" may be perceived as rude or confronting. Certainly the clinician's tone and attitude in asking any question is at least as important as the content and the timing of the question. After any elicitation question is asked, the clinician must be prepared for the common responses: "I don't know; you are the doctor," or "You tell me; I would not be here if I knew." The clinician must then communicate that he is not asking the patient to determine or control the treatment, but that the patient's wishes and hopes are still important to know so he can best understand the patient and provide the appropriate treatment.

Moving from the clinical to the experimental, we felt it was important to explore the assumption that serves as a basis for the above clinical recommendations to elicit patient requests: that patients do come with requests, whose expression depends on the sanctioning behavior of the clinician. In a series of studies (Eisenthal and Lazare 1976a, unpublished) we have shown that 99 percent of patients filling out a PRF will state at least one request that they strongly endorse, whereas only 69 percent of patients will verbalize a specific request using a structured pre-intake interview. In the natural setting of the clinical interview, we found that 63 percent of patients expressed specific requests. This group breaks down into 37 percent of patients who spontaneously emitted a specific request and 26 percent of patients who verbalized a request after the clinician's elicitation. The importance of the clinician's behavior in eliciting the request was emphasized by the significant increase in patient's verbalizations of specific requests following a second elicitation inquiry.

These findings support the view that most patients (63–69 percent) are predisposed to express specific requests in an intake interview. It is not clear to what degree the remaining 31–37 percent of patients have requests in mind but have not had sufficient sanction from the clinician to express their request, or do not have requests clearly formulated and need to have the experience of the clinical interaction to help them formulate in their minds exactly what they want. Similarly, one may ask whether the PRF, with its 99 percent endorsement, sanctions patients' expressing what they already have clearly formulated in mind, or whether it functions like the clinical interaction which crystallizes for a patient what had been a vague sense of what he wanted.

We attempted to identify which patients are most likely to express specific requests, since some patients do not state requests or state them in a nonspecific, general, or noncommittal form. The patients who tend to be specific can be characterized as (1) female, (2) coming to the clinic at their own instigation rather than at the suggestion of others, (3) being prior patients to the clinic, (4) having a complaint which is interpersonal or somatic rather than one which is vague, general, or situational. These data suggest that clinicians may need to help certain identifiable patient groups in formulating and expressing their requests. The process of negotiation, we believe, would be considerably less effectual without these specific request data.

Clinical Value of Eliciting and Responding to Patient Request

As we elicited requests, we became aware that gathering this data had (1) considerable diagnostic value and (2) a facilitative effect on the therapeutic flow of the interview. These two perspectives are illustrated clinically in eight case histories reported in two papers (Lazare et al. 1972, 1975a). As to the diagnostic aspect, the patient's statement of his request helps to define the problem more clearly, helps to focus on the priorities of the patient, and provides important clues on the most useful interventions. Without the elicitation of the request, the clinician is apt to mistakenly respond to a need he may feel the patient has or ought to have. For instance, the clinician may believe the patient may want and need the opportunity to ventilate and may therefore assume the role of a receptive but passive listener. Employing such a role could be insufficient and possibly harmful if the patient wanted and needed reality contact, control, or confession. The patient might have become more out of touch with reality or more out of control, or felt more guilty.

By distinguishing a wide variety of distinct requests or perceived treatment needs, clinicians can discard or go beyond the rubric of "supportive" and address specific patient needs with more precise clinical responses. In the past, diagnosing the need for supportive help often elicited vague clinical responses that often turned out not to be supportive.

These supportive requests were assumed to be made predominantly by patients of the lower social classes, while patients of the middle and upper social classes made "more sophisticated" requests, e.g., *psychodynamic insight* and *clarification*. This assumption has been used to explain why lower-class applicants to psychiatric clinics are less readily accepted for psychotherapy, are more likely to be assigned to less experienced psychotherapists, are judged as being less socially improved upon termination of treatment, and are more apt to terminate prematurely (Heine and Trosman 1960; Garfield and Wolper 1963; Borghi 1968).

To explore some of these assumptions, we examined the relationship between patient requests and social class (Frank, Eisenthal, and Lazare, unpublished). The major conclusion of this study was that patient requests are largely independent of social class. More specifically, patients from classes I–IV did not differ from each other in the kinds of help (requests) they wanted from the clinic. Class V patients wanted more active help (e.g., *social intervention, community triage*, and *administrative help*) and more authoritarian information (e.g., *psychological expertise*) than higher-class patients but just as much *psychodynamic insight* and *clarification*. Even with these class V differences in requests, social class never accounted for more than 5 percent of the variance in PRF scores. The important findings, it seems to us, are that lower-class patients want psychological interventions much more than had previously been assumed and that middle- and upper-class patients want much more of the so-called "supportive" interventions than has been previously assumed. These findings should help dispel the notion that the inequities in care provided to lower-class patients are a consequence of their having the "wrong" requests or expectations and that some requests are second-class because of the groups of patients who make them.

With regard to the clinical value of eliciting and responding to patient requests, we found the process particularly useful in facilitating the therapeutic flow of the interview. This could occur in several ways: First, by eliciting the request in an empathic manner, the clinician (1) diminishes the patient's need to engage in evasive activities meant to test the clinician's flexibility, interest, and concern; (2) conveys to the patient the collaborative nature of the interview; (3) facilitates the development of a therapeutic alliance; and (4) changes the focus of the interview toward the task. Second, by acknowledging or responding to the patient's request, the clinician encourages the patient to feel free to express more progressive requests. For example, a patient may not be able to ask for *social intervention* until the request for *control* or *reality contact* has been responded to. Failure to respond to the request may lead the patient to make a regressive request. For example, when the request for *psychodynamic insight* (a more progressive request) is not responded to, the patient may feel misunderstood and frustrated and ask for *advice* (a more regressive request). The language of "progressive" and "regressive" is meant to convey a hierarchy of requests which is dynamically influenced by the clinical interaction. This notion is currently under study. And finally, hearing the request often relieves the clinician of the fear that he will be overwhelmed by demands he cannot respond to. He is frequently surprised that patients do not want radical changes in character and symptomatology, that they do not want to become different human beings.

The Interview as a Clinical Negotiation

In the process of investigating patient requests, we observed that conflict between the clinician and patient is often present. Sometimes it is explicit, as in cases where the patient asks for medication and the clinician responds with a statement that another treatment is indicated. More usually the conflict is implicit, not immediately or directly apparent, as when the patient has a request he has not verbalized and the clinician is not about to grant the unstated request. An example would be a patient who wants to be hospitalized but neither verbalizes the request nor offers clinical data that would lead the clinician to spontaneously suggest hospitalization. As we pursued the nature and the extent of conflicts over requests, it became apparent that there were also conflicts over the definition of the problem, the illness attribution, the goals, the priorities in treatment, and important intangible matters such as self-esteem, honor, principles, trust, and saving face.

Given the wide variety of issues over which there could be conflict and the high probability that there would be conflict over at least some of them in any clinical encounter, we concluded that (1) *conflict is inherent in the relationship between clinician and patient* and (2) *conflict resolution by negotiation is a critical part of successful helping relationships.* Various aspects of conflict and/or negotiating behavior have been described by Freidson (1970) and Balint (1957) for the doctor-patient relationship and by Scheff (1968) and Levinson et al. (1967) for the psychotherapist-patient relationship.

By negotiation, we refer to a coming together or conferring over a source of conflict with the purpose of achieving some agreement (Onions 1953). In more operational terms it is "the process whereby two or more parties attempt to settle what each shall give and take, or perform and receive, in a transaction between them (Rubin and Brown 1975). The failure to negotiate successfully may be followed on the patient's part with dissatisfaction, noncompliance with treatment recommendations, changing physicians, and/or litigation. On the clinician's part, failure to negotiate may be followed by referral elsewhere or by the withholding of goodwill and support that would otherwise be offered.

The optimal goal of negotiation is to resolve conflict so that the clinician feels that he has done what he believes to be professionally appropriate while the patient feels he has received that which is in his best physical and psychological interest. Compromises are acceptable so long as they still provide enough satisfaction to make the relationship worthwhile and do not breach professional standards.

A number of influences on the negotiation process are identifiable. They include (1) the relative social status of both parties; (2) the relative intellectual, social, and fiscal resources of both parties; (3) the available alternatives to treatment; (4) the familiarity of each party with his role; (5) who does the asking and who has the power to refuse; (6) the site and physical arrangements for the negotiations; (7) fiscal arrangements; (8) the availability of third parties; (9) the answerability of each party to independent constituencies; (10) the therapeutic ideology of the clinician; and (11) the nature of the problem, request, and goals. Influences 1–6 indicate that clinician-patient negotiations are not between parties with equal power. The clinician is apt to have (1) a higher social status; (2) greater intellectual, social, and fiscal resources; (3) greater control over treatment alternatives; (4) more familiarity with his role; (5) the power to refuse the request; and (6) the opportunity to choose the site and make the physical arrangements for the negotiations.

In a study relevant to influences on the negotiation process, we investigated the role of the site, professional experience, and the nature of the request (Eisenthal, Ferrell, and Lazare 1976). We wondered how these three variables would influence the clinician's comfort in hearing a request (and we assumed that greater comfort facilitates successful negotiations). We found that, for psychiatric residents, (1) greater clinical experience was associated with greater comfort in hearing all requests; (2) the inpatient setting was related to greater comfort in hearing the majority of requests (clinician comfort is highest in the walk-in clinic for *community triage* and in the psychotherapy clinic for *psychodynamic insight*); and (3) there was greater comfort with requests that were psychological rather than nonpsychological and dynamic rather than nondynamic. Knowledge about comfort over hearing requests (and presumably the ability to negotiate over them) may be useful in decisions over where to train student clinicians and what to train them for.

In order to help the clinician to negotiate more effectively to attain goals which serve both parties, we are developing a series of strategies (Lazare, Eisenthal, and Frank, unpublished). We are also trying to identify and describe the clinical conditions under which each strategy will be useful. We have divided the negotiation process into five major sequential stages, each of which has identifiable negotiating strategies associated with it. The five major stages are (1) developing and sustaining an atmosphere for negotiation, (2) establishing the nature of the conflict, (3) general educative strategies, (4) specific strategies, and (5) end-state negotiations. In our experience thus far, the process of attaining the first two stages resolves conflicts in the vast majority of clinical situations. The remaining strategies are employed in the minority of cases where this initial resolution has not occurred.

We believe that the most sensitive and sought-after clinicians are the most effective negotiators. They sense the patient's worries, misconceptions about the illness, and hesitations about treatment. They create an atmosphere that encourages patients to present their perspective, on the one hand, and encourages them to hear the clinician's perspective, on the other hand. These clinicians know how to be forceful, but they also have learned how to compromise without losing their professional integrity.

Negotiations and Clinical Hypothesis

If we are to negotiate in a way that is meaningful and helpful to the patient, we must go beyond the clinician's psychiatric or medical diagnoses with their accepted treatments. This is because it is the clinician's task to treat not only disease but also illness behavior, including the patient's decision to become a patient. That someone has a passive-dependent personality disorder or a hysterical character is informative, but it is of little use in understanding why the patient is in the clinic, what he needs, and what the clinician might do to help. Even in medical settings, knowledge of diagnosis, particularly with chronic illness, is of little value in responding to illness behavior. In these situations it is often more important to provide emotional support and communication of information, since the medical diagnosis is already established.

The patient has a particular understanding of the problem, one or more goals, and a series of requests. Reaching an agreement with the patient over the definition of the problem and the reason for seeking help then becomes an essential preliminary task in the negotiation process. Without such agreement, the task of negotiating goals and requests can be seriously misdirected. How can the clinician and the patient proceed when the patient thinks his trouble is a restlessness with the situation in his life while the clinician believes the trouble is a neurotic depression, or when the patient thinks the problem is the need for a physical checkup while the clinician believes there is no suspected diagnosis to warrant a checkup?

In order to negotiate more responsively over the definition of the problem, the clinician must broaden his concept of diagnoses to an extended range of clinical hypotheses. These hypotheses explain human behavior in biological, social, psychological, and behavioral terms. An extended range of hypotheses has been proposed for the medical interview by the Royal College of General Practitioners (1972), and one for the psychiatric interview has been proposed by our group (Lazare 1973, 1976). In our proposal, each patient may be best understood by several of the following clinical hypotheses. PSYCHOLOGICAL: (1) Knowledge of the patient's *personality style* explains in part why he has come for treatment; (2) knowledge of the *precipitating event* and its dynamic meaning explains in part why the patient has come for treatment; (3) the patient's problem can be understood in part as a manifestation of *unresolved grief*; (4) the patient's problem can be understood in part as a *developmental crisis*; (5) the patient's problem can be understood in part in terms of *ego functioning and related psychodynamic issues*. SOCIAL: (6) *Cultural factors* influencing perceptions, beliefs, values, behavioral norms, and expectations give clues as to the choice, expression, and seriousness of symptomatology and explain in part the patient's reasons for seeking treatment; (7) the patient's problem can be understood in part as a result of a *change in the social space*; (8) *social isolation* explains in part the patient's problem; (9) the patient's problem can be understood in part as a *social communication*; (10) the patient's problem can be understood in part in terms of its *social impact*. BIOLOGICAL: (11) The patient's problem can be understood in part as an *affective disorder*; (12) the patient is suffering, in part, from *schizophrenia or other functional psychosis*; (13) the patient's problem can be understood in part as an *organic disease*; (14) the patient is suffering in part from *alcohol or drug abuse*; (15) the patient's problem can be understood in part in terms of *symptoms responsive to psychotropic agents*. BEHAVIORAL: (16) The problem can be partially understood in terms of *undesired behaviors*, their antecedent and reinforcing events, and specific treatment programs for these behaviors.

Let us apply these hypotheses to the first example. The patient complaining of restlessness with his life situation is a 40-year-old male who is contemplating ending his marriage and leaving a responsible job for something more fulfilling. In the midst of struggling with these decisions, he feels frustrated, powerless, and depressed. Affixing a label of depressive neurosis may help neither the clinician nor the patient. On the other hand, through the clinical hypothesis of a *developmental crisis* (perhaps combined with other hypotheses) both parties can better agree as to the complex series of developmental issues occurring around age 40 and then negotiate over goals and methods of treatment. In the second example, the patient requesting a physical checkup has just arrived in a town in which she has no friends or relatives. Although she suffers from hypertension, the disease is under control. In this situation, if the clinician uses the clinical hypothesis of *social isolation* rather than the medical diagnosis of "no acute medical problem," he can better understand the nature of the problem in terms that have meaning for the patient. The patient's request for a physical examination can then be understood as an attempt to establish social contact through the medical system. Negotiations over goals and methods can then proceed.

The Case Record

Negotiation between doctor and patient is at the heart of the clinical encounter. Yet the negotiation process is not discussed in clinical conferences, is not taught in any systematic manner, and is not recorded. In order to focus attention on this essential process, we have chosen to alter the clinical record on the assumption that if one has to write about it, one has to have thought about it. We propose three changes in the case record. First, instead of the 'Chief Complaint,'' we substitute the heading of "Patient Perspectives"—an expanded category composed of the request as well as the complaint, the definition of the problem, the illness attribution, and the goals. Second, the data of the history and the physical exam should be organized in such a way that if becomes clear how the clinical hypotheses are confirmed or refuted. Third, "Treatment Plan" is changed to "Negotiated Treatment Plan." Here the clinician indicates how he responded to the patient perspectives, what conflicts remain, and what treatment is planned (Lazare, Rubinstein, Keller, et al., unpublished). The use of such a record, we have found, has the impact of prescribing the clinical process.

Evaluation of a Negotiated Approach to Patienthood

At this stage of our work we can offer four pieces of indirect evidence to support the usefulness of the negotiated approach.

1. *This approach is useful in making clinical decisions to offer treatment.* To the best of our knowledge, the walk-in clinic referred to in this paper is the only outpatient setting that has shown that the decision to refer a patient into the clinic system is made independent of diagnosis or social class (Lazare et al. 1976). (Referral ensures further evaluation but does not guarantee treatment.) Previous studies have consistently shown that the upper classes and the healthier were preferentially referred to and accepted into the system. We believe our admission policy can be explained in part by the use of hypotheses which we find to be more relevant than most diagnoses, by a reliance on patient requests (which are for the most part independent of social class), and by the use of a negotiated approach which takes patients where they are rather than where the clinicians thinks they ought to be.

2. *This approach can promote patient satisfaction.* In evaluating the initial interview in the walk-in clinic from the patient's perspective, we found that patient satisfaction correlated better with indexes of a negotiated approach than with symptom relief or a belief that their feelings and problems were understood (Eisenthal and Lazare 1976). The indexes of the negotiated approach include (a) the patient's belief that the clinician helped him verbalize what it was that he wanted and (b) the patient's belief that he participated in the treatment decision. These findings persisted even when the patient did not receive the desired treatment plan. In a subsequent study evaluating the initial interview from the clinician's perspective, we found that the clinician believed that patient satisfaction was dominated by the desire for symptom relief. The clinician, therefore, does not accu-

rately perceive what most satisfies the patient (Eisenthal and Lazare 1977).

3. *This approach is useful in training.* We believe that the successful use of a walk-in clinic for training first-year residents in psychiatry can be accounted for, in part, by the availability of the conceptual framework described in this paper, which puts meaning and excitement into the clinical encounter. This setting provides the student with a unique opportunity to see large numbers of unscreened patients who present with a heterogeneous group of problems that do not easily lend themselves to official diagnostic categories or psychodynamic formulations. No other training center, to our knowledge, uses a walk-in setting for first-year resident training because of the frustration, fatigue, clinical uncertainty, and sense of helplessness in treating such a population. With the approach described in this paper, even when the diagnosis is unclear, a request can be elicited, several clinical hypotheses can be considered, the ensuing process and relationship can be understood as a negotiated process, and a sophisticated dialogue between the resident and supervisor can occur. The first-year training program in the walk-in clinic is [at this writing] in its ninth year, and it continues to enjoy the enthusiasm of its residents (Lazare and Eisenberg 1970; Lazare, Eisenthal, Keller et al., unpublished).

4. *The negotiated approach is being easily integrated into primary-care units.* Clinicians and teachers in these settings find these concepts valuable for clinical care and teaching. The material is currently included in the didactic presentations to residents in primary care. In addition, preliminary research in the Primary Care Practice at Massachusetts General Hospital suggests that there is a medical counterpart to the work described in this paper on requests and negotiations.

Criticism and Response

The work described in this paper has been subject to two major criticisms: (1) that it takes too much power away from the clinician and inappropriately gives it to the patient, and (2) that it inappropriately gives too much power to the clinician at the expense of the patient. Critics who take the first position often believe that patients do not have requests, or that the requests are irrelevant to clinical needs. They may fear that eliciting the patient's request puts the patient in the role of a shopper at a supermarket, who may take what he pleases. The clinician thereby dilutes his most effective source of influence, his legitimate authority. He further fears that he will find himself helpless and impotent as he opens up a Pandora's box of unending, complex, insatiable demands. These beliefs and fears are unnecessary. Patients do have requests, but the expression of requests does not bind the clinician to agree to fulfill them. They do make him more knowledgeable and encourage the patient in turn to be influenced by the clinician. The aim of negotiation is the maintenance of the highest professional standards, not their surrender. Finally, the expression of the request is usually a more modest statement of perceived needs than the clinician had anticipated.

Critics who take the second position argue that the physician already has too much power over patients and that the tools provided by the negotiation paradigm, particularly the strategies of negotiation, put the patient at an even greater disadvantage. We believe that the use of the negotiation concept—developing trust, establishing expertise, educating the patient, providing sample treatment—is part of the physician's job. If the physician thinks that surgical rather than medical intervention is the treatment of choice, it is his task to make the best possible case for his belief and thereby influence the patient. Should the physician not attempt to develop trust, establish his expertise, or educate the patient? What is really at issue, we believe, is not the physician's skill at negotiating but the possibility that he may influence patients to accept treatments that are not responsive to their needs or that may even be deleterious to their well-being. The solution to these abuses is not to discourage the negotiation process, which we regard as a part of the treatment, but to encourage patients to be more educated consumers and to encourage varied auditing of medical practice. (Both of these safeguards may well come from outside of the medical profession.) The negotiation process we describe and prescribe enhances the power of both parties and leads to better clinical care.

Appendix: Patient Requests and Sample Items

Administrative request. The patient is seeking administrative or legal assistance from the clinic to help him with his current dilemma. The specific request may be to provide a disability evaluation, a medical excuse to leave work, medical permission to return to work, permission to drive, admission to a hospital, or testimony in court. These powers are delegated by society to particular professionals or institutions. The power may be subsequently rescinded, or, as in the case of therapeutic abortions, may no longer be necessary.

Item: I need the clinic's authority to deal with a certain agency I am having trouble with.

Advice. The patient wants guidance about what to do in personal or social matters. He may already have formed an opinion but now wants professional advice. He wants to know the "right" things, the "best" thing, or the "wisest" thing to do. He may want the advice in order to have the clinician share the responsibility for a decision he is about to make.

Item: If someone could tell me the right thing to do about my personal affairs, I would be helped.

Clarification. The patient wants help to put his feelings, thoughts, or behavior in some perspective. He does not want to be told what to do but would rather take an active role in the therapeutic process. Often the patient wants the help to be able to make a decision. He wants to understand; he wants to see his choices. The patient usually sees his problem as being acute and not a part of an ongoing neurotic pattern.

Item: I want to clear things up, to make the best decision for myself.

Community triage. The patient is requesting information as to where in his community he can get the help he needs. He sees the clinic as an available source of the necessary information.

Item: I would like someone to tell me where in my community I can get help.

Confession. The patient feels guilty about what he has said, thought, or done and hopes that by talking to the therapist he will feel better. Specifically, the patient wants to be forgiven. He hopes the clinician (authority figure) will see the misdeed as medical or psychological in origin and therefore not bad.

Item: I want to confess to someone what I have thought or done.

Control. The patients is feeling overwhelmed and out of control. He may fear hurting himself or someone else, or going crazy. He is saying: "Please take over. I can no longer manage."

Item: I am losing my mind; I need help.

Medical. The patient sees his problem as being physical in origin, like any other medical condition, as opposed to psychological or situational in origin. He often refers to his problem as "nerves," or as a "nervous condition." The patient, accordingly, hopes for a medical kind of treatment, such as pills, ECT, hospitalization, or medical advice. He expects to take a passive role in the treatment.

Item: I want someone to examine me to figure out the cause of my nervous condition.

Psychological expertise. The patient believes that the source of his problem is psychological rather than physical or situational. He is asking the professional to provide an explanation as to why he thinks, feels, or acts the way he does. The patient anticipates playing a passive role in the interaction, contributing only that information which the expert requires.

Item: I want someone to tell me why I do the things I do.

Psychodynamic insight. The patient perceives his problem as psychological in origin, as evolving from his early development, and as having a repetitive quality. As a result, he is left feeling unhappy and unfulfilled, but not overwhelmed or out of control. He expects to take an active, collaborative role in taking about the roots of his problem and hopes that a better understanding of his problem will enable him to change.

Item: I think a lot of my problems are related to my past. I'd like to talk to someone so I can learn to overcome them.

Reality contact. The patient feels that he is losing hold of reality. He wants to talk to someone who is psychologically stable and "safe." The request is for the clinician to help him "check out" or "keep in touch with" reality so that he will feel he is thinking straight and not losing his mind.

Item: I want to talk to someone so I will feel sane.

Social intervention. The patient sees the problem as residing primarily in the people or situations around him. Because he feels that he does not possess the resources to effect the necessary change, he is asking the clinic to intervene on his behalf. He is asking not for the legal powers of the clinic but for its social influence.

Item: I want you to speak to the person or people who are giving me trouble.

Succorance. The patient is feeling empty, alone, not cared for, deprived, or drained. He wants the clinician to care, to be involved, to be comforting, to be warm and giving so that he can feel replenished and warm inside. It is not so much the content of the interchange that is requested as its affective quality of warmth and caring.

Item: I'm here because I need the warmth of human contact.

Ventilation. The patient would like to tell the clinician about various feelings and affect-laden experiences. The patient anticipates that "getting it out" or "getting it off his chest" will be therapeutic. He feels that he is carrying around a burden which he would like to leave with the clinician. In contrast to confession, the patient does not feel guilty and does not need or want forgiveness.

Item: I want to get some painful feelings out of my system.

Nothing. Patients who make no request are a heterogeneous group. They may have been referred without proper preparation; they may be psychotic; they may have problems but not be seeking help at this time; they may want help but be reluctant to state the problem; they may not need help; they may be in the wrong clinic.

Item: someone else brought me in here but I do not need psychiatric care.

References

Balint, M. 1957. *The Doctor, His Patient, and the Illness.* International Universities Press.

Borghi, J. 1968. Premature termination of psychotherapy and patient-therapist expectations. *American Journal of Psychotherapy* 22: 460–473.

Eisenthal, S., and Lazare, A. 1976a. Specificity of patient requests in the initial interview. *Psychological Reports* 38: 739–748.

Eisenthal, S., and Lazare, A. 1976b. Evaluation of the initial interview in a walk-in clinic: The patient's perspective on a "customer approach." *Journal of Nervous and Mental Disease* 162: 169–176.

Eisenthal, S., and Lazare, A. 1977. Evaluation of the initial interview in a walk-in clinic: The clinician's perspective on a "negotiated approach." *Journal of Nervous and Mental Disease* 164: 30–35.

Eisenthal, S., and Lazare, A. Expression of Patient Requests in the Initial Interview. Unpublished.

Eisenthal, S., Ferrell, R., and Lazare, A. 1976. Attitude of psychiatric residents to patient requests. *American Journal of Psychiatry* 143: 1079–1081.

Eisenthal, S., Frank, A., and Lazare, A. The Relationship of Patient Requests to Patient Expectations. Unpublished.

Eisenthal, S., Lazare, A., and Solomon, F. Patient Requests in a University Mental Health Service. Unpublished.

Frank, A., Eisenthal, S., and Lazare, A. Social Class Influences on Patient Requests in a Walk-in Psychiatric Clinic. Unpublished.

Freidson, E. 1970. *Profession of Medicine.* Dodd, Mead.

Garfield, S., and Wolper, M. 1963. Expectations regarding psychotherapy. *Journal of Nervous and Mental Disease* 137: 353–362.

Goin, M., Yamamoto, J., and Silverman, J. 1965. Therapy congruent with class-linked expectations. *Archives of General Psychiatry* 13: 133–137.

Goroll, A., Stoeckle, J., and Lazare, A. 1974. Teaching the medical interview: An experiment with first year students. *Journal of Medical Education* 49: 957–962.

Heine, R., and Trosman, H. 1960. Initial expectation of the doctor-patient interaction as a factor in continuance in psychotherapy. *Psychiatry* 23: 275–278.

Hill, J. A. 1969. Therapist goals, patient aims, and patient satisfaction in psychotherapy. *Journal of Clinical Psychology* 25: 455–459.

Lazare, A. 1973. Hidden conceptual models in clinical psychiatry. *New England Journal of Medicine* 288: 345–351.

Lazare, A. 1976. The psychiatric examination in the walk-in clinic: Hypotheses generation and hypotheses testing. *Archives of General Psychiatry* 33: 96–102.

Lazare, A., Cohen, F., Jacobson, A. M., et al. 1972. The walk-in patient as a "customer": a key dimension in evaluation and treatment. *American Journal of Orthopsychiatry* 42: 872–883.

Lazare, A., and Eisenberg, L. 1970. Psychiatric residency training: An outpatient first year program. *Seminars in Psychiatry* 2: 201–210.

Lazare, A., and Eisenthal, S. Patient Requests in a Walk-in Clinic: Replication of Factor Analysis in an Independent Sample. Unpublished.

Lazare, A., Eisenthal, S., and Frank, A. 1976. Disposition decisions in a walk-in clinic. *American Journal of Orthopsychiatry* 46: 503–509.

Lazare, A., Eisenthal, S., and Frank, A. Strategies of Negotiations in the Initial Psychiatric Interview. Unpublished.

Lazare, A., Eisenthal, S., Keller, M., et al. First Year Training in an Outpatient Department: An Eight Year Followup. Unpublished.

Lazare, A., Eisenthal, S., and Wasserman, L. 1975a. The customer approach to patienthood: Attending to patient requests in a walk-in clinic. *Archives of General Psychiatry* 32: 553–558.

Lazare, A., Eisenthal, S., Wasserman, L., et al. 1975b. Patient requests in a walk-in clinic. *Comprehensive Psychiatry* 16: 467–477.

Lazare, A., Rubinstein, J., Keller, M., et al. A Negotiated/Hypothesis Testing Case Record. Unpublished.

Levinson, D. J., Merrifield, J., and Berg, K. 1967. Becoming a patient. *Archives of General Psychiatry* 17: 385–406.

Onions, C. T. (ed.). 1953. *The Oxford Universal Dictionary.* Clarendon.

Overall, B., and Aronson, H. 1963. Expectations of psychotherapy in patients of lower socioeconomic class. *American Journal of Orthopsychiatry* 33: 421–430.

Royal College of General Practitioners. 1972. *The Future General Practitioner.* Lavenham.

Rubin, J. Z., and Brown, B. R. 1975. *The Social Psychology of Bargaining and Negotiation.* Academic.

Scheff, T. J. 1968. Negotiating reality: Notes on power in the assessment of responsibility. *Social Problems* 16: 3–14.

Williams, H. V., Lipman, R. S., Uhlenhuth, E. H., et al. 1967. Some factors influencing the treatment expectations of anxious neurotic outpatients. *Journal of Nervous and Mental Disease* 145: 208–220.

Wilson, N. C. 1973. The automated tri-informant goal-oriented progress note. *Journal of Community Psychology* 1: 302–306.

Index